Immunomodulatory and Cytotoxic Agents in Dermatology

BASIC AND CLINICAL DERMATOLOGY

Series Editors

ALAN R. SHALITA, M.D.

Professor and Chairman
Department of Dermatology
State University of New York
Health Science Center at Brooklyn
Brooklyn, New York

DAVID A. NORRIS, M.D.

Director of Research
Professor of Dermatology
The University of Colorado
Health Sciences Center
Denver, Colorado

1. Cutaneous Investigation in Health and Disease: Noninvasive Methods and Instrumentation, *edited by Jean-Luc Lévêque*
2. Irritant Contact Dermatitis, *edited by Edward M. Jackson and Ronald Goldner*
3. Fundamentals of Dermatology: A Study Guide, *Franklin S. Glickman and Alan R. Shalita*
4. Aging Skin: Properties and Functional Changes, *edited by Jean-Luc Lévêque and Pierre G. Agache*
5. Retinoids: Progress in Research and Clinical Applications, *edited by Maria A. Livrea and Lester Packer*
6. Clinical Photomedicine, *edited by Henry W. Lim and Nicholas A. Soter*
7. Cutaneous Antifungal Agents: Selected Compounds in Clinical Practice and Development, *edited by John W. Rippon and Robert A. Fromtling*
8. Oxidative Stress in Dermatology, *edited by Jürgen Fuchs and Lester Packer*
9. Connective Tissue Diseases of the Skin, *edited by Charles M. Lapière and Thomas Krieg*
10. Epidermal Growth Factors and Cytokines, *edited by Thomas A. Luger and Thomas Schwarz*
11. Skin Changes and Diseases in Pregnancy, *edited by Marwali Harahap and Robert C. Wallach*

12. Fungal Disease: Biology, Immunology, and Diagnosis, *edited by Paul H. Jacobs and Lexie Nall*
13. Immunomodulatory and Cytotoxic Agents in Dermatology, *edited by Charles J. McDonald*
14. Cutaneous Infection and Therapy, *edited by Raza Aly, Karl R. Beutner, and Howard Maibach*

ADDITIONAL VOLUMES IN PREPARATION

Immunomodulatory and Cytotoxic Agents in Dermatology

edited by
Charles J. McDonald
Brown University
Providence, Rhode Island

MARCEL DEKKER, INC. NEW YORK • BASEL • HONG KONG

Library of Congress Cataloging-in-Publication Data

Immunomodulatory and cytotoxic agents in dermatology/ edited by
Charles J. McDonald.
p. cm. — (Basic and clinical dermatology ; 13)
Includes bibliographical references and index.
ISBN 0-8247-9406-0 (alk. paper)
1. Dermatologic agents. I. McDonald, Charles J.
II. Series.
[DNLM: 1. Skin Diseases—drug therapy. 2. Immunosuppressive
Agents. 3. Antineoplastic Agents. 4. Anti-Inflammatory Agents.
5. Drug Monitoring. W1 CL69L v. 13 1997 / WR 140 I332 1997]
RL801.I46 1997
615'.778—dc21
DNLM/DLC
for Library of Congress

96-45655
CIP

The publisher offers discounts on this book when ordered in bulk quantities. For more information, write to Special Sales/Professional Marketing at the address below.

This book is printed on acid-free paper.

MARCEL DEKKER, INC.
270 Madison Avenue, New York, New York 10016

Current printing (last digit):
10 9 8 7 6 5 4 3 2 1

PRINTED IN THE UNITED STATES OF AMERICA

Preface

This text is intended to serve as an introduction to the use of immunomodulatory and cytotoxic drugs in current dermatological practice. It is designed to meet the increasing needs of dermatologists and other clinicians interested in becoming involved in the continuing care of patients with some of the most difficult-to-manage diseases. It should also provide the serious reader with sufficient background information on the chemistry, pharmacology, and toxicity of various drugs used to suppress inflammatory and immune responses. The general format introduces the reader through a series of condensed but very useful discussions to the chemistry, pharmacology, and toxicity of the most widely used drugs, as well as a variety of new and promising agents. A clear-cut knowledge of the material covered in these 12 chapters will enable the practitioner to administer these agents in a safe, effective manner.

The remaining 11 chapters on the treatment of specific dermatological diseases provide a better understanding of the *how* and *why* of therapy. Each author presents an extensive discussion of the individual agents used against human disease, with emphasis on the principal effect of the agent on cellular metabolism. The rationale for each agent's use is discussed, and where the literature is incomplete, plausible postulates are put forth.

Because monitoring is a most important area for the safe and successful use of drugs, a substantial portion of the text is devoted to drug monitoring in disease. Some drugs are treated as a group and some as individual agents.

Although this volume covers a broad spectrum of dermatological disease that may in some way be treated with immunomodulatory and cytotoxic drugs, some diseases have not been covered because the body of knowledge that relates to treatment is minuscule, published reports are few, or documentation is poor.

Scientific knowledge is advancing at a rapid pace, and new mechanisms of disease are being uncovered. Yet new, safe, and effective approaches to disease treatment do not necessarily follow. In our selective process, we have tried to present information that will prove of immediate use to the physician and those engaged in dermatological and pharmacological research.

Charles J. McDonald

Introduction
General Principles of Immunomodulatory and Cytotoxic Therapy

Charles J. McDonald
Brown University,
Providence, Rhode Island

Just over a decade ago, I published the following commentary. "The dermatologist now has at his/her disposal many effective therapeutic agents to complement the long and well-developed artistic practice of the specialty. No longer is it necessary to rely solely on the use of unscientific, ineffective, or marginally effective nostrums, poultices, and like substances in our treatment of dermatologic diseases. If our specialty is to benefit from advances in therapeutics, we, as dermatologists, have to become more familiar and more confident in our abilities as physicians to administer those remarkably effective agents now available (1)." On that occasion, I was commenting on the usefulness of a group of drugs then commonly referred to as cytotoxic or chemotherapeutic drugs. During the past decade intensive research has produced additional advances in the fields of immunology and inflammation, and immunopharmacology and immunotherapeutics, thereby adding immensely to the variety of methods and agents through which we may affect the course of dermatological disease.

To prepare the reader for the discussions that follow, this introduction offers a summary of certain principles of cytotoxic drug action common to a variety of agents and a simplified discussion of why diseases characterized by altered immunity and inflammation respond to immunomodulatory therapy. This preliminary discussion will aid in solidifying concepts being advanced by authors of the individual chapters.

The principal biological effect or lethality (cell kill) of each cytotoxic agent or class of agents is due in great measure to inhibition of one or more steps in the biosynthesis of deoxyribonucleic acid (DNA) and ribonucleic acid (RNA) within a variety of cell types. (Figure 1). Although the term "cell kill" is often used to describe the lethal effect of cytotoxic drugs, they do not kill cells directly but affect cell growth and division—and ultimately cell proliferation. For cells to grow and divide, a number of fundamental metabolic processes must take place continuously within the several phases of the cell cycle (Figure 2). DNA must be replicated without error once every cycle. This replication requires an adequate supply of purine and pyrimidine nucleosides (guanosine, adenosine, cytidine, uridine, and thymidine), the enzyme DNA polymerase, and an intact DNA template. Synthesis of protein is also necessary, not only for cell growth but also for cell replication. Proteins are formed through a series of complex polymerization reactions that take place on ribosomes within the cell cytoplasm. The sequence of nucleotides of messenger RNA determines how amino acids are positioned in the proper sequence, forming first polypeptides and then proteins. The process of protein formation requires template RNA, RNA polymerase, and messenger RNA. DNA acts as a template for the synthesis of complementary RNAs.

Some cytotoxic drugs, such as the alkylating agents, produce lethal effects principally through the formation of inter- and intrastrand cross-linking of DNA (causing inactivation of DNA) and subsequent depurination and hydrolysis of DNA at alkylated base positions. A number of specific intracellular enzymes are present that are capable of modifying the lethal effects of alkylation on DNA. These enzymes act principally to recognize the defective or alkylated base and effect its removal. This action opens the way for subsequent repair (2,3). Sometimes magnification of the original base damage occurs, particularly if the alkylated DNA is subjected to additional enzymatic attack without subsequent repair. The ability of a cell to effect repair is directly related to the lethality of the cytotoxic agent and to the ability of a cell to develop drug resistance.

The group of drugs known as antimetabolites cause cell death through a variety of mechanisms. They may substitute for a metabolite that is normally incorporated into a key molecule, thereby making the molecule functionally abnormal; they may compete successfully with a normal metabolite for occupation of the catalytic site of a key enzyme; or they may compete with a normal metabolite that acts on an enzyme regulatory site to alter the catalytic rate of the enzyme. Antimetabolites are synthetic substances (usually structural analogs) that, by their chemical nature, resemble naturally occurring essential metabolites. Through the action of antimetabolites, cell death generally occurs as a result of "unbalanced growth," that is, inhibition of DNA, RNA, or protein synthesis. An agent such as methotrexate (MTX), which affects to some degree DNA, RNA, and protein synthesis, can result in less unbalanced growth and possibly less cell kill. The addition of another cytotoxic antimetabolite, such as a purine base, to a regimen using MTX will often lead to an increase in the ability of MTX to

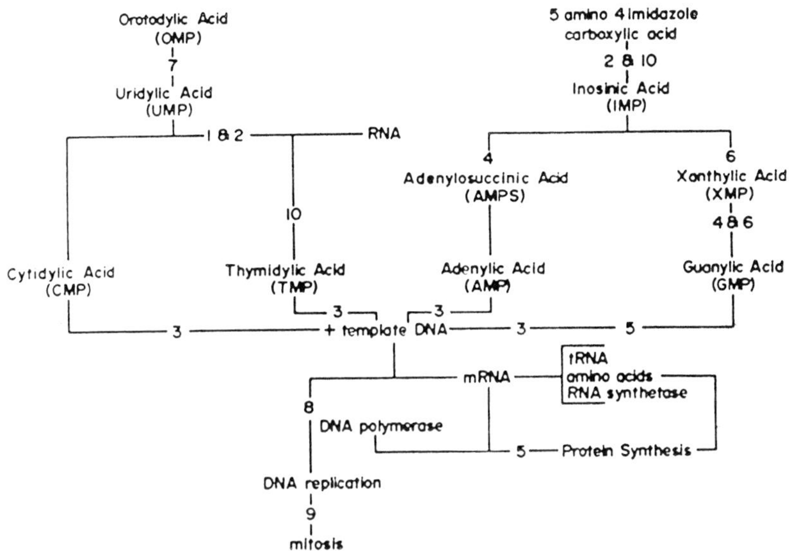

Figure 1 Proposed molecular site of action of the most commonly used chemotherapeutic agents. 1, FU group; 2, antifolics (methotrexate); 3, hydroxyurea; 4, mercaptopurine, azathioprine; 5, alkylating agents; 6, mycophenolic acid; 7, 6-azauridine; 8, bleomycins; 9, vinca alkaloids; 10, methotrexate. (From McDonald CJ. Cytotoxic Agents for use in Dermatology I, JAAD 1985:12, 753–775.)

kill cells in vitro. An example of the use of this kind of knowledge in the treatment of dermatologic disease is discussed in the chapter on psoriasis.

A few drugs, such as the antibiotic bleomycin, bind to DNA, acting in a manner somewhat analogous to the alkylating drugs, to effect cell kill. A few, such as the vinca alkaloids, act on the function of the mitotic spindle to cause mitotic arrest. However, it remains difficult to state how mitotic arrest causes cell kill. Because most cytotoxic actions occur at specific phases during a cell's cycle (Figure 2) and because drug cytotoxicity is confined principally to cells that are in the process of division, most cytotoxic drugs are considered cell cycle–specific. Some drugs, such as the alkylating agents, act on cells at any stage of the cell cycle and are thus not cell cycle–specific.

In many circumstances, target cells do not die as a result of cytotoxic drug action but instead may suffer from inhibition of a variety of metabolic processes. Inhibition can be total or partial. Partial inhibition may result in a reduction in the number of cells proceeding through a state of proliferation, or cell growth may cease. Cellular production of protein can be affected. If protein production ceases or is reduced, the amount available for manufacture of effector substance

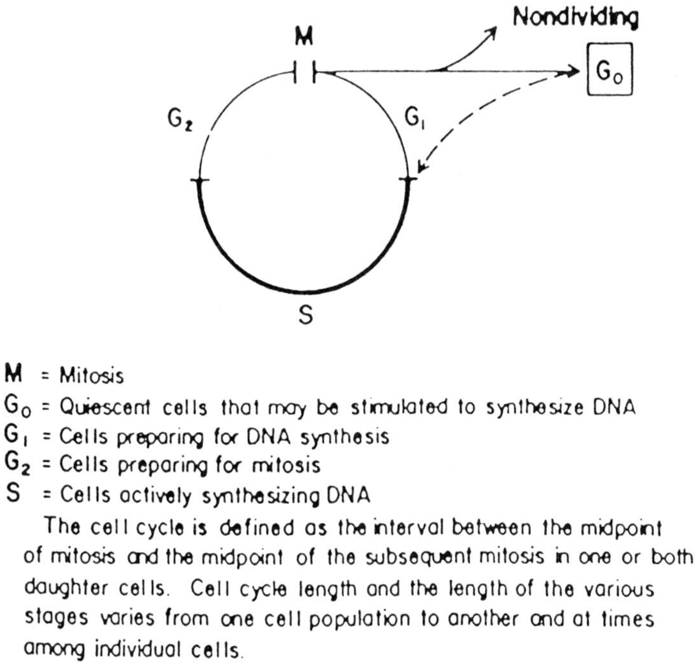

Figure 2 Cell cycle of continuously dividing, nondividing, and quiescent mammalian cells. (From McDonald CJ. Cytotoxic Agents for use in Dermatology I, JAAD 1985:12, 753–775.)

is reduced. Hence, cells that serve as a source of cytokines, lymphokines, growth factors, interferons, inhibitory factors, and the like are forced to cease production. In the absence of adequate amounts of effector substances normal inflammatory reactions are inhibited, or reactions that have resulted from cellular overactivity or overabundance of effector substances are impeded, and a return to normalcy results.

Diseases that are responsive to immunomodulatory and cytotoxic therapy include a wide variety, with very diverse etiologies and even more diverse manifestations. They include: the bullous diseases pemphigus vulgaris and bullous pemphigoid; the connective tissue diseases systemic lupus erythematosus, progressive systemic sclerosis, and dermatomyositis; and systemic vasculitis, periarteritis nodosa, leukocytoclastic angiitis, and Mucha-Habermann disease.

Parenthetically, the "T-cell diseases," such as mycosis fungoides lymphoma, Sézary's syndrome, and sarcoidosis, may very well be considered in this category.

Although each of the diseases in this group clinically manifests differently from the others, all are in some measure caused by, or associated with, abnormal thymus-derived (T cell) and/or bursa-derived (B-cell) lymphocyte function (4–20). To comprehend the action of immunosuppressive drugs in this group of diseases, it is of utmost importance to understand the series of events that occurs when an antigenic stimulus affects a host and a disease results.

The immune responses to antigenic stimulation are either humoral or cellular. Humoral immunity is mediated by B cells; it is immediate and results in the production of antibody. Cellular immunity is delayed and is mediated by T cells. The cellular response is often a cytotoxic response. T cells also take part in elicitation of the humoral response by acting as "effector"-type cells: they stimulate the production of antibodies by appropriate B cells, becoming in this set of circumstances "helper" T cells; they may also suppress the production of antibody ("suppressor" T cells). In the normal person, about 60–80% of the circulating lymphocytes in the peripheral blood are thymus-derived cells (T cells). The remainder are B lymphocytes. After formation in the bone marrow, B cells populate regional lymph nodes and other parts of the reticuloendothelial system. Mature inactive B cells reside mostly in the cortical and medullary portions of the lymph nodes and spleen. In the antigenically stimulated host, B cells enter a phase of active cell proliferation and, upon release from lymph nodes and spleen, enlarge and initiate production of antibodies. Plasma cells, abundant sources of antibody when antigenic stimulation is prolonged, are mature B cells that have lost the ability to divide. The complement system, which consists of a group of plasma/serum proteins, is often a necessary component in effecting antigen/antibody reactions in humoral immunity.

In the early stages of an immune response, and upon entry of a foreign antigen into the host, the antigen is, in most instances, immediately engulfed by macrophages/monocytes. The antigen is subjected to a series of processes that ultimately end in macrophage/monocyte "recognition" or "nonrecognition." Nonrecognition calls for signals to initiate specific T- and B-cell action: the synthesis of protein and nucleoprotein; cell division; the synthesis of antibody in humoral immunity; and the synthesis of lymphokines, monokines, and lympholytic substances in cellular immunity. The end result of these actions is initiation of an inflammatory or protective response. Failure to control the inflammatory response leads to a state of disease, inflammation or autoimmunity.

Cytotoxic and immunomodulatory drugs are used to effect control of inflammatory response that have continued unabated. They do this through their ability to affect purine and pyrimidine synthesis that in turn may inhibit nucleic acid synthesis and protein synthesis. As stated above, lymphocytes and monocyte/macrophages—the key mediators of immunity and inflammation, just as cells in other organ systems deprived of adequate nucleic acids or proteins and nucleoprotein—will not grow or replicate and produce new lymphocytes/monocytes (effectively depleting the lymphocyte/monocyte pool) and do not synthesize protein: thus antibody, monokine, lymphokine, and lympholytic substances are not synthesized. As in psoriasis chemotherapy, cytotoxic agents used as immunosuppressants act in a different or quantitative manner to affect rapidly dividing and actively synthesizing immunocytes (T- and B-lymphocytes) and monocyte/macrophages. That lymphocyte depletion results in effective immunosuppression has been demonstrated in studies showing successful organ transplantation after thoracic duct drainage, concomitant with depletion of the lymphocyte pool (21), and successful treatment of rheumatoid arthritis and systemic lupus erythematosus with the use of thoracic duct drainage (22).

There is evidence that some immunosuppressive agents display a very intense anti-inflammatory action that does not seem to correlate with immunosuppressive activity. Some cytotoxic agents act by reversibly altering lymphocyte membranes, by suppression of antigen recognition, and by altering macrophage function (23). Therefore, it is often difficult to ascribe the overall effect of an immunosuppressive drug solely to its action on DNA and lymphocyte kinetics. It is most important to stress that it is the *combined* immunosuppressive/anti-inflammatory-recognition-suppression action of the cytotoxic agents that makes them useful in diseases of altered immunity. This combined action may also account for the ability of these agents to effect a measurable therapeutic response without inducing leukopenia and lymphopenia.

What is the role in immunosuppression of specific cytotoxic agents such as azathioprine and cyclophosphamide? In vitro, the thiopurines have been shown principally to affect T-lymphocyte function. They may also inhibit B-cell function, but in general the effect appears to be more specific on the T-cell population.

Table 1 Adverse Reactions to Cytotoxic Drugs

Bone marrow suppression
Induction of lymphoma and leukemia
Infection
Hemorrhagic cystitis (Cytoxan)
Bladder carcinoma (Cytoxan)
Cardiomyopathy (Cytoxan)
Hepatic fibrosis and cirrhosis (methotrexate)
Pulmonary fibrosis (methotrexate and bleomycin)
Gonadal dysfunction
Bone necrosis
Dermatitis

Source: McDonald CJ. Cytotoxic Agents for use in Dermatology I, JAAD 1985:12, 753–775.

Table 2 Adverse Reactions to Systemic Corticosteroids

	No. patients	No. deaths/ % deaths*
Infection*	69	12/11
Pulmonary embolization*	13	3/3
Vascular thrombosis*	5	
Congestive heart failure*	2	2/2
Myocardial infarction*	2	2/2
Myopathy*	5	
Gastrointestinal bleeding*	12	
Osteoporosis*	31	
Psychologic and psychiatric*	35	
Glycosuria and hyperglycemia*	44	
Cushing's syndrome		
Anaphylaxis		
Adrenal suppression		
Panniculitis		
Electrolyte disturbances		
Posterior subcapsular cataracts		
Withdrawal syndrome		
Pseudotumor cerebri		
Hypertension		
Retarded growth		
Aseptic necrosis of bone		
Convulsions		
Fat deposition		
Hyperlipidemia		

* Source: Rosenberg FR, Sanders S, Nelson CT: Pemphigus: A 20-year review of 107 patients treated with corticosteroids. Arch Dermatol 112:962–970, 1976. (Reprinted with permission from McDonald CJ. Cytotoxic Agents for use in Dermatology I, JAAD 1985:12, 753–775.)

Thus, one would expect azathioprine to be most active in disorders of increased T-cell activity: delayed hypersensitivity, allograft rejection, and transplantation reactions. This specific drug–activity relationship does not always appear to hold true under clinical circumstances.

The alkylating agent cyclophosphamide appears to have two actions in the immune response that are dose-dependent (24). In high doses, it inhibits B-cell function. In chronic low doses, it inhibits T-cell function. When cyclophosphamide is given during cellular differentiation and proliferation, it kills large numbers of immunocompetent cells that are actively synthesizing nucleoprotein; this immunocytotoxic effect is often so intense that total destruction of a specific clone of antibody-producing cells may take place; immune tolerance then results.

T cells are also altered by high doses of cyclophosphamide, but they appear more sensitive to low-dose, chronic administration. Cyclophosphamide suppresses mouse phytohemagglutinin response and the production of macrophage migration inhibitory factor (MIF). Additionally, cyclophosphamide augments delayed hypersensitivity reactions, depending principally on the time of drug administration in the evolution of the immune response. Most often, if given prior to the administration of antigen, augmentation will occur.

Because there are capable physicians with an interest in the application of cytotoxic and immunomodulatory drugs in disease who have somehow been repulsed by the myriad stories (some real and many imagined) of the number and types of adverse reactions associated with the use of these drugs, it is germane to end this introduction with three relevant statements.

1. The number and severity of adverse reactions associated with the use of immunomodulatory and cytotoxic drugs are no greater than those experienced using long-term systemic corticosteroids. (Tables 1 and 2.)
2. The number and severity of acute and chronic adverse reactions can be sharply reduced by properly monitoring each individual patient.
3. If the occurrence of nonmelanoma skin cancer in the nontransplant patient is eliminated from consideration, immunomodulatory and cytotoxic agents do not cause an increased rate of cancer induction (24–26).

REFERENCES

1. McDonald CJ. Cytotoxic agents for use in dermatology I. JAAD 12:753–775, 1985.
2. Lehmann AR, Karran P. DNA repair. Int Rev Cytol 72:101–146, 1981.
3. Lee DE, Okorodudu AO, Lambert WWC, Lambert MW. Defective DNA endonuclease activity on anthramycin treated DNA in xeroderma pigmentosum and mouse melanoma cells. Biochem Biophys Res Commun 107:395–402, 1982.
4. Jordan RE, Trifthauser CT, Schroter AL. Direct immunofluorescent studies of pemphigus and bullous pemphigoid. Arch Dermatol 103:486–491, 1971.
5. Tappeiner G, Heine KG, Jordan RE. Presence of immuno complexes in pemphigus vulgaris serums as demonstrated by a Ciq binding assay. Clin Res 23:231, 1975.
6. Beutner EH, Chorzelski TP, Jordan RE. Autosensitzation in pemphigus and bullous pemphigoid. Charles C Thomas: Springfield, IL, 1970.
7. Schlitz JR. Pemphigus acantholysis: A unique immunological injury. J Invest Dermatol 74:359, 1980.
8. Singer KH, Sawka NJ, Samowitz HR. Lazarus GS. proteinase activation: A mechanism for cellular dyshesion in pemphigus. J Invest Dermatol 74:363–367, 1980.
9. Anhalt GJ, Labib RS, Voorhees JJ. et al. Induction of pemphigus in neonatal mice by passive transfer of IgG from patients with the disease. N Engl J Med 306:1189–1196, 1982.
10. Pehamberger H, Gschnait F, Konrad K. Holubar K. Bullous pemphigoid, herpes

gestationis and linear dermatitis herpetiformis: Circulating antibasement membrane zone antibodies: In vitro studies. J Invest Dermatol 74:105–108, 1980.

11. Koffler D, Agnello V, Thoburne R. et al. Systemic lupus erythematosus: prototype of immune complex nephritis in man. J Exp Med 134 (supl):169s-, 1971.
12. Koffler D, Carr R, Agnello V, et al. Antibodies to polynucleotides in human sera and genetic specificity and relation to disease. J Exp Med 134:294–312, 1971.
13. Fleischmajer R, Perlish JS, Duncan M. Scleroderma: A model for fibrosis, Arch Dermatol 119:957–962, 1983.
14. Soling J. Circulating immune complexes in LE scleroderma and dermatomyositis. Acta Derm Venereol (Stockh) 59:421–426, 1979.
15. deJesus DG, Clancy RL. Circulating T and B lymphocytes in progressive systemic sclerosis. J. Rheumatol 2:336–339, 1975.
16. Kondo H, Rabin BS, Rodnan GP. Cutaneous antigen-stimulating lymphokine production by lymphocytes of patients with progressive systemic sclerosis. J. Clin Invest 58:1388, 1976.
17. Stuart JM, Postlewaite AE, Kang AH. Evidence for cell mediated immunity to collagen in progressive systemic sclerosis. J Lab Clin Med 88:601, 1976.
18. Cochrane CG, Hawkins D. Studies on circulating immune complexes III. Factors governing the ability of circulating complexes to localize in blood vessels. J Exp Med 127:137, 1968.
19. Schroeter AL, Copeman PWM, Jordan RE, et al. Immunofluorescenceof cutaneous vasculitis. J Clin Invest 48:75a. 1969.
20. Cream JJ. Clinical and immunological aspects of cutaneous vasculitis. Q J Med 45:255, 1976.
21. Fish JC, Sarles He, Remmers AR Jr. et al. Renal transplantation after thoracic duct drainage. Ann Surg 193:752–756, 1981.
22. Paulus HE, Machleder HI, Clements PJ, et al. Prolonged thoracic-duct drainage in rheumatoid arthiritis and systemic lupus erythematosus. West J Med 130:309–324, 1979.
23. Boch JF. The pharmacological and immunological basis for the use of immunosuppressive drugs. Drugs 11:1–13, 1976.
24. Kinlen LJ, Sheil AG, Peto J, Doll R. Collaborative United Kingdom-Australasian study of cancer in patients treated with immunosuppressive drugs. Br Med J 2:1461–1466, 1979.
25. Penn I. Immunosuppression and skin cancer. Clin Plast Surg 7:361–368, 1980.
26. Marshall VC. Skin tumours in immunosuppressed patients. Aust NZ J Surg. 43:214–222, 1973.

Contents

Contributors

A. Razzaque Ahmed, M.D. Associate Professor, Department of Oral Medicine and Oral Pathology, Harvard School of Dental Medicine, Boston, Massachusetts

Joseph Alper, M.D. Department of Dermatology, Roger Williams Medical Center, Providence, Rhode Island

Jack L. Arbiser, Ph.D. Instructor, Department of Dermatology, and Fellow, Howard Hughes Medical Institute, Harvard Medical School, Boston, Massachusetts

Joseph R. Bertino, M.D. Chairman, Program of Molecular Pharmacology and Therapeutics, Memorial Sloan-Kettering Cancer Center, New York, New York

Marcia J. Browne, M.D. N.E. Hematology/Oncology Associates, Wellesley, Massachusetts

Jean-Claude Bystryn, M.D. Professor, Department of Dermatology, New York University Medical Center, New York, New York

Jeffrey P. Callen, M.D., F.A.C.P. Professor of Medicine (Dermatology), Chief, Division of Dermatology, Department of Medicine, University of Louisville School of Medicine, Louisville, Kentucky

Jeffrey W. Clark, M.D. Assistant Professor of Medicine, Harvard University, and Department of Hematology/Oncology, Massachusetts General Hospital, Boston, Massachusetts

David Friedman, M.D. Department of Dermatology, Roger Williams Medical Center, Providence, Rhode Island

Joan Guitart, M.D. Assistant Professor, Department of Dermatology, Northwestern University Medical School, Chicago, Illinois

Aditya K. Gupta, M.D., F.R.C.P.(C) Assistant Professor, Division of Dermatology, Department of Medicine, University of Toronto, Sunnybrook Health Science Centre, Toronto, Ontario, Canada

Joseph L. Jorizzo, M.D. Professor and Chairman, Department of Dermatology, Bowman Gray School of Medicine of Wake Forest University, Winston-Salem, North Carolina

Timothy M. Kuzel, M.D. Associate Professor, Department of Medicine, Northwestern University Medical School, Chicago, Illinois

Monica L. McCrary, M.D. Resident, Department of Dermatology, Medical College of Georgia, Augusta, Georgia

Charles J. McDonald Professor and Chairman, Department of Dermatology, Brown University, Providence, Rhode Island

Omeed M. Memar, Ph.D. Department of Microbiology and Immunology, University of Texas Medical Branch, Galveston, Texas

Shin Mineishi Assistant Professor, Department of Medicine, University of Wisconsin School of Medicine, Madison, Wisconsin

Narciss Mobini, M.D. Post-Doctoral Research Fellow, Department of Oral Pathology and Oral Medicine, Harvard School of Dental Medicine, Boston, Massachusetts

Samuel L. Moschella, M.D. Senior Consultant, Department of Dermatology, Lahey-Hitchcock Clinic, Burlington, Massachusetts

Ruth Oratz, M.D. Professor, Department of Dermatology, New York University Medical Center, New York, New York

Stephanie Pincus, M.D. Professor and Chair, Department of Dermatology, State University of New York at Buffalo, Buffalo, New York

Ron Prussick, M.D., F.R.C.P.(C) Division of Dermatology, Department of Medicine, University of Toronto, Sunnybrook Health Science Centre, Toronto, Ontario, Canada

Leslie Robinson-Bostom, M.D. Assistant Professor of Medicine, Department of Dermatology, Brown University, Providence, Rhode Island

Daniel N. Sauder, M.D., F.R.C.P.(C)., F.A.C.P. Professor and Chief, Division of Dermatology, University of Toronto, Sunnybrook Health Science Centre, Toronto, Ontario, Canada

Gulnar M. Shivji, B.Sc. Division of Dermatology, Department of Medicine, University of Toronto, Sunnybrook Health Science Centre, Toronto, Ontario, Canada

Stephen K. Tyring, M.D., Ph.D. Professor, Department of Dermatology, Microbiology and Immunology, and Internal Medicine, University of Texas Medical Branch, Galveston, Texas

Alan B. Weitberg, M.D. Chairman, Department of Medicine, and Chief, Division of Hematology/Oncology, Roger Williams Medical Center, Associate Professor of Medicine and Director, Medical Oncology, Brown University School of Medicine, Providence, Rhode Island

Stephen E. Wolverton, M.D. Clinical Associate Professor, Department of Dermatology, Indiana University Medical Center, Indianapolis, Indiana

Sharon Zellis, D.O. Resident, Department of Dermatology, Philadelphia College of Osteopathic Medicine, Philadelphia, Pennsylvania

1
Alkylating Agents

Charles J. McDonald
Brown University, Providence, Rhode Island

I. CHEMISTRY

Alkylating agents, among which are the nitrogen mustards mechlorethamine and cyclophosphamide, are compounds that are capable of forming highly reactive chemical intermediates, such as carbonium ions, which in turn interact with a variety of molecules possessing nucleophilic centers (reactive protons). Alkylating drugs that undergo strongly electrophilic chemical reactions through the formation of carbonium ion intermediates form strong covalent linkages (alkylation) with nucleophilic moieties such as hydroxyl, carboxyl, imidazole, sulfhydryl, phosphate, and amino groups. The cytotoxic effect of the alkylating agents most likely correlates with their ability to form cross-stranded covalent linkages. It has been proposed that the alkylating drugs exert their most significant biological effects through alkylation of the purine base, guanine, at the 7-nitrogen of adenine or the 3-nitrogen of cytosine. To be of biological significance, alkylation must take place while purine bases are attached to nucleic acid chains. Biochemical abnormalities that may result from alkylation include (a) abnormal base pairing of guanine and thymine residues, leading to genetic miscoding; (b) abnormal pairing of two guanine residues with the resultant incompatible cross-linking of two nucleic acid chains; (c) pairing of a guanine residue to a protein, thus causing the abnormal linkage of a nucleic acid and a protein; (d) depurination of the DNA chain leading ultimately to chain scission; and (e) labilization and opening of the imidazole ring of quanine. Bifunctional alkylating agents that have two drug reactive sites are most effective in inducing cross-linking. Interestingly, agents having more than two alkylating sites do not appear to have comparable or greater cross-linking ability. Although reactive intermediates of alkylating agents may attack any molecule possessing reactive protons, it appears that the

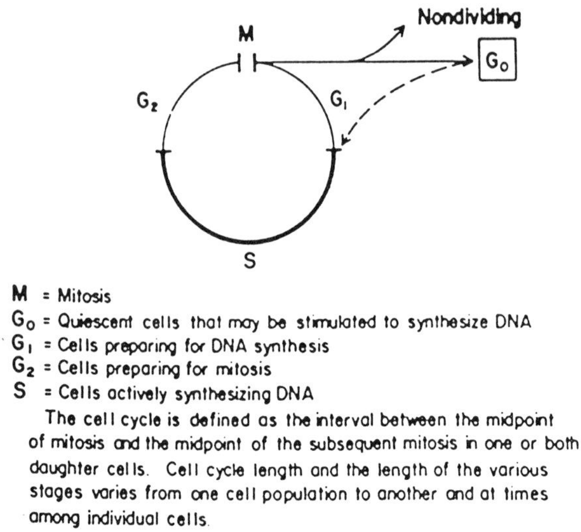

Figure 1 Cell cycle of continuously dividing, nondividing, and quiescent mammalian cells. (Reprinted with permission from McDonald CJ. Cytotoxic Agents for use in Dermatology I JAAD 1985;12, 753–775).

most important target molecule is DNA. Attacks on other macromolecules, such as ribonucleoproteins and proteins, seem less significant. The reactions that have been cited herein may all lead to abnormal nucleic acid functions that ultimately result in cell death (the cytotoxic effect) (1).

While alkylating agents exert their most profound effects on rapidly dividing or proliferating cells, they retain the propensity to "alkylate" cells at any stage of the cell replication cycle. Cells affected most appear to be those in late G_1 or S. Cytotoxicity becomes manifest when a specific cell enters the S phase and cannot progress beyond the G_2 phase of the cycle (Figure 1). Although alkylating drugs are primarily toxic to the cell, that is, promoting cell death through depurination and chain scission, they are also capable of causing permanent modifications in DNA that are nonlethal but may result in transmission of the damaged DNA to subsequent generations, thereby initiating mutagenesis and carcinogenesis.

II. PHARMACOLOGY

Although the drugs in this group act biochemically by alkylation, they differ in chemical and physical properties, pharmacological disposition, biological effects, and efficacy in specific diseases. The discussions on pharmacological properties will be limited to those two agents most commonly used in the treatment of dermatological disease, mechlorethamine and cyclophosphamide.

Mechlorethamine (Mustargen) was the first alkylating agent to be tested in human malignancy (Figure 2). This topically applied drug has been used widely in the treatment of the cutaneous T-cell lymphoma, mycosis fungoides (2). Efforts to treat psoriasis with topical mechlorethamine have proven to be considerably less successful. Parenterally administered drug has also been used to treat mycosis fungoides (3), other systemic lymphomas, and autoimmune disease (4).

Mechlorethamine is effective when administered by mouth, by the parenteral route, or when applied topically. Severe local gastrointestinal reactions that often occur after oral administration, as well as erratic intestinal absorption, require in most situations the use of the intravenous or the topical route. Intravenous mechlorethamine rapidly undergoes chemical transformation, combining with water or other reactive cell components within minutes after administration. Transformation proceeds so rapidly and completely that less than 0.1% of a given dose can be recovered in the urine.

In an effort to achieve greater drug selectivity for neoplastic tissue while reducing the incidence of adverse drug effects, cyclophosphamide (Cytoxan) was developed. By altering slightly the chemical structure of mechlorethamine, cyclophosphamide can be formulated. Cyclophosphamide has been used in dermatology principally as an immunosuppressive agent. It is considered one of the

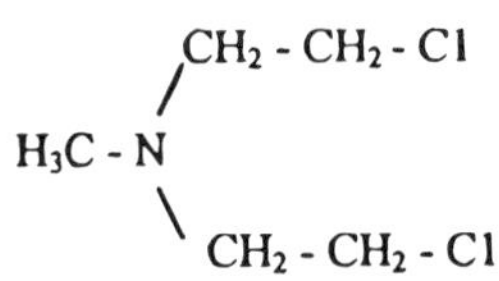

Mechlorethamine

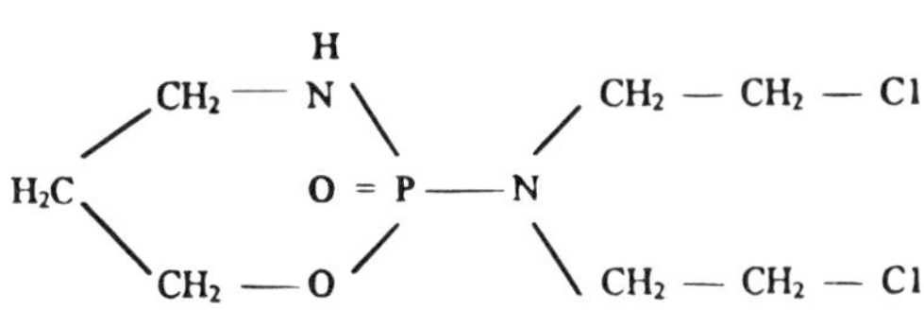

Cyclophosphamide

Figure 2 The nitrogen mustards most commonly used in dermatological disease.

most effective of the commonly used immunosuppressive drugs. Cyclophosphamide has also been used to treat mycosis fungoides lymphoma. In this disease it is usually used systemically and in combination with other cytotoxic drugs.

Unlike mechlorethamine, cyclophosphamide does not evoke severe local reactions in the gastrointestinal tract and, therefore, can be administered by mouth as well as by the intravenous route. Cyclophosphamide remains inactive in the body until it is metabolically activated in the liver by the cytochrome P_{450} mixed function oxidase system. Several toxic and nontoxic metabolites of cyclophosphamide are formed subsequent to metabolic activation. Within the liver cyclophosphamide is converted to 4-hydroxycyclophosphamide and aldophosphamide. These compounds are oxidized further to the active mustard phosphoramide and the inactive mustards nornitrogen mustard, carboxyphosphoramide, and acrolein. The cytotoxicity of cyclophosphamide is related in great part to the activity of 4-hydroxycyclophosphamide and phosphoramide mustard (5).

There is considerable variation in plasma concentration of active cyclophosphamide metabolites after drug administration. Plasma half-life may vary from 1.5–9 h. Generally less than 25% of unmetabolized cyclophosphamide appears in the urine (6,7). A number of factors are responsible for variations in plasma concentration, such as obesity, liver failure, renal failure, and prior administration of barbiturates.

III. MECHLORETHAMINE

A. Indications

In the treatment of leukemias, lymphomas, and solid tumors the use of mechlorethamine has been superseded by other more user-friendly alkylating drugs. Treatment of mycosis fungoides lymphoma may be the sole indication for use of mechlorethamine. Topical mechlorethamine (0.25%) is often quite effective in inducing remissions in patients with eczematous and plaque-type mycosis fungoides. Remissions may be expected in 80–100% of patients with disease in these two stages. Nodules, ulcers, and tumors, as well as internal disease, do not regularly respond to topical application of mechlorethamine.

B. Method of Use in Dermatological Disease

For use in topical therapy (principally of mycosis fungoides), a single vial containing 10 mg of mechlorethamine is mixed with 10 ml of water, which, in turn, is mixed with 40 ml of equal parts of water and propylene glycol. Propylene glycol may be omitted (water is an acceptable substitute) but in my experience propylene glycol serves as an excellent vehicle for mechlorethamine, dispersing the drug more evenly over the skin surface than does a plain water-based mixture.

This mixture (approximately 0.20–0.25% concentration) is then applied directly to the entire skin surface. If "contact dermatitis" results at any time from the initial 0.25% concentration of drug, a series of sequential dilutions are then made. The concentration of drug that causes the least cutaneous reaction is then selected for continuous use. Mechlorethamine diluted in this manner and then refrigerated has a half-life of more than 3 d (8,9).

Parenteral mechlorethamine can be expected to induce remissions in up to 50–75% of patients with mycosis fungoides. Eczematous, plaque, and nodular disease respond better than tumor-ulcerative disease. Because there are limits to the total amount of drug any single patient may be given by this route, induced remissions are difficult to maintain.

Parenteral mechlorethamine may be given as a single bolus of 10 mg mixed with 10 ml of water for sterile injection. When administered in this manner, mechlorethamine should be injected into the tubing of a rapidly flowing intravenous infusion rather than directly into a vein. Mechlorethamine may also be given as a continuous infusion over an 8-h period. When given as a series of 8-h infusions the usual total dose is 0.4–0.8 mg/kg of body weight, or 28–56 mg in a 70-kg individual. Small fractions of the total dose, not to exceed 2 mg, are given daily over a period of 28–30 d. This regimen, although cumbersome and in almost all cases requiring continuous hospitalization, is particularly effective in the management of mycosis fungoides lymphoma (3). Care must be taken to protect the intravenous solution from light exposure during the course of administration. When administered as a continuous infusion, the contents of a single vial are mixed with sterile water for injection, and the appropriate amount (usually 2 mg) is withdrawn and mixed with 250–500 ml of 5% dextrose and water. Each day the new mixture is infused over an 8-h period until myelosuppression or clearing of the disease occurs. In some patients, this regimen may be used up to 30 d without provoking serious systemic toxicity.

IV. CYCLOPHOSPHAMIDE

A. Indications

Cyclophosphamide is principally used for its immunosuppressive properties in a variety of dermatologic diseases. It is indicated in the treatment of severe autoimmune bullous diseases as pemphigus vulgaris, pemphigus erythematosus, pemphigus foliaceous, bullous and cicatricial pemphigoid, severe nonresponsive bullous erythema multiforme, progressive systemic sclerosis, the renal disease of systemic lupus erythematosus, cutaneous (leucocytoclastic) vasculitis, dysproteinemias, and in combination with a variety of cytotoxic agents for the treatment of late stage cutaneous T-cell lymphoma. Cyclophosphamide is not indicated for the treatment of psoriasis and other hyperproliferative diseases.

B. Method of Use in Dermatological Disease

When used for immunosuppression, cyclophosphamide may be given by the oral or parenteral route. The usual total daily dosage is 2–3 mg/kg divided into three equal doses. In my experience, it is rarely necessary to exceed a total daily dose of 150 mg. Doses above 200 mg/d are almost invariably associated with myelosuppression. Myelosuppression is an unwanted and unnecessary adverse effect. *It should always be remembered that it is not necessary to cause myelosuppression in order to produce an immunosuppressive effect with any drug.*

Cyclophosphamide administered by the parenteral route may be given in doses similar to those administered by the oral route. Investigators have also shown that relatively large doses of cyclophosphamide (5–9 mg/kg/d) given in short daily bursts over a period of 7–15 d may be effective in the treatment of proteinuric lupus neuropathy (10). Total drug dosages are between 1.5 and 5 g. This regimen should not be attempted by one inexperienced in the use of cytoxic drugs. When used, the patient must be hospitalized and all of the support systems necessary to cope with the severely myelosuppressed patient should be available.

V. DRUG TOXICITY

Local reactions to mechlorethamine are rather frequent after topical application and intravenous administration. Topical application may be followed by contact irritation and vesiculation. Contact irritation and allergy are believed to occur in a high percentage of patients. Cutaneous irritation may be avoided by using a "nonpolar" vehicle for topical application (11). Desensitization may be accomplished by use of topical and systemic techniques (12,13). A number of experienced therapists have concluded that the best therapeutic responses to mechlorethamine are induced in patients who develop cutaneous "irritation/sensitivity" reactions while being treated. Irritation/sensitivity reactions are undesirable in psoriatic patients because of the potential to develop a diffuse isomorphic (Koebner) response.

Increased skin pigmentation is another undesirable side effect of topical mechlorethamine administration, occurring principally in clinically active disease sites (14). Prolonged use of topical mustard may induce skin cancer (15).

Toxicity after the systemic administration of either mechlorethamine or cyclophosphamide includes bone marrow suppression and gastrointestinal mucosa ulcerations. Nausea, vomiting, and diarrhea may occur in the absence of mucosal injury. Amenorrhea, azoospermia, and long-lasting sterility may occur after prolonged treatment. High doses of mechlorethamine may produce seizures, salivation, and miosis. Erythema, induration, tenderness, and sloughing of the skin may occur after infiltration of parenterally administered mechlorethamine.

The use of cyclophosphamide can be associated with the development of alopecia, which in some cases may become permanent, and with sterile hemorrhagic cystitis. The metabolites acrolen, phosphoramide mustard, and chloroacetaldehyde have all been proposed as the agents responsible for cyclophosphamide associated hematuria (5,16). The onset of hemorrhagic cystitis may be minimized or prevented by encouraging a large daily fluid intake and frequent voiding. Hemorrhagic cystitis may be ameliorated with the agent sodium 2-mercaptoethanesulfone (Mesena). Mesena apparently reacts with the toxic metabolites of cyclophosphamide and deactivates them. Bladder carcinoma occurs rarely, and in most cases is believed to follow chronic, untreated hemorrhagic cystitis. Frequently obtained urinalyses may give early warning of hemorrhagic cystitis. Very high doses of cyclophosphamide may cause myocardial and hepatic injury. Drug dosages of this magnitude are almost never indicated in the treatment of dermatological diseases.

Both mechlorethamine and cyclophosphamide are potentially mutagenic and teratogenic.

REFERENCES

1. Colvin OM. The alkylating agents. In: Chabner B, ed. Pharmacological principles of cancer treatment. Philadelphia: W. B. Saunders, 1982:276–308.
2. Vonderheid EC. Topical mechlorethamine chemotherapy. Consideration on its uses in mycosis fungoides. Int J Dermatol 1984; 23:180–186.
3. Van Scott EF, Grekin DA, Kalmanson JD, et al. Frequent low doses of intravenous mechlorethamine for late-stage mycosis fungoides lymphoma. Cancer, 1980; 36:1613–1618.
4. DeVita VT Jr, Canellous GP, Mosley JH III. A decade of combination chemotherapy of advanced Hodgkin's Disease. Cancer 1972; 30:1495–1504.
5. Colvin M, Hilton J. Pharmacology of cyclophosphamide and metabolites. Cancer Treatment Rep 1981; 65:89–95.
6. Bagley CM, Bostick FW, DeVita VT. Clinical pharmacology of cyclophosphamide. Cancer Res 1973; 33:226–233.
7. Jardine I, Fenselau C, Appler M, Kan MN, Brundett RB, Colvin M. Quantification by gas chromatography chemical ionization. Mass spectrometry of cyclophosphamide, phosphoramide mustard, and nor-nitrogen mustard in the plasma and urine of patients receiving cyclophosphamide therapy. Cancer Res 1978; 38:408–415.
8. Inch WR, McCredie JA. Effect of aging aqueous nitrogen mustard on white blood cell count, body weight and Walker 256 tumor in the rat. Can J Biochem Physiol 1963; 41:417–425.
9. Taylor JR, Halprin KM, Levine V, et al. Mechlorethamine hydrochloride solution and ointment. Arch Dermatol, 1980; 116:783–785.
10. Dinant HJ, Decker JL, Klippel JH, et al. Alternative modes of cyclophosphamide and azathioprine therapy in lupus nephritis. Ann Intern Med 1982; 96:728–736.

11. Price NM, Deneau DG, Hoppe RT. The treatment of mycosis fungoides with ointment-based mechlorethamine. Arch Dermatol 1982; 118:234–237.
12. Purdy MJ. Topical mustine hydrochloride and psoriasis: A follow-up study. Australas J Dermatol 1975; 16:13–16.
13. Van Scott EJ, Kalmanson JO. Complete remission of mycosis fungoides lymphoma induced by topical nitrogen mustard (HN_2). Cancer 1973; 32:18–30.
14. Epstein E Jr, Ugel AR. Effects of topical mechlorethamine on skin lesions of psoriasis. Arch Dermatol 1970; 102:504–506.
15. Kravitz P, McDonald CJ. Topical nitrogen mustard induced carcinogenesis. Acta Dermatol Venereol (Stockh) 1978; 58:421–425.
16. Brock N, Pohl J, Stekar J. Studies on the urotoxicity of oxazaphosphorine cytostatics and its prevention. I. Experimental studies on the urotoxicity of alkylating agents. Eur J Cancer Clin Oncol 1981; 17:596–607.

2
Methotrexate

Joseph R. Bertino
Program of Molecular Pharmacology and Therapeutics, Memorial Sloan-Kettering Cancer Center, New York, New York

Shin Mineishi
University of Wisconsin School of Medicine, Madison, Wisconsin

I. CHEMISTRY

Methotrexate (MTX; 2-4-diamino-N10-methylpteroylglutamic acid) is used widely as an antineoplastic, antiinflamatory, and immunosuppressive agent (1–5). It is a "classic" antimetabolite, in that the structure of the compound is only slightly different from the metabolite, folic acid; that is, an amino group substitution for the hydroxyl at position 4 and a methyl group substitution for a hydrogen at position 10 (Figure 1). Like folic acid, MTX is a weak organic acid. The pure compound is a yellow or yellowish-orange crystalline material that decomposes without melting at approximately 200°C. Its disodium salt is highly soluble in aqueous solution above pH 7.0. Purity may be assessed by high-performance liquid chromatography (HPLC)(6), and concentrations of MTX may be measured by ultraviolet absorption in 0.1 N NaOH. Sensitive and specific assays for low concentrations of MTX (10^{-6}–10^{-9} M) in serum and cerebrospinal fluid have been described (7).

II. MECHANISM OF ACTION

A. Transport

MTX accumulates in mammalian cells by an active, carrier-mediated transport process (8). The drug competes with 5-methyltetrahydrofolate (5-MeFH4) for

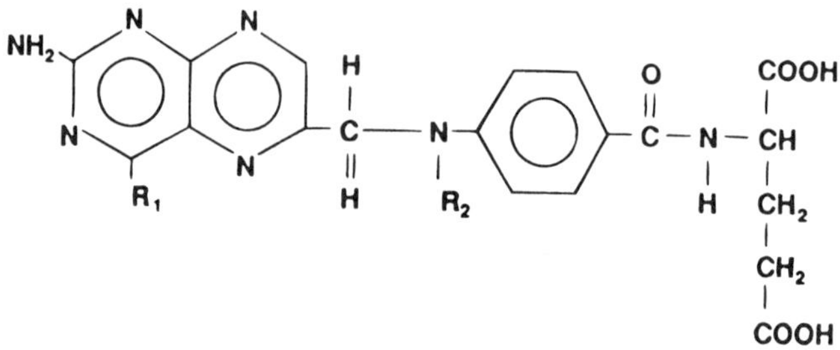

	R_1	R_2
Folic Acid	OH	H
Aminopterin	NH_2	H
MTX	NH_2	CH_3

Figure 1 Structure of methotrexate, aminopterin, and folic acid.

uptake into cells. 5-MeFH4 is the major form of serum folate, and influx of this reduced folate, as well as folinic acid (leucovorin-LV, or 5-formyltetrahydrofolate) will be decreased in the presence of high extracellular concentrations of MTX. Thus, very large doses of LV are required to reverse MTX toxicity when the extracellular concentration of this antifolate is high ($>10^{-6}$ M). Therefore, an important principle to be followed to reverse MTX toxicity is to use sufficiently large amounts of LV in order to obtain more than 10-fold higher concentrations of LV than MTX. This ratio will both prevent further uptake of MTX by cells, as well as allow influx of LV into cells in the presence of a high extracellular concentration of MTX. Only when the extracellular MTX concentration is decreased to less than 10^{-8} M will the physiological level of folates allow DNA synthesis to recover (9).

B. Polyglutamylation

Recently, polyglutamylation has been elucidated as an important determinant of MTX sensitivity (10–14). A single enzyme, folylpolyglutamate synthetase (FPGS) is responsible for adding glutamates in gamma-carboxyl linkage to both folate coenzymes and MTX and other analogs with a glutamate moiety (15). This enzyme adds up to seven or eight additional glutamates to folate or MTX. As a consequence of this polyglutamylation, efflux is markedly reduced, and MTX as well as folates are retained in the cells (16). Cells able to form long-chain MTX polyglutamates are thus more susceptible to MTX cytotoxicity, especially to short-time infusions of this drug (17,18).

Fortunately, neither gastrointestinal mucosa nor bone marrow progenitor cells polyglutamate MTX readily (19,20). Thus, for short-time exposures, cells in S phase during exposure to MTX are killed, but cells not in S phase (e.g., stem cells in G0) and unable to form long-chain polyglutamates are not, as MTX effluxes rapidly when the extracellular MTX concentration decreases.

C. Inhibition of Dihydrofolate Reductase

MTX is a potent inhibitor of a key enzyme in thymidylate biosynthesis, dihydrofolate reductase (DHFR) (1–5). This inhibition is the major mechanism of action of MTX. Inhibition of this enzyme activity by MTX leads to a decreased production of tetrahydrofolate, which in turn leads to a deficiency of N5–N10-methylene FH4, the one carbon donor for thymidylate biosynthesis (Figure 2). This "thymineless" state causes inhibition of DNA synthesis, and cell death ensues. MTX and its polyglutamates, as well as polyglutamates of dihydrofolate, also inhibit purine biosynthesis. Although MTX is a tight-binding inhibitor of DHFR, MTX in molar excess to the target enzyme, DHFR, is required to shut off tetrahydrofolate synthesis completely (21,22). Inasmuch as DHFR is in excess in most cells, only a small fraction of the total enzyme need remain catalytically functional to maintain the intracellular reduced folate pool (2,23).

D. Mechanisms of Resistance

Four major mechanism of resistance to MTX have been described in experimental tumors: an increase in DHFR activity, almost always due to amplification of the DHFR gene (24,25), a decrease in uptake of MTX due to either reduced influx or decrease in formation of polyglutamates (or increased hydrolysis of polyglutamates) (26–28), or mutations that result in an altered DHFR with decreased

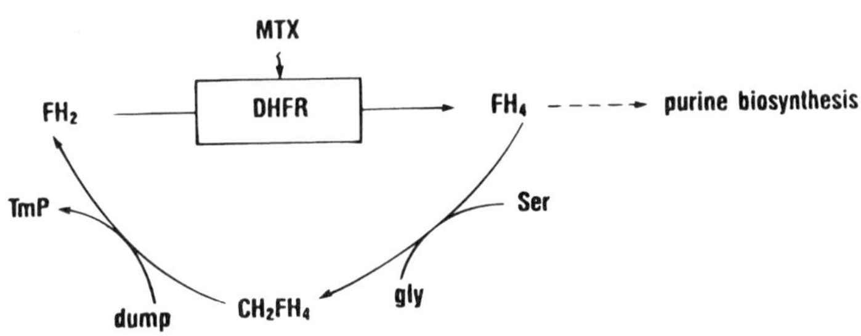

Figure 2 Mechanism of action of methotrexate (MTX). Methotrexate competes with reduced folates [5 $MeFH_4$ and 5-formyl FH_4 (leucovorin)] for uptake. Intracellularly, MTX rapidly combines with the enzyme dihydrofolate reductase (DHFR), thus blocking tetrahydrofolate synthesis and subsequently thymidylate biosynthesis and purine biosynthesis. Free MTX is polyglutamylated and as a consequence is retained in cell.

binding to DHFR (29–32). Recent studies have linked mutations or absence of the tumor suppresser gene, *p53,* with gene amplification (33,34). Of interest is the lack of resistance that occurs in normal cells as a consequence of repeated dosing with MTX.

III. PHARMACOLOGY

A. Absorption

Although MTX is believed to be well absorbed after low doses ($<$15 mg/m^2), recent studies have shown variability in absorption, even at these low doses (35,36). Absorption decreases with increasing oral doses. After oral administration, MTX levels in blood peaks in 1–2 hr. Food, nonabsorbable antibiotics, bile salts, and a shortened intestine transit time may decrease the rate and extent of absorption (37,38). Intra- and interpatient variability is significant.

B. Distribution

After IV administration, disappearance from plasma can be fitted to a triphasic curve. The initial phase (α-phase or distribution phase) has a $t_{1/2}$ of 30–45 min, and distribution volume of 18% (0.18L/kg body weight). The second phase (β-phase or renal clearance phase) has a $t_{1/2}$ of 3–4 h. A terminal phase ($t_{1/2} \approx 10$ h), may be the result of enterohepatic circulation of the drug. This prolonged terminal phase may contribute to the toxicity of this drug when plasma concentrations are maintained for a long period of time at greater than 10^{-8} M. Organ distribution and retention of MTX reflects the presence or absence of specific transport systems, the level of DHFR in each tissue, and the amount of conversion to polyglutamates. The organs that retain highest amount of MTX are the liver and kidneys. Patients with pleural effusion or peritoneal fluid may accumulate the drug in these "third spaces" (39), and systemic toxicity may result from delay in the plasma clearance of the drug. Entry of MTX across physiological barriers, that is, into cerebrospinal fluid and testis, is slow and limited. With conventional doses of MTX (5–100 mg/m^2), cytocidal CSF levels are not achieved, but with high doses of MTX (0.5–20 g/m^2), CSF levels are cytotoxic and may contribute to the therapeutic efficacy of high-dose regimens when CNS or meningeal disease is present.

C. Metabolism

At low doses of MTX, little metabolism of MTX occurs, except for a small amount of 2-4-diaminopteroate formation, a result of bacterial metabolism of MTX in the colon. With higher doses of MTX, 7-OH-MTX is formed, chiefly in the liver (40–43). Large amounts of this metabolite are found in plasma and urine (7–30% of total drug excreted) during the second 12 h after administration of high-dose MTX. This metabolism is caused by aldehyde oxidase, an enzyme found at high concentration in the liver. The 7-OH compound is a much less active inhibitor of DHFR, therefore this metabolism clearly is an inactivation of the drug. This metabolite is much less soluble in water, so vigorous hydration and alkalization of the urine is required to avoid the precipitation of this compound as well as MTX in renal tubules when high-dose regimens are used.

D. Excretion

MTX excretion is primarily renal. At conventional doses the drug is excreted mostly unchanged within first 24 h. At very low plasma concentrations, MTX may be reabsorbed by renal tubules. At higher concentrations, MTX may be actively secreted by tubules as well as filtered. After parenteral administration, only a small fraction (1–2%) is found in stool as unchanged drug and metabolites.

Most of the MTX excreted in the bile is reabsorbed. Fecal elimination after oral administration is proportional to the dose: for example, at a dose of 30 mg/ m^2, 4–6% is found in feces, and at 80 mg/m^2, 28.6% is eliminated in the stool.

E. Drug Interactions

Several drugs have been shown to potentially increase or decrease MTX toxicity based mainly on in vitro work. Salicylate and sulfa drugs displace MTX from plasma proteins, leaving more free drug available to tissues and for renal excretion, and may enhance the toxicity of MTX. Weak organic acids, like probenecid and salicylates, may diminish renal tubular excretion (44,45). Antibiotics may interfere with bacterial flora metabolizing the drug, and may decrease reabsorption. Dilantin may interact with MTX, and there is some evidence that it may enhance MTX toxicity. Allopurinol may decrease therapeutic efficacy in experimental tumor cells, probably by increasing the purine pools available for salvage (46). The clinical importance of these interactions are not well understood.

Recently, severe reactions have been reported between MTX and nonsteroidal antiinflammatory drugs, presumably due to decreased excretion of MTX secondary to the competition for renal excretion (47,48).

Vincristine may augment the toxicity of MTX by increasing uptake of this drug. Cephalothin and hydrocortisone may decrease its uptake. An important interaction between MTX and L-asparaginase has been exploited clinically and leads to enhanced therapeutic effects in patients with acute lymphocytic leukemia (ALL). L-asparaginase, a protein synthesis inhibitor, prevents MTX cytotoxicity when used concomitantly with this drug. If used as a "rescue," however, administered 24 h after MTX dosage, asparaginase will relieve toxicity to normal tissue, but (ALL) cells will not be rescued because they are asparagine autotrophs, that is they cannot synthesize asparagine and thus depend on an exogenous supply of this compound (49).

IV. CLINICAL INDICATIONS

MTX has been used widely for the treatment of neoplastic diseases, including choriocarcinoma, malignant lymphoma, acute leukemias, breast cancer, and GI malignancies. As an immunosuppressive agent, it is used for prophylaxis of graft-versus-host disease after bone marrow transplantation. As an antiinflammatory/immunosuppressive agent, it is used in the treatment of rheumatoid arthritis, psoriasis, and dermatomyositis. In these circumstances the drug is usually administered weekly or biweekly in low doses, p.o. The mechanism of this therapeutic effect in low, relatively nontoxic doses in these inflammatory diseases is not known.

V. ADVERSE REACTIONS

Self-renewing tissues, that is, bone marrow and epithelial cells, are at risk for damage by MTX. Duration of the exposure to MTX is an important factor in determining the level of toxicity as well as the dose. Very large doses of MTX ($20 g/m^2$) can be tolerated well if rescued by large doses of LV 6–24 h later (3,4). When plasma concentrations of 10^{-6} M or higher are maintained for more than 48 hs, irreversible toxicity may occur. A safe guideline for using MTX at high doses is to use LV rescue when the MTX level exceeds 10^{-8} M at 36 h. The amount of LV used should be proportional to the blood level of MTX. Low-dose oral therapy (2.5–12.5 mg) weekly is well tolerated by rheumatoid arthritis (RA) patients, and in one large outpatient study ($N = 183$), only seven patients had therapy discontinued due to side effects (50).

A. Hematological Toxicity

All three lineages of bone marrow cells are affected by MTX, but usually neutropenia predominates. Recovery after single doses of MTX is usually rapid, occurring 14–21 d after the nadir, which is about 10 d after injection. With the use of hematopoietic growth factors, the period of neutropenia may be lessened. Marrow toxicity is dose related, but there is a significant variability between patients. Subclinical folate deficiency due to poor nutrition, impaired renal function, or stressed marrow due to previous x-ray treatment, chemotherapy, or infection may predispose the marrow and gastrointestinal tract to toxicity. Young patients usually tolerate this drug well, presumably because of good renal function.

B. Gastrointestinal Toxicity

Gastrointestinal toxicity is relatively rare with low-dose MTX treatment. Mucositis may be seen 2–7 d after MTX administration. This is usually an early sign of MTX toxicity, and treatment should be discontinued and complete healing should be allowed before the next dose is administered. Nausea, anorexia, and less commonly, vomiting may be seen, but usually with higher doses. Diarrhea may also occur, and in toxic doses may progress to severe bloody diarrhea.

C. Nephrotoxicity

Conventional doses of MTX, not requiring LV, usually do not cause nephrotoxicity, except for rare idiosyncratic reactions. With high doses of MTX with LV rescue, renal toxicity is much more common, and may result in delayed clearance of MTX and systemic toxicity. It is believed that nephrotoxicity is due to the precipitation of MTX and its less soluble metabolite, 7-OH MTX, to the renal tubules, as well as the direct effect of the drug on the tubules (43). The use of vigorous hydration and alkalization of the urine to increase the solubility of MTX and 7-OH MTX has proven to be effective in preventing this event. In most instances the renal impairment is reversible if appropriate action is taken to improve elimination of the drug and high doses of LV are administered. These patients should be carefully monitored and LV should be continued until the plasma concentration of MTX becomes less than 10^{-8} M.

D. Hepatotoxicity

Several days after high-dose administration of MTX, acute elevation of liver enzymes (SGOT) commonly occurs. This usually returns to normal rapidly and does not appear to predict chronic liver toxicity. Severe acute hepatic toxicity is rarely seen with either conventional or high-dose regimens. Low-dose continuous or weekly treatment with MTX has been associated with portal fibrosis and in some patients frank cirrhosis (51,52). This complication is reported in patients with psoriasis, rheumatoid arthritis, and ALL treated with long-term oral MTX. Predisposing factors are duration of therapy, alcoholism, and psoriasis. An intermittent schedule with pulse therapy may decrease the risk of this complications (53). In RA patients significant hepatic toxicity requiring discontinuation of therapy is reported to be less than 4% with the oral pulse intermittent schedule.

E. Pulmonary Toxicity

Pulmonary toxicity due to MTX has been described, although it is uncommon. It may even occur in patients who are receiving low-dose oral MTX for RA (54,55). The clinical picture usually consists of cough, dyspnea, fever, and hypoxia. The chest x-ray reveals a patchy interstitial infiltrate. Pneumocystis carinii pneumonia must be ruled out, especially in patients also receiving steroids. Histological exam may show diffuse interstitial lymphocyte infiltrates, giant cells, and noncaseating granulomas. In some patients a peripheral eosinophilia is observed, raising the possibility that this is an allergic pneumonitis. The process may progress to fibrosis, and it is important to discontinue the drug while the pulmonary toxicity is reversible. Some patients may be retreated with MTX without recurrence of the problem.

F. Skin Toxicity

Skin toxicity to MTX occurs in 5–10% of patients, consisting of an erythematous rash, characteristically noted on the neck and upper trunk. The rash may be pruritic and relatively insignificant, and usually lasts for several days. In other instances, especially when related to other signs of severe MTX toxicity, it may progress to severe bullous formation and desquamation (56).

G. Neurotoxicity

Neurotoxicity from MTX can be acute, subacute, or chronic. An acute toxic syndrome has been observed after intrathecal administration and consists of headache, fever, and meningismus lasting several hours and pleocytosis that may mimic bacterial infections. This syndrome is the most common of the neurological syndromes associated with intrathecal MTX administration and appears to be related to high cerebrospinal fluid (CSF) concentrations of the drug.

A subacute form of central nervous system (CNS) toxicity has also been observed after intrathecal administration. In this instance more severe signs of motor dysfunction are noted, such as paraplegia, cerebellar dysfunction, and cranial nerve palsies and seizures, usually after two or more doses of the drug per week (57).

In addition to the neurotoxicity associated with intrathecal MTX administration, patients receiving high-dose intravenous MTX ($>$50 mg/m^2) after radiation therapy to the brain ($>$2000 rads) have developed a necrotizing leukoencephalopathy associated with progressive neurological deterioration. This may begin insidiously and progress to severe neurological impairment (dementia, ataxia, seizures, and coma) (58,59).

H. Other Side Effects

MTX is known to cause abortions, especially if administered during the first trimester of pregnancy. However, there is no report of higher than normal incidence of fetal abnormalities in women who have been successfully treated with MTX for choriocarcinoma. These women also have not had a higher than normal incidence of secondary malignancies. Thus far there is no evidence that MTX has any mutagenic or carcinogenic effects.

Osteoporosis has been reported with chronic low-dose MTX administration (60). Fever, seizure, recall of radiation toxicity or phototoxicity, and anaphylactoid reactions have been reported with high-dose administration (61). Pleuritic and left upper quadrant pain, presumably due to splenic capsule inflammation, has been reported after treatment with moderately high-dose regimens.

In patients receiving low doses of MTX for the treatment of psoriasis and rheumatoid arthritis, the drug is generally well tolerated. In one study in patients with rheumatoid arthritis, 50% of the patients were still taking the drug after 5 y (62). Major toxic events leading to drug discontinuation occurred in only 13 of 152 patients, and were mainly gastrointestinal (nausea, vomiting) and skin toxicity (10 of 13). Minor toxicities were seen in 34 of 152 patients, and as expected, these were primarily gastrointestinal, skin rash; mucositis and leukopenia were less commonly observed (62).

REFERENCES

1. Jolivet J, Conan KH, Curt GA. The pharmacology and clinical use of methotrexate. N Engl J Med 1983; 309:1094.
2. Allegra CJ. Antifolates. In: Cancer chemotherapy: Principles and practice. Chabner BA, Collins JM, ed. Lippincott, Philadelphia: 1990:110.
3. Bertino JR. Clinical pharmacology of methotrexate. Med Pediatr Oncol 1982; 10:401.
4. Ackland SP, Schilsky, RL. High-dose methotrexate: A critical reappraisal. J Clin Oncol 1987; 12:2017.
5. Bertino JR. Ode to methotrexate. J Clin Oncol 1993; 11:5.
6. Catterji DC, Gallelli JF. High pressure liquid chromatography analysis of methotrexate in the presence of its degradation products. J Pharm Sci 1977; 66:1212.
7. Falk LC, Clark DR, Kalman SM, Long TF. Enzymatic assay for methotrexate in serum and cerebrospinal fluid. Clin Chem 1976; 22:784.
8. Sirotnak FM. Correlates of folate analog transport: Pharmacokinetics and selective antitumor action. Pharmacol Ther 1982; 257:1890.
9. Chabner B, Young R. Threshold methotrexate concentrations for DNA synthesis of normal and tumorous target tissues. J Clin Invest 1973; 52:1804.
10. Fry DW, Anderson LA, Borst M, Goldman ID. Analysis of the role of membrane transport and polyglutamation of methotrexate in gut and Ehrich tumor in vivo as factors in drug sensitivity and selectivity. Cancer 1983; 43:1087.

11. Jolivet J, Schilisky RL, Bailey BD, Drake JC, Chabner BA. Synthesis, retention, and biological activity of methotrexate polyglutamates in cultured human breast cancer cells. J Clin Invest 1982; 70:351.
12. Matherly LH, Barlowe CK, Goldman ID. Antifolate polyglutamylation and competitive drug displacement of dihydrofolate reductase as important elements of leucovorin rescue in L1210 cells. Cancer Res 1986; 46:588.
13. Schilisky RL, Bailey BD, Chabner BA. Methotrexate polyglutamate synthesis by cultured human breast cancer cells. Proc Natl Acad Sci USA 1980; 77:2919.
14. Whitehead VM, Rosenblatt DS, Vuchich MJ, Scuster JJ, White A, Beaulieu D. Accumulation of methotrexate and methotrexate polyglutamates in lymphoblasts at diagnosis of childhood acute lymphoblastic leukemia: A pilot prognostic factor analysis. Blood 1990; 76:44.
15. McGuire JJ, Hsieh P, Coward JK, Bertino JR. Enzymatic synthesis of folypolyglutamates. J Biol Chem 1980; 255:5776.
16. Balinska M, Galivan J, Coward JK. Efflux of methotrexate and its polyglutamate derivatives from hepatic cells in vitro. Cancer Res 1981; 41:2751.
17. Curt GA, Jolivet J, Bailey BD, Carney DN, Chabner BA. Synthesis and retention of methotrexate polyglutamates by human small cell lung cancer. Biochem Pharmacol 1984; 33:1682.
18. Curt GA, Jolivet J, Carney DN, Bailey BD, Drake JC, Clendenin NJ, Chabner BA. Determinants of the sensitivity of human small-cell lung cancer cell lines to methotrexate. J Clin Invest 1985; 76:1323.
19. Fabre I, Fabre G, Goldman ID. Polyglutamation, an important element in methotrexate cytotoxicity and selectivity in tumor versus murine granulocyte precursor cells in vitro. Cancer Res 1984; 44:3190.
20. Kozumi S, Curt GA, Fine RL, Griffin JD, Chabner BA. Formation of methotrexate polyglutamates in purified marrow myeloid precursor cells from normal human bone marrow. J Clin Invest 1985; 75:1008.
21. Sirotnak FM, Donsbach RC. The intracellular concentration dependence of antifolate inhibition of DNA synthesis in L1210 leukemia cells. Cancer Res 1974; 34:3332.
22. White CJ, Loftfield S, Goldman ID. The mechanism of action of methotrexate: III. Requirement of free intracellular methotrexate for maximal suppression of (14C) formate incorporation into nucleic acids and protein. Mol Pharmacol 1975; 11:287
23. Bertino JR. The general pharmacology of methotrexate. In: Wilke WS, ed. Methotrexate therapy in rheumatic diseases. New York: Marcel Dekker, 1989:11.
24. Alt FW, Kellems RE, Bertino JR, Schimke RT. Selective multiplication of dihydrofolate reductase genes in methotrexate-resistant variants of cultured murine cells. J Biol Chem 1978; 253:1357.
25. Srimatkandada S, Medina WD, Cashmore AR, Whyte W, Engel D, Moroson BA, Franco CT, Dube SK, Bertino JR. Amplification and organization of dihydrofolate reductase genes in human leukemia cell line, K-562, resistant to methotrexate. Biochemistry 1983; 22:5574.
26. Fischer GA. Defective transport of amethopterin (methotrexate) as a a mechanism of resistance to the antimetabolites in L5178Y leukemic cells. Biochem Pharmacol 1962; 11:1233.

27. Rosowsky A, Wright JE, Cucchi CA, Boeheim K, Frei E III. Transport of fluorescent antifolate by methotrexate-sensitive and methotrexate-resistant human leukemic lymphoblasts. Biochem Pharmacol 1986; 35:356.
28. Henderson GB, Tsuji JM, Kumar HP. Transport of folate compounds by leukemic cells: Evidence for a single influx carrier for methotrexate, 5-methyltetrahydrofolate, and folate in CCRF-CEM human lymphoblasts. Biochem Pharmacol 1987; 36:3007.
29. Flintoff WF, Essani K. Methotrexate resistant chinese hamster ovary cells contain a dihydrofolate reductase with an altered affinity for methotrexate. Biochemistry 1980; 19:4321.
30. Goldie JH, Dedhar S, Krystal G. Properties of a methotrexate-insensitive variant of dihydrofolate reductase from methotrexate-resistant L5178Y cells. J Biol Chem 1981; 256:11629.
31. Dicker AP, Waltham MC, Volkenandt M, Schweitzer BI, Otter GM, Schmid FA, Sirotnak FM, Bertino JR. Methotrexate resistance in an in vivo mouse tumor due to a non-active-site dihydrofolate reductase mutation. Proc Natl Aced Sci USA 1993; 90:11797.
32. Banerjee D, Schweitzer BI, Volkenandt M, Li M, Waltham MC, Mineishi S, Bertino JR. Mutant human dihydrofolate reductase as dominant selectable markers in chinese hamster ovary cells. Gene, in press.
33. Livingston L, White A, Sprouse J, Livanos E, Jacks T, Tlsty TD. Altered cell cycle arrest and gene amplification potential accompany loss of wild-type p53. Cell 1993; 70:923.
34. Yin Y, Tainsky MA, Bischoff FG, Strong LC, Wahl GM. Wild-type p53 restores cell cycle control and inhibits gene amplification in cells with mutant p53 allele. Cell 1992; 70:937.
35. Balis FM, Savitch JL, Bleyer WA. Pharmacokinetics of oral methotrexate in children. Cancer Res 1983; 34:2342.
36. Chungi VS, Bourne DWA, Dittert LW. Drug absorption: Kinetics of GI absorption of methotrexate. J Pharm Sci 1978; 67:560.
37. Said HM, Hollander D. Inhibitory effect of bile salts on the enterohepatic circulation of methotrexate in the unanesthetized rat: Inhibition of methotrexate intestinal absorption. Cancer Chemother Pharmacol 1986; 16:121.
38. Steinberg SE, Campbell CL, Bleyer WA, Hillman RS. Enterohepatic circulation of methotrexate in rats in vivo. Cancer Res 1982; 42:1279.
39. Wan SH, Hufman DH, Azarnoff DL, Stephens R, Hoogstraten B. Effect of route of administration and effusion on methotrexate pharmacokinetics. Cancer Res 1974; 34:3487.
40. Lankelma J, van der Klein E. The role of 7-hydroxyl methotrexate during methotrexate anticancer chemotherapy. Cancer Lett 1980; 9:133.
41. Sonneveld P, Schultz FW, Nooter K, Hahlen K. Pharmacokinetics of methotrexate and 7-hydroxymethotrexate in plasma and bone marrow of children receiving low-dose oral methotrexate. Cancer Chemother Pharmacol 1986; 18:111.
42. Stewart AL, Margison JM, Wilkinson PM, Lukas SB. The pharmacokinetics of 7-hydroxymethotrexate following medium-dose methotrexate therapy. Cancer Chemother Pharmacol 1985; 14:165.

43. Jacobs SA, Stoller RG, Chabner BA, Jones DG. 7-hydroxymethotrexate as urinary metabolite in human subjects and rhesus monkey receiving high dose methotrexate. J Clin Invest 1976; 57:534.
44. Aherne GN, Prall E, Marks V, Mould G, White WF. Prolongation and enhancement of serum methotrexate concentrations by probenecid. B. M. J. 1978; 1:1097.
45. Liegler DG, Henderson ES, Hahn MA, Oliverio VT. The effect of organic acids on renal clearance of methotrexate in man. Clin Pharm Ther 1969; 10:849.
46. Grindey GB. The effect of allopurinol on the therapeutic effects of methotrexate. Cancer Res 1975; 35:1702.
47. Singh RR, Malaviya AV, Pandey JN, Guleria JS. Fatal interaction between methotrexate and nonsteroidal antiinflammatory drugs. Lancet 1986; 1:8480.
48. Thyss A, Milano G, Kuber J, Namer M, Schneider M. Clinical and pharmacokinetic evidence of a life-threatening interaction between methotrexate and ketoprofen. Lancet 1986; 1:256.
49. Esterhoy RJ, Wiernik PH, Grove WR, Markus SD, Wesley MN. Moderate dose methotrexate, vincristine, asparaginase and dexamethasone for the treatment of adult acute lymphocytic leukemia. Blood 1982; 59:334.
50. Zeiders RS. Oral methotrexate therapy in rheumatoid arthritis. Arthritis Rheum 1982; 25(suppl):565.
51. Mackenzie AH. Adverse hepatic effects of methotrexate therapy. In: Wilke WS, ed. Methotrexate therapy in rheumatic diseases. New York: Marcel Dekker, 1989:179.
52. Zachariae H, Kragballe K, Soggaard H. Methotrexate-induced cirrhosis. Br J Dermatol 1980; 102:407.
53. Dahl MGC, Gregory MM, Scheuer PJ. Methotrexate hepatotoxicity in psoriasis-comparison of different dose regimens. B. M. J. 1972; 1:654.
54. St. Clair EW, Rice JR, Syndersman R. Pneumonitis after low dose methotrexate therapy in rheumatoid arthritis. Arch Intern Med 1985; 145:2035.
55. Carson CW, Cannon GW, Egger JM, Ward JR, Clegg DO. Pulmonary disease during the treatment of rheumatoid arthritis with low dose pulse methotrexate. Semin Arthrit Rheum 1987; 16:186.
56. Doyle LA, Berg C, Bottino G, Chabner BA. Erythema and desquamation after high-dose methotrexate. Ann Inter Med 1983; 98:611.
57. Bleyer WA, Drake JC, Chabner BA. Neurotoxicity and elevated cerebrospinal fluid methotrexate concentration in meningeal leukemia. N Engl J Med 1973; 289:770.
58. Shapiro WR, Allen JC, Horten BC. Chronic methotrexate toxicity to the central nervous system. Clin Bull Memorial Sloan-Kettering 1980; 10:49.
59. Pelan-Ramu N, Poplack DG, Blei CL, Herdt JR, Vermess M, Dichiro G. Computer-assisted tomography in methotrexate encephalopathy. J Comput Assist Tomogr 1977; 1:216.
60. Nesbit M. Acute and chronic effects of methotrexate on hepatic, pulmonary, and skeletal systems. Cancer 1976; 37:1048.
61. Goldberg NH, Romolo JL, Austin EH, Drake J, Rosenberg SA. Anaphylactoid type reactions in two patients receiving high-dose intravenous methotrexate. Cancer 1978; 41:52.
62. Alarcon GS, Tracy IC, Blackburn WD Jr. Methotrexate in rheumatoid arthritis. Arthrit Rheum 1989; 32:671.

3
Pyrimidine Analogs

Marcia J. Browne
N.E. Hematology/Oncology Associates, Wellesley, Massachusetts

Jeffrey W. Clark
Harvard University and Massachusetts General Hospital, Boston, Massachusetts

Pyridimine analogs are antineoplastic agents that are structurally and chemically similar to naturally occurring compounds required for the synthesis of pyrimidines. Inhibition of key enzymes in the pyrimidine synthetic pathway or misincorporation into the DNA molecule by these compounds interferes with DNA synthesis resulting in strand breaks or premature chain termination.

I. 5-FLUOROURACIL

5-Fluorouracil (5-FU) is a commonly used antimetabolite synthesized by Heidleberger and colleagues in 1957 (1). This drug was rationally developed because of the observation that rat hepatoma cells utilize uracil for nuclear acid synthesis more efficiently than do nonmalignant rat intestinal mucosa cells (2). This finding suggested that pathways utilizing uracil differ in normal and malignant cells and may be an exploitable target for antineoplastic chemotherapy. 5-FU has become useful in the treatment of solid tumors including colorectal, breast, and head and neck cancers. In the dermatological field, it has been used topically or intralesionally for premalignant skin disease, specifically actinic keratoses (3), and for keratoacanthomas (4–6), arsenical keratoses, warts (7–9), psoriasis (10,11), and porokeratoses (12). The use of 5-FU systemically for dermatological diseases is evolving.

A. Chemistry

5-FU is an analog of the pyrimidine uracil with a fluorine atom substituted for hydrogen at the 5-carbon position of the pyrimidine ring (see Figure 1). Most mammalian cells obtain thymidine-5′-triphosphate (dTTP), a key precursor for DNA synthesis, from 2′-deoxyuridine-5′-monophosphate (dUMP) via the enzyme thymidylate synthetase, which replaces the hydrogen at the 5-carbon position with a methyl group to form thymidine-5′-monophosphate (dTMP). The fluorine atom in 5-FU is slightly bulkier than the hydrogen atom in uracil but does not prevent the conversion of 5-FU to the nucleoside FdURD and ultimately to the nucleotide FdUMP, a reaction essential to the antitumor activity of this compound (13). FdUMP is also a substrate for thymidylate synthetase, but the carbon-fluorine bond is more stable, thereby preventing substitution of the methyl group, and ultimately inhibits enzyme function (14). 5-FU is more soluble in aqueous solutions than its natural pyrimidine analog and is stable in solution at physiologic pH for weeks (14).

B. Mechanism of Action

5-FU is rapidly transported across cell membranes sharing the same transport system as uracil (13) and requires intracellular activation for its cytotoxic activity. There are two primary mechanisms of action capable of causing cell injury and death: inhibition of thymidylate synthetase and incorporation into RNA (see Figure 2).

Intracellularly, 5-FU is metabolized to fluorouridine monophosphate (FUMP) and subsequently converted to fluorouridine triphosphate (FUTP) and fluorodeoxyuridine–monophosphate (FdUMP), the active nucleotide forms. FdUMP inhibits thymidine synthetase (TS), the only de novo source of thymidylate in the cell, by binding tightly to TS and preventing formation of thymidylate. Thymidylate is an essential precursor to dTTP, one of four deoxyribonucleotides required for DNA synthesis (15,16).

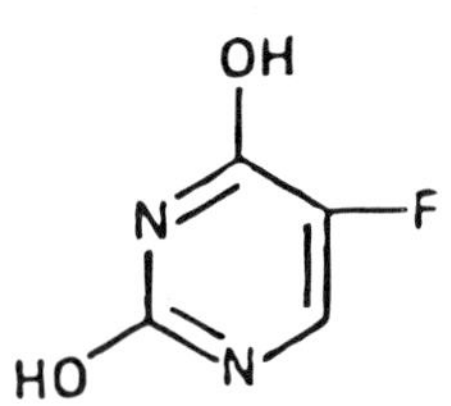

FU

Figure 1 Structure 5-fluorouracil.

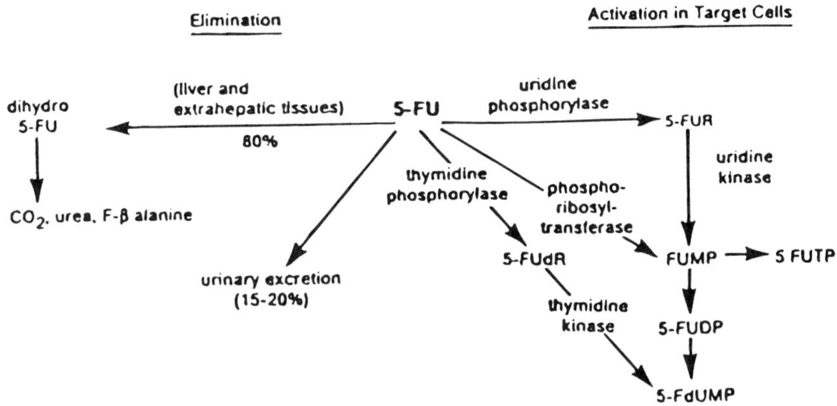

Figure 2 Pathways of 5-fluorouracil elimination and activation.

The second mechanism of action involves FUTP incorporation into RNA, which interferes with RNA processing and function and therefore cell viability (17–19).

Recent data suggest that 5-FU incorporation into DNA may produce single-strand breaks that also contribute to the drug's cytotoxicity (20,21).

C. Pharmacology

1. Absorption and Distribution

5-FU is usually administered intravenously. Bioavailability after oral administration is highly variable due to erratic absorption and variable first-pass metabolism in the liver (22,23). Less than 75% of a dose reaches the systemic circulation after oral administration, with peak plasma concentrations reaching a maximum of 5–200 μM within 1 h of administration (24). Bioavailability appears to increase with increasing dose. The clinical response rate to oral 5-FU is lower than that to intravenous 5-FU (25) and therefore oral 5-FU is rarely used.

5-FU penetrates well into the cerebrospinal fluid (CSF) and extracellular "third space" fluids such as pleural effusions or ascites when administered by the intravenous route (13). CSF concentrations of 1×10^{-8} lasting 12 h can be obtained with conventional doses of 5-FU. Attainable CSF concentrations of 5-FU depend on the schedule of administration, and more CSF exposure is provided by bolus delivery than slow infusion (26).

Peak plasma levels of 0.1–1.0 mM are obtained following intravenous administration of conventional doses of 10–15 mg/kg (27), but rapid breakdown by dihydropyrimidine dehydrogenase in the liver and other tissues leads to a rapid decrease in plasma levels. The plasma half-life of 5-FU is 6–20 min, but there may be considerable variability between patients. The volume of distribution (V_D) for 5-FU is 12–38% (median 22%) of total body weight (28,23).

2. Excretion

More than 80% of 5-FU is eliminated by metabolic conversion of dihydrofluorouracil (DHFU) by dihydropyrimidine dehydrogenase. Approximately 15% is excreted unchanged in the urine. Persons deficient in dihydropyrimidine dehydrogenase (an uncommon disorder) have greatly increased toxicity when treated with 5-FU (29). Further metabolism of DHFU to alpha-fluoroureidoproprionic acid, α-fluoro-β-alanine, and carbon dioxide occurs. The primary sites of metabolism are kidney, liver, white blood cells, and gastrointestinal mucosa. Because metabolism occurs in extrahepatic sites, dose reduction of 5-FU is not necessary in patients with liver dysfunction.

3. Clinical Dermatological Use

Although topical 5-FU is widely used for a variety of dermatological conditions (e.g., psoriasis, premalignant squamous cell lesions, and squamous cell carcinomas) nontopical use of pyrimidines has a more limited role. However, there are a number of current clinical uses for nontopical pyrimidines, and a number of analogs of these agents are potential candidates for therapeutic utility in dermatology in the future.

5-FU can be given intralesionally for a variety of conditions (see above for discussion). Historically, systemic chemotherapy has been felt to have limited value against unresectable or metastatic squamous cell carcinomas of the skin. However, a recent (albeit with a small number of patients) study suggests that there is a reasonable response rate to the combination of 5-FU and cisplatin given systemically for this disease (30). Other combinations (such as 5-FU combined with bleomycin) have been less extensively studied for this purpose, but given their activity against other squamous cell carcinomas are also worth considering (31). This is an area requiring further study for this purpose or possibily for adjuvant therapy for individuals with cutaneous squamous cell carcinomas at high risk of recurrence or dissemination. Clearly, 5-FU is of potential use for the treatment of patients with cutaneous metastases from any tumor (such as breast cancer) against which it has activity. Although 5-FU itself has limited activity against melanoma (except possibly for topical application in selected patients, presumably by stimulating an immune reaction), there are a number of preclinical models that suggest that it may be effective in combinations with other approaches such as immunomodulation or hyperthermia for treating melanoma (32–36).

Systemically administered 5-FU also appears to have a role in the treatment of recalcitrant psoriasis (37,38). In a study by Alper et al. (37), nine patients received 191 courses of 5-FU in combination with either methotrexate or azauridine. Eight of nine patients experienced at least 50% clearing of their disease, three showing this response within 4 wk and the remaining five responding within 8 wk. Finally, there are a number of pyrimidine analogs that have greater activity in preclinical testing against melanoma than 5-FU itself and which may be clinically useful in the future.

4. Adverse Reactions

The main toxic effects of 5-FU (see Table 1) are on rapidly dividing tissues, primarily the gastrointestinal mucosa and the bone marrow. The toxicity of 5-FU may present a broad spectrum and appears to be related to the dose, route, and the schedule of administration.

Myelosuppression occurs more frequently following bolus intravenous therapy rather than infusion and may be the dose-limiting toxicity. The nadir of granulocytopenia and thrombocytopenia usually occurs between the tenth and fourteenth day following the first administration of the drug. If this nadir occurs concomitantly with diarrhea, the potential of overwhelming sepsis is increased because disruption of the normal integrity of the gut lining can facilitate entry of enteric organisms into the bloodstream.

Gastrointestinal toxicity may be severe and life threatening and can include involvement at any level of the gastrointestinal tract. Stomatitis and diarrhea are the most frequent side effects. Stomatitis may consist only of erythema and mild tenderness or may be manifested by ulcerations, necrosis, and severe dysphagia or retrosternal pain. Diarrhea is usually mild at clinically used doses but can be profuse and/or bloody. In combination with nausea, vomiting, or dysphagia, diarrhea may lead to severe dehydration requiring hospitalization. A history and physical exam, with special attention to the presence of mouth soreness or watery diarrhea, should be performed on all patients before each dose of 5-FU to determine whether the drug can be safely given. The presence of even mild mucositis and diarrhea may preclude administration of the drug. Supportive care with adequate hydration and electrolyte replacement should be given if diarrhea occurs. Antidiarrheal agents alone are ineffective in the setting of moderate to severe diarrhea from 5-FU (39,40).

Toxicities to the skin include alopecia (which occasionally can progress to total hair loss), dermatitis, nail changes (41) (hyperpigmentation and onycholysis), increased pigmentation (42,43), and photosensitivity. Increased tanning and sunburn reactions can occur due to enhanced reactions to ultraviolet light. An enhancement of cutaneous toxicity from therapeutic radiation therapy can be seen with 5-FU and may be manifested by erythema, or in severe cases, progression to

Table 1 Toxicities of 5-FU

Hematological
Leukopenia
Thrombocytopenia
Gastrointestinal
Stomatitis
Mucositis
Diarrhea
Dermatological
Alopecia
Nail changes
Dermatitis
Hyperpigmentation
Photosensitivity
Inflammation of actinic keratoses
Enhancement of radiation effects
Neurological
Cerebellar ataxia
Somnolence
Upper motor neuron signs
Cardiotoxicity/Pulmonary
Angina
Supraventricular tachycardia
Ventricular tachycardia
Congestive heart failure
Reversible cardiomyopathy
Myocardial infarction
Sudden death
Ophthalmological
Conjunctivitis
Epiphora
Blepharitis
Tear-duct stenosis
Cicatricial ectropion

vesicles and desquamation within 7 d of the initiation of radiation. Less common side effects include hyperpigmentation localized to the skin over a vein that has been used for administration of 5-FU (44), atrophy of the skin, hand-foot syndrome (45) (which is usually associated with continuous infusion intravenous therapy), and an inflammatory reaction in actinic keratoses (which can be used for therapeutic benefit). An allergic contact dermatitis from topical 5-FU can occur.

Acute neurological symptoms including somnolence, upper motor neuron signs, and cerebellar ataxia can occasionally be seen, most particularly in patients receiving high dose intensity or intracarotid administration of 5-FU for head and neck cancer (46,47). The neurological toxicity may be due to fluorocitrate, a neurotoxic metabolite of 5-FU (48). Other possible mechanisms include disruption of the blood-brain barrier, which has been shown in the canine model to produce neurotoxicity associated with edema and foci of hemorrhagic necrosis.

Cardiotoxicity is an infrequently described side effect of 5-FU. Cardiac manifestations that have been described include angina, supraventricular tachycardia, ventricular tachycardia, congestive heart failure, reversible cardiomyopathy, myocardial infarction, and sudden death (49–51). Clinically, patients have complained of chest pain in temporal association with administration of 5-FU, often associated with electrocardiographic and serum enzyme changes. Observations suggest that the presence of coronary artery disease does not contribute to 5-FU-induced cardiotoxicity (51). The syndrome is usually reversible and responds favorably to the discontinuation of 5-FU followed by conventional therapy for angina and congestive heart failure.

5-FU is associated with significant ocular toxicity that includes conjunctivitis, blepharitis, tear-duct stenosis, excessive lacrimation, epiphora, and cicatricial ectropian (52–54). The acute inflammatory response is reversible when 5-FU is discontinued early after the appearance of the toxicity, but progression of the inflammation may result in the need for surgical correction of dacrostenosis or ectropion.

II. CYTARABINE

Cytarabine (cytosine arabinoside; ara-C) is an antimetabolite that has important clinical activity against leukemias and lymphomas, including cutaneous leukemic lesions. Originally isolated from the sponge *Cryptothethya crypta* (55), this arabinose nucleoside is now produced synthetically.

A. Chemistry

Cytarabine is an arabinoside nucleoside whose chemical structure differs from the naturally occurring deoxyribonucleosides by the presence of a Beta-OH group in the 2′ position of the sugar (see Figure 3). Cytarabine is the most active cytotoxic agent of this class, although several arabinose nucleosides have antitumor and antiviral activity.

B. Mechanism of Action

Cytarabine acts as an analog for the nucleoside deoxycytidine and inhibits DNA function in several ways (see Figure 4) (56). Firstly, cytarabine competitively inhibits DNA polymerase alpha after undergoing phosphorylation to form ara-

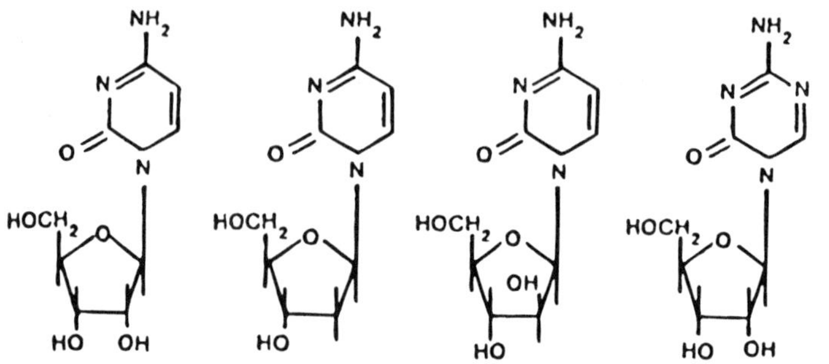

CYTIDINE DEOXYCYTIDINE CYTOSINE ARABINOSIDE 5-AZACYTIDINE

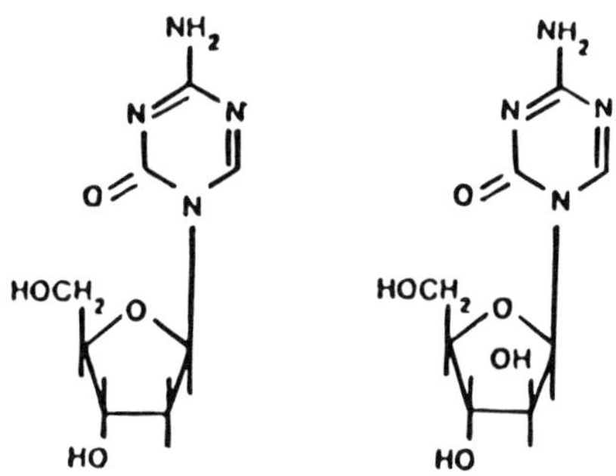

5-AZA-2′-DEOXYCYTIDINE 5-AZA-CYTOSINE ARABINOSIDE

Figure 3 Structure of cytidine analogs with antitumor activity.

CTP, thereby interfering with DNA synthesis. Although this contributes to the cytotoxic effects of ara-C, the most important correlate with cytotoxicity is the incorporation of cytarabine into DNA. A linear relationship exists between the amount of cytarabine incorporated and the log of cell kill. The incorporated cytarabine inhibits template function and chain elongation (57). Cytarabine also appears to cause abnormal duplication of limited portions of DNA (58). The reduplication of segments increases the possibility of recombination, crossover, and gene amplification. Cytarabine kills cells selectively during the S phase of the cell cycle.

C. Pharmacology

1. Absorption

Cytarabine is transported across cell membranes by a carrier-mediated process that is shared by other nucleosides including deoxycytidine. It is converted to

1-β-Arabinofuranosylcytosine in leukemia

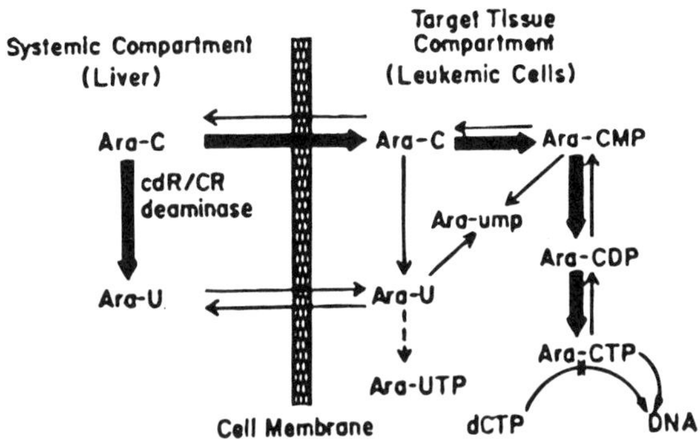

Figure 4 Metabolic pathway of ara-C. Heavy arrows indicate major pathway.

its active form, ara-CTP by the action of three enzymes: deoxycytidine (CdR) kinase, deoxycytidylate (dCMP) kinase, and nucleoside diphosphate (NDP) kinase (see Figure 4) (56). Following intravenous administration, cytarabine is rapidly deaminated by cytidine deaminase forming an inactive product, ara-UMP. The gastrointestinal mucosa and liver have high concentrations of cytidine deaminase and therefore oral administration of cytarabine results in much lower plasma levels than does intravenous administration. Three- to tenfold higher doses must be given to achieve a comparable effect and therefore cytarabine is not given by the oral route.

2. Distribution

Cytarabine is transported by active transport and distributes quickly into total body water (59,60). Increases in plasma cytarabine concentrations are proportional with increasing dose. Cytarabine crosses into the central nervous system (CNS) and reaches steady-state levels at 20–40% of those found simultaneously in plasma during continuous intravenous infusion (61).

3. Excretion

The plasma half-life is 7–20 min and the plasma concentration declines rapidly. More than 70% of the administered drug is excreted in the urine as ara-U, an inactive metabolite. Because of rapid deamination of cytarabine, ara-U becomes the predominant form of cytarabine within minutes of drug administration. The formation of ara-U takes place primarily in plasma, liver, and granulocytes (62).

At high rates of infusion, the deamination reaction becomes saturated and cytarabine plasma levels rise rapidly leading to serious toxicity (16).

4. Clinical Indications

Systemic ara-C is useful for the treatment of patients with cutaneous lesions of sensitive malignancies, such as leukemias and lymphomas. It is also one of the agents that can be given intrathecally for carcinomatous meningitis due to metastatic melanoma. As discussed above, there are a number of pyrimidine analogs that have shown activity against melanoma in preclinical testing and these may be developed for clinical therapy in the future.

5. Adverse Reactions

The primary determinants of cytarabine toxicity are drug concentration and duration of drug exposure. The main side effects are myelosuppression and gastrointestinal injury (see Table 2).

Neutropenia and thrombocytopenia are the main manifestations of hematological toxicity. Anemia may occur and megaloblastic changes are seen in both the red and white blood cell precursors.

Table 2 Toxicities of Cytarabine

Hematological
Leukopenia
Thrombocytopenia
Anemia
Megaloblastic changes
Gastrointestinal
Nausea
Vomiting
Diarrhea
Mucositis
Ileus
Dermatological
Neutrophilic eccrine hydradenitis
Neurological
Cerebellar ataxia
Slurred speech
Confusion
Coma
Pulmonary
Noncardiogenic pulmonary edema
Streptococcus viridans pneumonia
Ophthalmological
Conjunctivitis
Anaphylaxis

Gastrointestinal symptoms include nausea, vomiting, and diarrhea which can occur during drug administration. Oral mucositis may be severe in patients receiving more than 5 d of treatment. Injury to the lower GI tract may manifest as diarrhea, bleeding, ileus, abdominal pain, and protein-losing enteropathy. Reversible intrahepatic cholestasis occurs in about 25% of patients but is not usually an indication for discontinuing the drug. Pancreatitis has been seen in a small number of patients (63).

Neurological toxicity is seen in 20% of patients receiving high-dose cytarabine. This is seen particularly in patients over 50 y of age. Symptoms include slurred speech, ataxia, confusion, and coma (64). Although the toxicity is reversible in the majority of cases, fatal outcomes have been observed. The neurological toxicity appears to be more common in patients with abnormal serum creatinine levels, despite the fact that ara-C is eliminated primarily by metabolism and not by renal excretion.

Conjunctivitis, responsive to topical steroids, is a frequent side effect of cytarabine (65). Other uncommon but reported side effects of cytarabine include neutrophilic eccrine hydradenitis manifested by plaques and nodules usually during the second week after high-dose administration (66,67), anaphylaxis (68), a painful hand-foot syndrome, and pulmonary complications including noncardiogenic pulmonary edema (69), and *Streptococcus viridans* pneumonia (70).

III. FLUCYTOSINE

Flucytosine (5-FC) is a fluorinated pyrimidine analog of cytosine. It was synthesized as a potential antineoplastic drug but was not found to have significant antitumor activity. In 1964, the activity of flucytosine against murine cryptococcus was reported (71), and in 1968, flucytosine was first used in humans to treat candidiasis and cryptococcus (72,73). It is now used solely as an antifungal agent. Flucytosine (especially in combination with amphotericin B) has activity against cutaneous or systemic fungal infections with cutaneous manifestations.

A. Chemistry

Flucytosine has a fluorine group substituted at the 5-carbon position of cytosine (see Figure 5). It is a white powder, moderately soluble in water and very stable in dry storage.

B. Mechanism of Action

Flucytosine is taken up by fungal cells by means of the fungi-specific enzyme cytosine permease. There are two pathways by which flucytosine exerts an

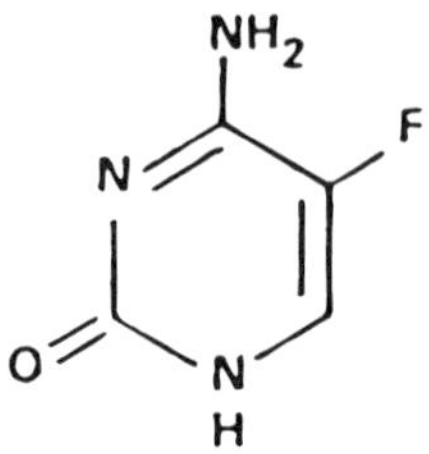

5-Fluorocytosine
(5-FC)

Figure 5 Structural formula of 5-fluorocytosine (5-FC).

antifungal effect. After uptake into the fungal cell, flucytosine is deaminated to 5-FU by cytosine deaminase and is subsequently converted through several intermediate steps to 5-fluorodeoxyuridine monophosphate (F-dUMP), which inhibits DNA synthesis through the inhibition of thymidylate synthetase (74).

The second mechanism of action involves the conversion to 5-FU and subsequently to 5-fluoridine triphosphate, which is incorporated into the fungal RNA resulting in inhibition of protein synthesis (75). A study using ^{19}F nuclear magnetic resonance spectroscopy has confirmed these mechanisms (76).

C. Pharmacology

1. Absorption

More than 90% of orally administered drug is absorbed from the gastrointestinal tract. Absorption is rapid but can be delayed by food, antacids, and renal insufficiency (77). Peak plasma levels are attained within 1–2 h in patients with normal renal function (78). It is primarily given orally although it has been used intravenously primarily in Europe.

2. Distribution

The volume of distribution approaches that of total body water. Flucytosine is poorly bound to proteins. Concentrations in the cerebrospinal fluid are about 74% of simultaneous serum concentrations (77). Flucytosine also penetrates peritoneal fluid (79), vitreous, and inflamed joints (80).

3. Excretion

The half-life of flucytosine in the serum of patients with normal renal function is 3–5 h but can be significantly prolonged in patients with renal failure (81).

Excretion is predominantly by glomerular filtration by the kidney and is linearly correlated with the creatinine clearance. Flucytosine is cleared by both hemodialysis and peritoneal dialysis, although more readily by the former (82). Guidelines for dosing flucytosine in patients with renal compromise have been suggested (83). Abnormal hepatic function has no effect on the half-life.

D. Clinical Indications

Flucytosine is used solely as an antifungal agent and is useful in combination with amphotericin B in the treatment of several deeply invasive mycoses. During the last several years there has been a dramatic increase in the number of fungal infections in immunocompromised hosts. Because of the dose-limiting nephrotoxicity of amphotericin B, improved clinical outcome in some mycoses with combination therapy, and the paucity of effective antifungal compounds, interest in flucytosine has been renewed.

Flucytosine is effective in combination with amphotericin B in cryptococcal meningitis (84,85) and is now the standard induction regimen in this disease (86,87). The combination is also effective in AIDS-related cryptococcosis (88). It is effective in the treatment of disseminated candidiasis (89,90), although there is a propensity for the development of resistance when used as monotherapy. The combination of amphotericin B and flucytosine should be used preferentially for candida meningitis, hepatosplenic candidiasis, and candidal endocarditis, endophthalmitis, and peritonitis, especially when these are caused by other species of candida besides *albicans.*

Dermatological indications include treatment of chromoblastomycosis caused by dermatiaceous molds. Treatment of this disease has been hampered by the paucity of effective antifungal agents and by in vitro resistance of these molds to amphotericin B. Two studies, one in the United States (91) and one in Brazil (92), have shown flucytosine to have significant activity as a sole therapy for chromoblastomycosis, with an overall cure rate of 72% being documented. Resistance to monotherapy with flucytosine appears to correlate with the size of the lesion and the duration of the therapy.

Flucytosine is also effective against aspergillus but has not been effective in blastomycosis, coccidiomycosis, histoplamosis, or sporotrichosis.

E. Adverse Reactions

Flucytosine has relatively few side effects when given alone in patients with normal renal function. Rash and diarrhea are the most common side effects and

Table 3 Adverse Reactions

Rash
Diarrhea
Bone marrow aplasia
Hepatic necrosis
Enterocolitis

hepatic dysfunction is seen in about 5% of patients (see Table 3). Flucytosine has, however, been associated with bone marrow aplasia (93,94), hepatic necrosis, and enterocolitis (95,96). Myelosuppression and hepatotoxicity appear to be concentration-dependent in most patients. These toxicities may be avoidable if flucytosine levels are kept at less than 100 mg/ml and are reversible with either a reduction in drug dosage or temporary discontinuation of the drug (97). In patients who are receiving combination therapy, amphotericin-induced renal insufficiency may exacerbate toxicities (98).

REFERENCES

1. Heidelberger C, Chaudhuari NK, Danenberg P, et al. Fluorinated pyrimidines: a new class of tumor inhibitory compounds. Nature 1957; 179:663–666.
2. Rutman RJ, Cantarow A, Paschki. KE Studies on 2-acetylaminofluorene carcinogenesis: III. The utilization of uracil-2-C^{14} pre-neoplastic rat liver. Cancer Res 1954; 14:119–126.
3. Breza T, et al. Noninflammatory destruction of actinic keratoses by fluorouracil. Arch Dermatol 1976; 121:1258.
4. Odom RB, Odette DK. Treatment of keratoacanthomas with intralesional 5-fluorouracil. Arch Dermatol 1978; 114:1779.
5. Goette DK, Odom RB. Successful treatment of keratoacanthomas with intralesional fluorouracil. J Am Acad Dermatol 1980; 2:212.
6. Goette DK. Treatment of keratoacanthoma with topical fluorouracil. Arch Dermatol 1983; 119:951.
7. Hursthouse MW. A controlled trial on the use of topical 5-fluorouracil on viral warts. Br J Dermatol 1975; 92:93.
8. Gonsalves JC. 5-Fluorouracil in the treatment of common warts of the hands: a double-blind study. Br J Dermatol 1975; 92:89.
9. Lockshin NA. Flat facial warts treated with 5-fluorouracil. Arch Dermatol 1979; 115:929.
10. Ljunggren B, Moller H. Topical use of fluorouracil in the treatment of psoriasis. Arch Dermatol 1972; 106:263.
11. Tsuji T, Sugai T. Topically administered fluorouracil in psoriasis. Arch Dermatol 1972; 105:208.

12. Dupre A, Cvistol B. Mibelli's porokeratosis of the lips. Arch Dermatol 1978; 114:1841.
13. Grem JL. Fluorinated pyrimidines, In: Cancer chemotherapy. Chabner BA, Collins JM, eds. JB Lippincott Philadelphia: 1990:180.
14. Diasio RB, Harris BE. Clinical pharmacology of 5-fluorouracil. Clin Pharmacokinet 1989; 16:215–237.
15. Bosch L, Harbers, E, and Heidelberger C. Studies on fluorinated pyrimidines: V. Effects of nucleic acid metabolism in vitro. Cancer Res 1958; 18:335–343.
16. Chu E, Takimoto CH. Antimetabolites. In: eds. Principles and Practice of Oncology. Devita VT, Hellman S, Rosenberg SA, Philadelphia: J.B. Lippincott, 1993: 358–374.
17. Wilkinson DS, Tisty TD, Hanas RJ. The inhibition of ribosomal RNA synthesis and maturation in Novikoff hepatoma cells by 5-fluoroduidine. Cancer Res 1975; 35:3014–3020.
18. Pinedo HM, Peters GF. Fluorouracil: biochemistry and pharmacology. J Clin Oncol 1988; 6:1653–1664.
19. Harbers E, Chaudhuri NK, Heidelberger C. Studies on fluorinated pyrimidines: VIII. Further biochemical and metabolic investigations. J Biol Chem 1959; 234:1255–1262.
20. Tanaka M, Yoshida S, Saneyoshi M, et al. Utilization of 5-fluoro-2′-deoxyuridine triphosphate and 5-fluoro-2′-deoxycytidine triphosphate in DNA synthesis by DNA polymerases alpha and beta from calf thymus. Cancer Res 1981; 41:4132–4135.
21. Ingraham HA, Tseng BY, Goulian M. Mechanism for exclusion of 5-fluorouracil from DNA. Cancer Res 1980; 40:998–1001.
22. Bruckner HW, Creasey WA. The administration of 5-fluorouracil by mouth. Cancer 1974; 33:14–18.
23. Cohen JL, Irwin LW, Marshall OJ, et al. Clinical pharmacology of oral and intravenous 5-fluorouracil (NSC-19893). Cancer Chemother Rep 1974; 58:723–731.
24. Fraile RJ, Baker LH, Buroker TR, et al. Pharmacokinetics of 5-fluorouracil administered orally by rapid intravenous and slow infusion. Cancer Rcs 1980; 40:2223–2228.
25. Hahn RG, Moertel CG, Schutt J, et al. A double-blinded comparison of intensive course 5-fluorouracil by oral versus intravenous route in the treatment of colorectal carcinoma. Cancer 1975; 35:1031–1035.
26. Kerr IG, Zimm S, Collins JM, et al. Effect of intravenous dose and schedule on cerebrospinal fluid pharmacokinetics of 5-florouracil in the monkey. Cancer Res 1984; 44:4929–4932.
27. Schilsky RL. Antimetabolites. In: The chemotherapy source book. Perry MC, ed. Baltimore: Williams and Wilkins, 1992:306–308.
28. Finch RE, Bending MR, Lant AF. Plasma levels of 5-fluorouracil after oral and intravenous administration in cancer patients. Br J Clin Pharmacol 1979; 7:613–617.
29. Diasio RB, Schuetz JD, Wallace HJ, et al. Dihydrofluorouracil, a fluoracil catabolite with antitumor activity in murine and human cells. Cancer Res 1985; 45:4900–4903.
30. Khansur T, Kennedy A. Cisplatin and 5-fluorouracil for advanced locoregional and metastatic squamous cell carcinoma of the skin. Cancer 1991; 67:2030–2032.
31. Aoki H, Mieno K, Amino K, Miura S, Ohtaki K, Satoi Y, Shikata J. Problems with topical therapies for extensive squamous cell carcinoma of the buttocks. Gan To Kagaku-Ryoho 1991; 11:1955–1957.

32. Ryanb RF, Krementz ET, Litwin MS. A role for topical 5-fluorouracil therapy in melanoma. J Surg Oncol 1988; 4:250–256.
33. Maehara Y, Sakaguchi Y, Kusumoto T, Kusumoto H, Sugimachi K. Potentiation of 5-fluorouracil cytotoxicity by combining hyperthermia and dipyridamole in vitro. Anticancer Res 1989; 9(4):967–969.
34. Gazit Z, Weiss DW, Shouval D, Yechezkeli M, Schirrmacher V, Notter M, Walter J, Kedar E. Chemoadoptive immunotherapy of nude mice implanted with human colorectal carcinoma and melanoma cell lines. Cancer Immunol Immunother 1992; 35(2):135–144.
35. Driscoll JS, Marquez VE, Plowman J, Liu PS, Kelley JA, Barchi JJ Jr. Antitumor properties of 2 (1H)-pyrimidinone riboside (zebularine) and its fluorinated analog. J Med Chem 1991; 34(11):3280–3284.
36. Yamagami K, Fujii A, Arita M, Okumoto T, Sakata S, Matsuda A, Ueda T, Saski T. Antitumor activity of 2′-deoxy-2′-methylidenecytidine, a new 2′-deoxycytidine derivative. Cancer Res 1991; 1:51(9):2319–2323.
37. Alper JC, Wiemann MC, Rueckl FS, McDonald CJ, Calabresi P. Rationally designed combination chemotherapy for the treatment of patients with recalcitrant psoriasis. J Am Acad Dermat 1985; 13:568–577.
38. Abernethy DR, Alper JC, Wienamm MC, McDonald CJ, Calabresi P. Oral 5-fluorouracil in psoriasis: pharmacokinetic-pharmacodynamic relationships. Pharmacol 1989; 39:78–88.
39. Ansfield FJ, Schroeder JM, Curreri AR. Five years clinical experience with 5-fluorouracil. JAMA 1962; 181:295–299.
40. Hohn DC, Rayner AA, Economou JS. Toxicities and complications of implanted pump hepatic arterial and intravenous floxiuridine infusion. Cancer 1986; 57:465–470.
41. Bianch L, Iraci S, Tomassoli M, et al. Coexistence of apparent transverse leukonychia (Muehrcke's lines type) and longitudinal melanonychia after 5-fluorouracil/-adriamycin/cyclophosphamide chemoptherapy. Dermatol 1992; 185:216–217.
42. Svetislava SJ, Bonner MW, McCollough M, et al. Unusual serpentine hyperpigmentation associated with 5-fluorouracil. J Am Acad Dermatol 1991; 25:905–908.
43. Perlin E, Ahlgren JD. Pigmentary effects from the protracted infusion of 5-fluorouracil. Int J Dermatol 1991; 30:43–44.
44. Umstead GS, Fryer NL, Decker DA. Local tissue reaction to intravenous fluorouracil and leucovorin, DICP. Ann Pharmacol 1991; 25:249–250.
45. Fabian CA, Molina R, Slavik M. Pyridoxine therapy for palmar-plantar erythrodysesthesia associated with continuous 5-fluorouracil infusion. Invest New Drugs 1990; 8:57–63.
46. Weiss HD, Walder MD, Wiernik P. Neurotoxicity of commonly used antineoplastic agents. N Engl J Med 1974; 291:75–80.
47. Kaplan RS, Wiernik P. Neurotoxicity of antineoplastic agents. Semin Oncol 1982; 9:103–130.
48. Koenig H, Patel A. A biochemical basis for fluorouracil toxicity. Arch Neurol 1970; 23:155–160.

49. Gradishar WJ, Vokes EE. 5-Fluorouracil cardiotoxicity: A critical review. Ann Oncol 1990; 1:409–414.
50. Freeman NJ, Costanza ME. 5-Fluorouracil-associated cardiotoxicity. Cancer 1988; 61:36–45.
51. Robben NC, Pippas AW, Moore JO. The syndrome of 5-fluorouracil cardiotoxicity. Cancer 1993; 71:493–508.
52. Haidak DJ, Hurwitz BS, Yeung KY. Tear-duct fibrosis (dacrostenosis) due to 5-fluorouracil. Ann Intern Med 1978; 88:657.
53. Fraunfelder FT, Meyer SM. Ocular toxicity of antineoplastic agents. Ophthalmology 1984; 90:1–3.
54. Griffith JD, Garnick MB. Eye toxicity of cancer chemotherapy. Cancer 1981; 48:1539–1549.
55. Bergmann W, Feeney R. Contributions to the study of marine products: XXXII. The nucleosides of sponges. J Org Chem 1951; 16:981–987.
56. Rustum YM, Raymakers RA. 1-B-Arabinofuranosylcytosine in therapy of leukemia: Preclinical and clinical overview. Pharm Ther 1992; 56:307–321.
57. Chabner BA. Cytidine analogues. In: Chabner BA, Collins JM, eds., Cancer chemotherapy. Philadelphia: J.B. Lippincott, 1990.
58. Woodcock DM, Fox RM, Cooper IA. Evidence for a new mechanism of cytotoxicity of 1-B-D-arabinofuranosylcytosine. Cancer Res 1979; 39:1418–1424.
59. van Prooijen R, van der Kleijn E, Haanen C. Pharmacokinetics of cytosine arabinoside in acute leukemia. Clin Pharm Ther 1977; 21:744–750.
60. Wau SH, Huffman DH, Azarnoff DL, et al. Pharmacokinetics of 1-B-D-arabinofuranosylcytosine in humans. Cancer Res 1974; 34:392–397.
61. Ho DH, Frei E III. Clinical pharmacology of 1-B-D-arabinofuranosylcytosine. Clin Pharm Ther 1971; 12:944–954.
62. Bolwell BJ, Cassileth PA, Gale RP. High dose cytarabine: A review. Leukemia 1988; 2:253–260.
63. Altman A, Dinndorf P, Quinn J. Acute pancreatitis in association with cytosine arabinoside therapy. Cancer 1982; 40:1384–1386.
64. Herzig RH, Hines JD, Herzig GP. Cerebellar toxicity with high dose cytosine arabinoside. J Clin Oncol 1987; 5:927–932.
65. Hopen G, Mondino BJ, Johnson BL, et al. Corneal toxicity with systemic cytarabine. Am J Optham 1981; 91:500–506.
66. Castleberry RP, Crist WM, Holbrook T. The cytosine arabinoside syndrome. Pediatr Oncol 1981; 9:257–261.
67. Flynn TC, Harris TJ, Murphy GF, et al. Neutrophilic eccrine hidradenitis: A distinctive risk associated with cytarabein therapy and acute leukemia. J Am Acad Dermatol 1984; 11:584–590.
68. Rassiga AL, Schwartz HJ, Forman WB, et al. Cytarabine-induced anaphylaxis: Demonstration of antibody and successful desensitization. Arch Intern Med 1980; 140:425–426.
69. Anderson BS, Luna MA, Yee C, et al. Fatal pulmonary failure complicating high-dose cytosine arabinoside therapy in acute leukemia. Cancer 1990; 65:1079–1084.

70. Kern W, Kurrle E, Schmeiser T. Streptococcal bacteremia in adult patients undergoing aggressive chemotherapy: A review of 55 cases. Infection 1990; 18:138–145.
71. Grunberg E, Titsworth E, Bennett M. Chemotherapeutic activity of 5-fluorocytosine. Antimicrob Agents Chemother 1964; 1963:1566068.
72. Tassel D, Madoff MA. Treatment of *Candida* sepsis and *Cryptococcus* meningitis with 5-fluorocytosine. JAMA 1968; 206:830–832.
73. Utz JP, Tynes BS, Shadomy HJ, et al. 5-Fluorocytosine in human cryptococcosis. Antimicrob Agents Chemother 1969; 1968:344–346.
74. Diasio RB, Bennett JE, Myers CE. Mode of action of 5-fluorocytosine. Biochem Pharm 1978; 27:703–707.
75. Polak A, Scholer HJ. Mode of action of 5-fluorocytosine and mechanisms of resistance. Chemotherapy 1975; 21:113–130.
76. Chouini-Lalanne N, Malet-Martinao MC, Martineo R, et al. Study of the metabolism of flucytosine in *Aspergillus* species by ^{19}F nuclear magnetic resonance spectroscopy. Antimicrob Agents Chemother 1989; 33:1939–1945.
77. Bennett J. Antifungal agents. In: Mandell, Douglas, Bennett, eds., Basic principles in the diagnosis and management of infectious diseases. New York: John Wiley, 1990.
78. Block ER, Bennett JE. Pharmacological studies with 5-fluorocytosine. Antimicrob Agents Chemother 1972; 1:476–482.
79. Muther RS, Bennett WM. Peritoneal clearance of amphotericine-B and 5-fluorocytosine. West J Med 1980; 133:157–160.
80. Levinson DJ, Silcos DC, Rippon JW, et al. Septic arthritis due to nonencapsulated *Cryptococcus neoformans* with coexisting sarcoidosis. Arthrit Rheum 1974; 17:1037–1047.
81. Cutler RE, Blair AD, Kelly MR. Flucytosine kinetics in subjects with normal renal function. Clin Pharm Ther 1978; 24:333.
82. Polak A. Pharmacokinetics of amphotericin-B and flucytosine. Postgrad Med J 1979; 55:667–670.
83. Daneshmend TK, Warnock DW. Clinical pharmacokinetics of systemic antifungal drugs. Clin Pharmacokinet 1983; 8:17–42.
84. Utz JP, Garriques IL, Sande MA. Therapy of cryptococcosis with a combination of flucytosine and amphotericin-B. J Infect Dis 1975; 132:368–373.
85. Bennett JE, Dismukes WE, Duma RJ. A comparison of amphotericin-B alone and combined with flucytosine in the treatment of cryptococcal meningitis. N Engl J Med 1979; 301:126–131.
86. Zuger A, Louie E, Holzman RS. Cryptococcal disease in patients with the acquired immunodeficiency syndrome: Diagnostic features and outcome of treatment. Ann Intern Med 1986; 104:234–240.
87. Schumtzhard E, Vejajjiva A. Treatment of cryptococcal meningitis with high-dose, long-term combination of amphotericin-B and flucytosine. Am J Med 1988; 85:737–738.
88. Chuck SL, Sande MA. Infections with *Cryptococcus neoformans* in the acquired immunodeficiency syndrome. N Engl J Med 1989; 321:794–799.
89. Eilard T, Alestig K, Wahlen P. Treatment of disseminated candidiasis with 5-fluorocytosine. J Infect Dis 1974; 130:155–159.

90. Vandevelde AG, Mauceri AA, Johnson JE. 5-fluorocytosine in the treatment of mycotic infections. Ann Intern Med 1972; 77:43–51.
91. Lopes CF, Alvarenga RJ, Cisalpino EO, et al. Six year's experience in the treatment of chromomycosis with 5-fluorocytosine. Int J Dermatol 1978; 17:414–418.
92. Lopes CF. Recent developments in the therapy of chromoblastomycosis. Bull Pan Am Health Org 1981; 15:58–64.
93. Meyer R, Axelrod JL. Fatal aplastic anemia resulting from 5-fluorocytosine. JAMA 1974; 228:1573.
94. Bryan CS, McFarland JA. Cryptococcal meningitis: Fatal marrow aplasia from combined therapy. JAMA 1978; 239:1068–1069.
95. Harder EJ, Hermans PE. Treatment of ungal infections with flucytosine. Arch Intern Med 1975; 135:231–237.
96. Terrell CL, Hermans PE. Antifungal agents used for deep-seated mycotic infections. Mayo Clin Proc 1987; 62:1116–1128.
97. Francis P, Walsh T. Evolving role of flucytosine in immunocompromised patients: New insights into safety, pharmacokinetics and antifungal therapy. Clin Infect Dis 1992; 15:1003–1018.

4
Purine Analogs

David Friedman
Roger Williams Medical Center, Providence, Rhode Island

Joseph Alper
Roger Williams Medical Center, Providence, Rhode Island

I. AZATHIOPRINE

A. Chemistry

Azathioprine (AZA) is a thiopurine with the chemical name 6-(1-methyl-4-nitro-5-imidazolythio)purine (1). It is structurally closely related to 6-mercaptopurine (6-MP) with the addition of an imidazole group at the single sulfur atom (2). 6-MP was originally synthesized as a derivative of hypoxanthine. Azathioprine was then synthesized in 1961 with the hope that the addition of the imidazole group would delay metabolism and increase effectiveness.

About 70% of the drug is first metabolized to 6-MP (2). This occurs by nonenzymatic cleavage of the sulfur bond, producing methyl-4-nitro-5-imidazole and mercaptopurine (1). This reaction can be facilitated by sulfhydral-containing agents such as glutathione (2). Up to 12% of the drug can also be converted to hypoxanthine and other metabolites. The next steps in metabolism are not yet clearly defined, in spite of active research for over 20 years. The 6-MP is either broken down to 6-thiouric acid (6-TU) by xanthine oxidase (XO) or is further transformed in cells to thioinosinic acid and 6-thioguanine nucleotides (TGN) (3). Many enzymes are required for conversion to these metabolites. Genetic variations in activity of one of these enzymes, thiopurine methyltransferase (TPMT), is probably responsible for some of the variation in sensitivity to AZA in different individuals (1). Also, hypoxanthine phosphoribosyltransferase

(HPRT), which is needed for initial cleavage of 6-MP, has varying activity in different tissues (1). This may explain the differential effects and toxicity in various organs of the body.

B. Mechanism of Action

AZA is used clinically for two effects: immunosuppression and myelosuppression. The first of these is relatively well understood, but not so much the latter. Immunosuppression is the most common use for the drug in dermatology.

Myelosuppression is mediated primarily by incorporation of TGN into nucleated cells. There are several of these substances including 6-thioguanosine-5′-diphosphate and 6-thioguanosine-5′-triphosphate. Since these are purine analogs, formation of both adenylic acid and guanylic acid is impaired (3). The interference with synthesis of these two nucleic acids, however, is not enough to explain all the cytotoxicity of AZA (4). The direct incorporation of TGN, 6-thioguanosine into RNA and deoxythioguanosine into DNA, is probably the major cause of cellular inhibition (4). This effect alone is probably more important in patients with oncological rather than dermatological diseases.

The immunosuppressive action may also occur as a result of cellular inhibition. Because direct incorporation of TGN into DNA occurs, rapidly dividing cells are the primary target for AZA. Both T and B lymphoblasts seem to be most susceptible (5). Therefore, AZA is considered a phase-specific drug. Cell-mediated and humoral responses are impaired because of this effect early during cell proliferation. In contrast, the drug has little effect on established immune responses (5). Although cellular inhibition can easily explain the immunosuppressive effects of AZA, other mechanisms may exist (1,6). The variety of other effects include interference with synthesis of interleukin-2, interference with antigenic triggering on the basis of the reactive thiol groups, and a suppressive activity at the surface membrane (1).

Since AZA is initially metabolized to 6-MP, it would seem that either drug could be given with equal effect. This does not seem to be the case. AZA was originally synthesized with an added imidazole side group to 6-MP to delay metabolic degradation of the drug. The result was supposed to be a drug with longer duration of action (2). This may, indeed, be the case, but there are still no definitive data to suggest exactly how this occurs (7).

It is probably safe to say that all the details of the mechanism of action of AZA are not yet known. This is surprising since the drug has been extensively used and actively studied for more than 20 years.

C. Pharmacology

1. Absorption

AZA is very well absorbed from the gastrointestinal tract. Peak plasma concentration is achieved within 2 h of an oral dose (8). AZA seems to be better absorbed than 6-MP. About 12% of an oral dose of AZA is found in the stool, while 22% of 6-MP is found (2).

2. Distribution

After an oral dose, AZA is widely distributed in all body fluids except the central nervous system (9). About 30% of the drug is bound to plasma proteins, the rest is rapidly metabolized to a variety of intermediates as described above. Thus, the plasma half-life is quite short—about 1.9 h (1). Impaired renal function does not appear to alter the plasma levels of either AZA or 6-MP (1). Rather, the variations in metabolism and cell concentrations appear to be related to genetic differences in enzyme activity needed for drug breakdown.

Although AZA is rapidly cleared from serum, it persists in other body tissues. The concentration in red blood cells (RBCs) gives a readily available tissue in which to measure TGN levels. Some authors have found good correlation between RBC levels of TGN and drug effect or toxicity (6), while others have not (3). All authors agree, however, that there is wide variability in how different patients concentrate TGN in their RBCs. Some patients have rapidly increasing levels (with attendant leukopenia), while others concentrate RBC TGN more slowly (3). In either case, single-day dosing makes good sense because of this "reservoir" effect in body tissues.

3. Excretion

As outlined above, AZA is rapidly metabolized after absorption from the gut. Many of these metabolites are incorporated into rapidly dividing cells. Some, however, are degraded to inactive or partially active metabolites. Approximately 50% is excreted via the kidneys as inactive forms within 24 h of an oral dose (2). Some of these metabolites have been identified as glutathione-imidazole or cysteinyl-imidazole adducts (10). Mercaptoimidazole is formed after formation of the glutathione or cysteinyl adduct which is the primary urinary imidazole excreted in man. Since most of the urinary metabolites are inactive, increased toxicity of the drug does not occur in the presence of renal failure.

D. Clinical Indications

As implied by the preceding discussion, the immunosuppressive effects of AZA would be most useful in dermatological diseases whose pathogenesis is, at least in part, caused by autoimmune mechanisms. The antimitotic effect of the drug is more useful in patients with oncologic disease. I have found AZA to be most useful, in general, as a "steroid-sparing" drug, since lower doses of each of these may be used, avoiding some of the adverse effects of both.

The use of AZA in a variety of dermatological diseases has been reported and reviewed (9). The diseases for which it has been employed include pemphigus, pemphigoid, systemic lupus erythematosus, dermatomyositis, Behçet's disease, and vasculitis (9). These are only a few of the more common disorders for which AZA has been shown to be effective. In essentially all of these diseases, the main use of AZA is to allow reduction of the dose of corticosteroids. Treatment of chronic eczema with AZA may not be justified given the potential side effects (see below).

I have experience using AZA has been used in one other disease the treatment of that may take advantage of its antimitotic effect—psoriasis. In some patients, AZA by itself has produced improvement when no other pharmacological agent has worked. It has also been used in combination with 5-fluorouracil or hydroxyurea with gratifying results. These comments are purely anecdotal. However, it does point out that the antimitotic effect may be useful in certain dermatological conditions. Of course, others who feel that psoriasis is an immunological disease may believe that any beneficial effect in psoriasis is due to the immunosuppressive effect of AZA.

E. Adverse Reactions

Different toxicity from AZA occurs depending on the individual. There are potentially several factors to explain this phenomenon. Myelosuppression is the most common adverse effect. This tends to be dose related and is not seen in dermatological patients as much as in patients with renal transplants. At the usual dose used in dermatological patients (100–200 mg/d), it has rarely caused significant myelosuppression.

Thrombocytopenia and pancytopenia have rarely been seen in dermatological subjects but may occur (9).

An increased susceptibility to skin cancer is seen primarily in renal transplant patients (11). Both premalignant lesions (actinic keratoses, Bowen's disease) and malignant tumors (squamous cell carcinoma, basal cell carcinoma, and malignant melanoma) are seen with increased frequency in these patients (11). The malignant tumors are usually very aggressive and can be a leading cause of morbidity and mortality. This is particularly true in areas near the equator or in patients who have other risk factors for cutaneous malignancy—Celtic ethnic origin, blue eyes, fair complexion (11). It is interesting that exposure to sun following renal transplant does not seem to be a risk factor in developing skin cancer (11). The increased risk for skin cancer in renal transplant patients seems to be related to increased levels of TGN in the red blood cells of these patients (12). Of interest is that 6-thioguanine oxidation is maximal when exposed to UV light between 320 and 360 nm (12). This is the UVB range which is responsible for cutaneous carcinogenesis.

Malignancies other than skin have also been reported with increased frequency in renal transplant patients. These include a variety of lymphomas, carci-

5

Antiviral Agents

Monica L. McCrary
Medical College of Georgia, Augusta, Georgia

Omeed Memar and Stephen K. Tyring
University of Texas Medical Branch, Galveston, Texas

I. INTRODUCTION

Many antiviral agents have become increasingly used in dermatological practice, both due to the explosion of new agents available (e.g., famciclovir, valaciclovir, lamivudine, saquinavir, ritonavir, indinavir) and the rapidly increasing prevalence of some viral diseases (e.g., AIDS, genital herpes, genital warts) with dermatological manifestations. Historically, the vast majority of antiviral drugs were against herpes viruses. However, the onset of HIV infection in the early 1980s has led to the development of multiple antiretroviral agents. Both the antiherpes and antiretroviral drugs consist primarily of nucleoside (either purine or pyrimidine) analogs that either act to inhibit viral DNA polymerase (the former) or viral reverse transcriptase (the latter). Recently however, the first of a group of anti-HIV drugs that act by inhibiting HIV protease received FDA approval (saquinavir, ritonavir, indinavir), and they will undoubtedly be quickly followed by others. Currently there are many antiviral agents with novel mechanisms of action under development or being clinically evaluated, including nucleotide analogs and agents that act by stimulating the host's own immune system to recognize and destroy viruses or virally infected cells (interferon alpha, imiquimod, therapeutic vaccines).

II. NUCLEOSIDE ANALOGS

A. Acyclovir (Zovirax)

Acyclovir was the first safe, systemic antiherpes drug approved by the FDA and is now the most widely prescribed antiviral drug in the world (see Figure 1). It is a purine analog that is phosphorylated to the monophosphate form by virus-encoded thymidine kinase (TK) (1,2). It is then converted to the diphosphate form from the monophosphorylated species by cellular guanylate kinase, and subsequently acted upon by other cellular enzymes, resulting in acyclovir triphosphate (3). This compound competively inhibits viral DNA synthesis (4) and inactivates viral DNA polymerase (5). Acyclovir is converted to the monophosphate form mostly in TK+ herpes-infected cells and not in uninfected cells, and thus exhibits specific activity against herpes simplex types 1 and 2 (HSV-1 and -2), Epstein-Barr virus (EBV), and varicella zoster virus (VZV) (6) since all of these express TK. (Unfortunately, this in vitro efficacy against EBV has not proven to be of clinical significance). Finally, unlike the previously mentioned viruses, cytomegalovirus (CMV) does not express TK and shows no in vitro response to acyclovir. However, acyclovir does appear to suppress CMV replication and therefore may be used in the prophylaxis against CMV in individuals at high risk (7).

Acyclovir is now available in topical, oral, and intravenous forms. Topical acyclovir is indicated only for the treatment of the first outbreak of genital herpes and has shown little effect against herpes labialis or recurrent genital herpes. Intravenous acyclovir is used for therapy of immunocompromised patients with acute herpes zoster, disseminated herpes simplex, or for severe acute trigeminal zoster. The oral form is by far the most widely used, and is prescribed for genital herpes (both suppressive and episodic use), herpes labialis, chickenpox (primary varicella), and shingles (varicella zoster).

Acyclovir has established itself as the model of antiviral therapy because of its low incidence of side effects (nausea, headache, and reversible renal dysfunction at high doses) and high specificity. Many of the newer antivirals have used acyclovir as a pattern for their mechanism of action. However, although very successful, its use for the decrease of asymptomatic viral shedding (8) and suppression of recurrent herpetic infections (9) has been limited by its relatively high cost, frequent dosing, and low bioavailability (15–20%).

B. Famciclovir (Famvir)

Famciclovir is a novel nucleoside analog approved for the treatment of acute herpes zoster and for episodic therapy for recurrent genital herpes. Its active form is penciclovir, which exhibits a structure, potency, selectivity, and antiviral spectrum very similar to that of acyclovir (Figure 1). Like acyclovir, it also requires viral encoded thymidine kinase for the conversion to its monophosphate. By the action of cellular enzymes, the monophosphate is phosphorylated to penciclovir-triphosphate, which inhibits viral DNA polymerase and therefore viral replication (10). In addition, penciclovir has also been found to have good activity in cell culture against HSV types 1 and 2 and against varicella zoster

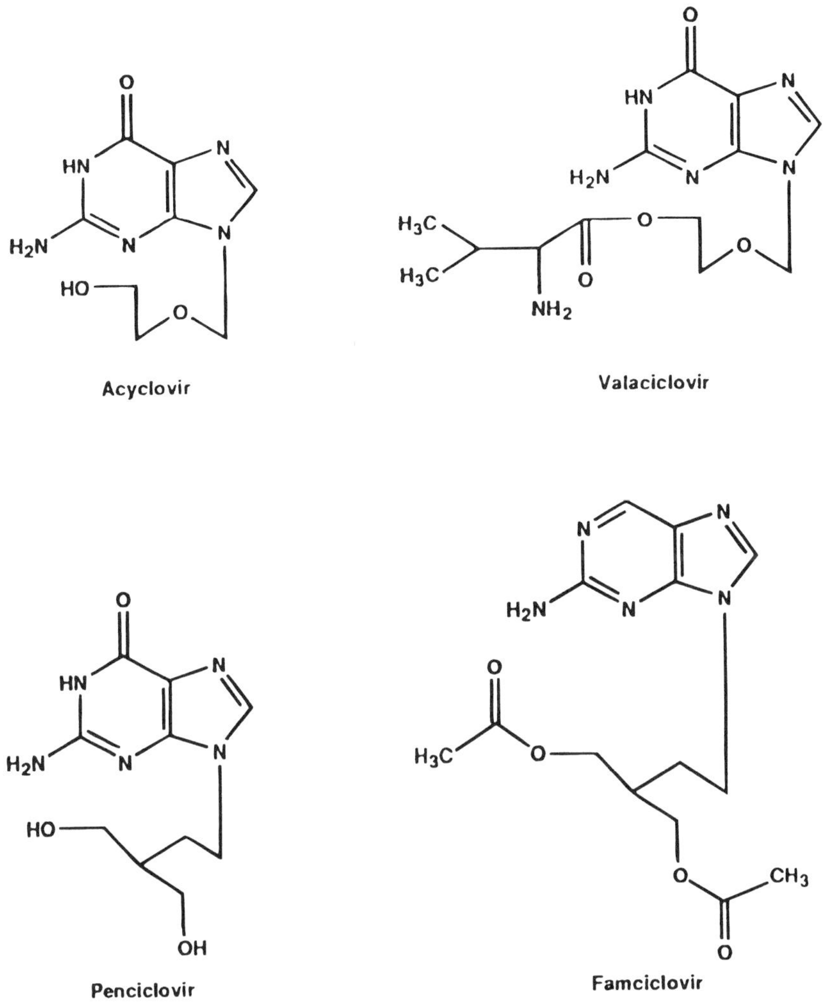

Figure 1 Molecular structure of acyclovir, valaciclovir, penciclovir, and famciclovir.

virus. In contrast to acyclovir, however, it has a longer intracellular half-life (11,12) (and therefore may be dosed less frequently) and a higher bioavailability (77%). Similar to acyclovir, famciclovir is rarely associated with significant side effects (13). Interestingly, it has been found that inhibition of HSV-2 replication occurs at low doses of penciclovir and new viral replication does not occur for many hours, even when the compound is removed from the culture medium, which seems to be a unique property of penciclovir (14). Efficacy of penciclovir has been demonstrated against EBV in vitro (15), but clinical trials of famciclovir or penciclovir have not been reported with EBV infection. Of perhaps the greatest significance, however, was a study by Tyring et al. (16) that found that famciclovir significantly reduces the duration of postherpetic neuralgia (PHN), particularly in those persons at higher risk for PHN (people who are 50 years of age or older) (13).

C. Valaciclovir (Valtrex)

Valaciclovir was approved for the treatment of acute herpes zoster and for episodic therapy of recurrent genital herpes in 1995. A valine ester of acyclovir (Figure 1), it acts as a prodrug, being converted to acyclovir after oral administration, and allows higher blood acyclovir levels to be obtained (approximately three to five times higher). Both the mode of action and the spectrum of antiviral activity are identical to those of acyclovir, and studies comparing valaciclovir to acyclovir showed valaciclovir, 1 g twice daily or 500 mg twice daily, to be superior to placebo and to acyclovir, 200 mg five times daily, in the episodic treatment of recurrent genital herpes simplex infections. In addition, valaciclovir was equivalent to acyclovir in its safety profile (16,17). Valaciclovir, 1 g three times daily, was found to be superior to acyclovir, 800 mg five times daily, in the treatment of herpes zoster. It hastened the resolution of zoster-associated pain (including postherpetic neuralgia), reduced analgesic use, and accelerated the loss of abnormal sensations in a double-blind, multicenter trial. Finally, valaciclovir and acyclovir were found to be similar in their safety, effectiveness on duration of new lesion formation, and time to crusting/healing (18).

D. Idoxuridine (IDU, Herplex, Stoxil)

Idoxuridine is a pyrimidine analog that resembles thymidine. It is phosphorylated to the triphosphate form within cells and then incorporates into newly synthesized DNA. This makes the DNA molecule unstable and fragile. It was first synthesized in 1959 (19), and it has inhibitory effects against nearly every DNA virus. It was the first antiviral medication to receive FDA approval for the treatment of herpes keratitis and is still indicated for the treatment of this condition.

E. Trifluridine (Viroptic)

Trifluridine is a fluorinated pyrimidine deoxynucleoside [2′-deoxy-5-(trifluoromethyl)uridine] which is phosphorylated to a triphosphate form and incorporates into newly synthesized viral DNA (and to some extent into cellular DNA) and disrupts viral replication. While its mechanism of action is not completely understood, it is active against HSV-1 and -2, CMV, vaccinia, and some strains of adenovirus (20). However, it is currently only indicated for the treatment of HSV-1 and -2 primary keratoconjunctivitis and recurrent epithelial keratitis.

F. Vidarabine (Vira A, Ara-A)

Vidarabine (9-B-D-arabinofuranosyladenine) exerts its effect by interrupting viral DNA synthesis by acting as an organic analog of the purine nucleoside adenosine. Vidarabine is indicated for the treatment of herpes keratitis and keratoconjunctivitis. When used systemically, however, it has been shown to be quite neurotoxic. Therefore, since acyclovir has been found to be superior in the treatment of HSV and VZV infections (21), vidarabine is not routinely used systemically.

G. Ganciclovir (Cytovene)

Ganciclovir is a nucleoside analog also known as 9-(1,3-dihydroxy-2-propoxymethyl)guanine. It differs from acyclovir structurally only by the addition of a hydroxymethyl group on the 3′-position of the acyclic side chain. Unlike acyclovir however, it is 100 times more effective against CMV-infected cells in vitro (22). While the mechanism against CMV is not completely understood, it is known that the active triphosphate form of ganciclovir is made by a CMV-specific protein kinase (23). The triphosphate form then incorporates itself into newly synthesized CMV DNA and inhibits CMV DNA synthesis by both inhibiting CMV DNA polymerase and inducing premature chain termination. Luckily, ganciclovir is specific for CMV-infected cells. CMV retinitis affects approximately 40% of patients with AIDS, and is the most common cause of vision loss in this group. Therefore, the use of ganciclovir for treatment and prophylaxis of CMV retinitis and other CMV infections is increasing. Recently, a study showed that a combination of ganciclovir and foscarnet was more effective than either drug alone in treating recurrences of CMV retinitis (24).

H. Sorivudine (BV-ara-U)

Sorivudine [1-B-D-arabinofuranosyl-E-5-(2-bromovinyl)uracil] is a synthetic acyclic deoxythymidine nucleoside analog that is currently undergoing clinical trials and has not yet received FDA approval. Like acyclovir and famciclovir, it is transported into infected cells and converted to a monophosphate analog. However, unlike these drugs, which require a cellular kinase to be converted to diphosphate analogs, sorivudine requires a virus-encoded thymidine kinase for the second step of phosphorylation. Then a cell-specific kinase is required to produce the triphosphate analog. It is believed that the specificity of this two-step activation by virus-encoded kinases and the absence of incorporation into host-cell DNA may give sorivudine a lower toxic potential for normal cells.

Particularly exciting is the fact that sorivudine exhibits approximately 1000-fold greater inhibitory action against VZV in vitro than does acyclovir (25). Unfortunately, its development was hindered by the deaths of several chemotherapy patients in Japan who received soruvidine for the treatment of their shingles. It is believed that the principal metabolite of sorivudine, BVU-uracil, may potentiate the effects of 5-fluorouracil and its derivatives by inhibition of the enzyme dihydropyrimidine dehydrogenase (DPD), which is required to metabolize 5-fluorouracil and its derivatives. Therefore, sorivudine should not be given to patients taking 5-fluorouracil.

III. REVERSE TRANSCRIPTASE INHIBITORS

A. Azidothymidine (AZT, Zidovudine, Retrovir)

Azidothymidine is a thymidine that lacks a 3′-hydroxy group and was the first HIV-specific antiviral approved by the FDA for treatment of HIV infection. It is converted to the monophosphate form upon entry into cells by cellular thymidine kinase. It is then converted to the diphosphate form by cellular thymidylate kinase and then to the triphosphate form by other cellular enzymes. This triphosphate form inhibits replication of some retroviruses, including HIV, by interfering with the viral reverse transcriptase. In this manner, AZT blocks infectivity and the cytopathic effects of HIV (26). It is indicated in HIV-positive adults with CD4 counts of less than 500/mm^3 and in HIV-positive children older than 3 mo, and is considered the drug of choice in fighting HIV infection. In addition, it has been shown to decrease the transmission of HIV to infants born to HIV-infected mothers and the risk of HIV acquisition after exposure by needle stick in health care workers. The most frequent side effect of AZT is bone marrow suppression.

B. Zalcitabine (DDC, HIVID)

Zalcitabine acts as a synthetic pyrimidine nucleoside analog. It is indicated for use in combination therapy in the treatment of HIV infections, and is approved for use with AZT for patients with HIV who are deteriorating by both clinical and immunological parameters (CD4 < 300/mm^3). Side effects include peripheral neuropathy and occasionally pancreatitis.

C. Didanosine (DDI, Videx)

Didanosine is another reverse transcriptase inhibitor, being indicated for those patients with HIV who either are unable to tolerate AZT or who have become refractory to its effects. The most significant adverse effect of DDI is pancreatitis.

D. Stavudine (d4T, Zerit)

Stavudine is another nucleoside analog and reverse transcriptase inhibitor that is indicated for use in HIV-positive patients who either have some contraindication to the use of the other antiretroviral drugs or who have experienced profound clinical or immunological deterioration while on them. It has shown efficacy in preventing the decline of CD4 counts in HIV-infected patients, and in one randomized double-blind trial was shown to be more effective than AZT. The major side effect of stavudine therapy is peripheral neuropathy, which affects 15–21% of patients.

E. Lamivudine (3TC. Epivir)

Lamivudine is another nucleoside analog and inhibitor of HIV reverse transcriptase that was recently approved for combination use with AZT in patients who have developed resistance to AZT alone. Together with AZT, it decreases viral load and HIV resistance to AZT and helps to increase and maintain CD4 cell counts (27). However, when used alone, drug resistance develops quickly, and only transient increases in CD4 cell counts and decreases in viral load were seen (28). So far the drug seems to have few adverse effects (e.g., occasional headache, nausea, fatigue).

IV. NUCLEOTIDE ANALOGS

A. Cidofovir (HPMPC)(Vistide)

Cidofovir is an acyclic nucleoside phosphonate (i.e., nucleotide analog) also known as [(S)-1-a(3-hydroxy-2-phosphonyl methoxypropyl) cytosine]. It has shown efficacy against a wide spectrum of viral diseases in animal models (29), including HSV-1 keratitis (TK+ and TK−) (30). It has recently received FDA approval for therapy of CMV infections; currently clinical trials are under way to determine its effectiveness against HSV, and HPV (human papillomavirus) infections in humans.

V. IMMUNOMODULATORY AGENTS

A. Interferon-α (Alferon, Intron, Roferon)

Interferons act by upregulating proteins that inhibit transcription and translation (31). Specifically, interferon α upregulates the expression of MHC class I antigens and thus may facilitate the recognition of virally infected cells by the host's immune system. Interferon-α was shown to have significant efficacy both in the treatment of Kaposi's sarcoma (response rate of approximately 40%) (32) and condyloma acuminata, as well as for therapy of hepatitis B and hepatitis C infections. Not only is IFN-α approved for the treatment of these four conditions as well as hairy cell leukemia, it was most recently approved for adjuvant therapy following surgery in patients with malignant melanoma free of disease but at high risk for systemic recurrences. In a double-blind, placebo-controlled study it was demonstrated that intralesional IFN-α resulted in 62% elimination of warts, while placebo showed only 21% elimination (33). The best results, however, were obtained when IFN-α was used in conjunction with laser excision (34). Reported side effects of IFN-α include fever, myalgia, lethargy, and headaches (35).

B. Imiquimod (IQ)

Imiquimod is a heterocyclic amine. It acts by stimulating human peripheral mononuclear cells to release a variety of cytokines such as interleukin (IL)-1, IL-6, IL-8, tumor necrosis factor alpha, and interferon alpha. Imiquimod is currently undergoing clinical trials in the treatment of genital herpes and genital warts and is currently pending FDA approval for the treatment of anogenital warts. Imiquimod decreased the number of genital herpes lesions when used in combination with acyclovir compared to imiquimod alone (36) in an animal model. In addition, a 90% reduction in wart area was seen after the topical application of 5% IQ cream in a clinical trial testing its efficacy in genital and perianal warts. No serious adverse effects have been noted, but mild local skin irritation is commonly observed with use of imiquimod (37).

VI. THERAPEUTIC VACCINES

Currently, several therapeutic vaccines are under development for the treatment of such viral diseases as genital herpes and condyloma acuminata. The first successful use of a therapeutic vaccine to modify the course of a viral disease was obtained by Strauss et al. (38), who were able to decrease the recurrence rate of outbreaks of genital herpes by 33% using a recombinant glycoprotein vaccine. In addition, Wiltz et al. (39) were able to decrease the recurrence rate of condyloma acuminata to 4.6% with a combined regimen of autogeneous vaccination and excision.

VII. PROTEASE INHIBITORS

A. Saquinavir (Invirase)

Saquinavir is one of a new class of anti-HIV drugs known as protease inhibitors, and it was the first of these agents to receive FDA approval. It is a synthetic peptide-like substrate analog that acts by inhibiting the activity of HIV protease and thus prevents the cleavage of viral polyproteins, a step necessary for the generation of functional proteins in HIV-infected cells. It is a highly specific inhibitor of HIV-1 and -2 proteases and was found to help increase and sustain CD4 cell counts in combination use with AZT (40). The most frequently reported adverse effects with its use are diarrhea, nausea, and abdominal discomfort.

B. INDINAVIR (Crixivan)

C. RITONAVIR (Norvir)

Other recently approved protease inhibitors include indinavir (Crixivan) and ritonavir (Norvir), which lower HIV RNA levels and increase CD4 counts (used alone or in combination with AZT) (41). Recently, an exciting announcement was made by Dr. Emilio Emini at the Third Conference on Retroviruses and Opportunistic Infections. He reported that when indinavir was used in triple combination with AZT and 3TC, HIV became undetectable in the blood of 85% of patients. However, nephrolithiasis has been reported with the use of indinavir. Also at this conference, an announcement was made by Dr. John Leonard that in a study that involved 1100 patients, 13% receiving ritonavir died or suffered further progression of severe AIDS compared with 27% receiving placebo. In addition, the death rate was 4.8% among patients receiving ritonavir compared to 8.4% among patients receiving placebo.

VIII. OTHERS

A. Docosanol (Lidakol)

N-Docosanol (behenyl alcohol) is a 22-carbon straight-chain fatty acid whose mechanism of action apparently involves altering the cell membrane so as to impede viral fusion and entry into the cell (42,43). Found in many commercially available cosmetics, docosanol has shown antiviral activity against a number of viruses including HSV-1 and -2, CMV, and RSV in vitro. In phase 2 clinical studies comparing the use of docosanol 10% cream to placebo, docosanol reduced healing time in the treatment of herpes labialis (44).

B. Foscarnet (Foscavir, Phosphonophormic Acid)

Unlike most of the nucleoside analogs, forscarnet sodium is not dependent on the presence of thymidine kinase (TK) and is active without any activation or phosphorylation. As a result, it is active against TK-herpes strains, and it is an important tool in the fight against increasing drug resistance. Specifically, it has been found to be effective against TK-strains in AIDS patients (45). It is an organic analog of inorganic pyrophosphate that prevents viral replication by reversibly inhibiting viral DNA polymerase (46). In addition, it inhibits viral reverse transcriptase and therefore could have potential as an anti-HIV agent. However, currently it is only approved for the treatment of CMV retinitis and other CMV infections in immunocompromised patients and for therapy of acyclovir-resistant herpes infections.

REFERENCES

1. Fyfe JA, et al. Thymidine kinase from herpes simplex virus phosphorylates the new antiviral compound 9-(2-hydroxyethoxymethyl)guanine. J Biol Chem 1978; 253:8721–8727.
2. Littler E, et al. Identification of an Epstein-Barr virus-encoded thymidine kinase. EBMO 1986; 5:1959–1966.
3. Miller WH, Miller RL. Phosphorylation of acyclovir (acylguanosine) monophosphate by GMP kinase. J Biol Chem 1980; 255:7204–7207.
4. Derse D, et al. Inhibition of purified human and herpes simplex virus-induced DNA polymerases by 9-(2-hydroxyethoxymethyl)guanine triphosphate: effects on primer-template function. J Biol Chem 1989; 256:11447–11451.
5. Furman PA, St Clair MH, Spector T. Acyclovir triphosphate is a suicide inactivator of the herpes simplex virus polymerase. J Biol Chem 1984; 259:9575–9579.
6. O'Brien JJ, Campoli-Richards DM. Acyclovir—an updated review of its antiviral activity, pharmacokinetic properties, and therapeutic efficacy. Drugs 1989; 37:233–309.
7. Meyers JD. Prevention and treatment of cytomegalovirus infection after marrow transplantation. Bone Marrow Transplant 1988; 3:95–104.
8. Wald A, et al. Suppression of subclinical shedding of herpes simplex virus type 2 with acyclovir. Ann Intern Med 1996; 124 (1):8–15.
9. Goldberg LH, et al. The acyclovir study group. Long-term suppression of recurrent genital herpes with acyclovir. A 5-year benchmark. Arch Dermat 1993; 129:582–587.
10. Vere Hodge RA, Perkins RM. Mode of action of 9-(4-hydroxy-3-hydroxy methylbut-l-yl)guanine (BRL 39123) against herpes simplex virus in MRC-5 cells. Antimicrob Agent Chemother 1989; 33:223–229.
11. Earnshaw DL, et al. Mode of antiviral action of penciclovir in MRC-5 cells infected with herpes simplex virus type 1 (HSV-1), HSV-2, and varicella zoster virus. Antimicrob Agent Chemother 1992; 36:2747–2757.
12. Standring-Cox R, et al. Prolonged activity of penciclovir against varicella-zoster virus in cell culture. 7th International Conference on Antiviral Research. Charleston, South Carolina, 27 February–4 March 1994. Poster 114.
13. Tyring SK, et al. Famciclovir for the treatment of acute herpes zoster: effects on acute disease and postherpetic neuralgia. Ann Intern Med 1995; 123:89–96.
14. Weinberg A, Bate BJ, Masters HB. Interscience Conference on Antimicrobial Agents Chemotherapy, 1991; abstract 1231.

15. Boyd MR, et al. Antiherpes virus activity of 9-(4-hydroxy-3-hydroxy-methoxymethylbut-1-yl) guanine (BRL 39123) in cell culture. Antimicrob Agents Chemother 1987; 31:1238–1242.
16. Tyring SK, et al, and the Valaciclovir International Study Group. A randomised, placebo-controlled comparison of oral acyclovir and valaciclovir HCL in patients with recurrent genital herpes infections. J Infect Dis (submitted).
17. Spruance SL, et al. and the Valaciclovir HSV Study Group. A large scale placebo-controlled trial of peroral valaciclovir for episodic treatment of recurrent herpes genitalis. Arch Intern Med 1996; 156:1729–1735.
18. Beutner KR, et al. Valaciclovir compared with acyclovir for improved therapy for herpes zoster in immunocompetent adults. Antimicrob Agent Chemother 1995; 39:1546–1553.
19. Prusoff WH. Synthesis and biological activities of iododeoxyuridine, an analog of thymidine. Biochem Biophys Acta 1959; 32:295–296.
20. Spector SA, Tyndall M, Kelley E. Inhibition of human cytomegalovirus by trifluorothymidine. Antimicrob Agent Chemother 1983; 23:113–118.
21. Safrin S, et al. Foscarnet therapy for acyclovir-resistant mucocutaneous herpes simplex virus infection in 26 AIDS patients: preliminary data. J Infect Dis 1990; 161:1078–1084.
22. Biron KK, et al. Metabolic activation of the nucleoside analogue 9-{[2-hydroxy-1-1(hydroxymethyl) ethoxy]methyl}guanine in human diploid fibroblasts infected with human cytomegalovirus. Proc Natl Acad Sci USA 1985; 82:2473–2477.
23. Sasadeusz JJ, Sacks SL. Systemic antivirals in herpes virus infections. Dermat Clin 1993; 11:171–185.
24. The studies of ocular complications of the AIDS Research Group in collaboration with the AIDS Clinical Trials Group. Combination foscarnet and ganciclovir therapy vs monotherapy for the treatment of relapsed cytomegalovirus retinitis in patients with AIDS: the cytomegalovirus retreatment trial. Arch Opthalmol 1996; 114:23–33.
25. Straus SE. Shingles. Sorrows, Salves, and Solutions. JAMA 1993; 269:1836–1839.
26. Mitsuya H, et al. 3′-Azido3′ deoxythymidine (BW A509U): an antiviral agent that inhibits the infectivity and cytopathic effect of human T-lymphotropic virus type III; /lymphadenopathy-associated virus in vitro. Proc Natl Acad Sci USA 1985; 82:7096–7100.
27. Larder BA, et al. Potential mechanism for sustained antiretroviral efficacy of AZT-3TC combination therapy. Science 1995; 269:696–699.
28. Schuurman R, et al. Rapid changes in human immunodeficiency virus type 1 RNA load and appearance of drug-resistant virus populations in persons treated with lamivudine (3TC). J Infect Dis 1995; 171:1411–1419.
29. DeClercq E, et al. A novel selective broad-spectrum anti-DNA virus agent. Nature 1986; 323:464–467.
30. Maudgal PC, DeClercq E. (S)-1-(3-hydroxy-2-phosphonylmethoxypropyl) cytosine in the therapy of thymidine kinase-positive and -deficient herpes simplex virus experimental keratitis. Invest Opthalmol Vis Sci 1991; 32:1816–1820.
31. Gresser I. Biologic effects of interferons. J Invest Dermato 1990; 95:66s–71s.

32. Krown SE, et al. Preliminary observations on the effect of recombinant leukocyte A interferon in homosexual men with Kaposi's sarcoma. N Engl J Med 1983; 308:1071–1076.
33. Friedman-Kien AE, et al. Natural interferon alpha for treatment of condylomata acuminata. JAMA 1988; 259:533–538.
34. Reid R, et al. Superficial laser vulvectomy. V. Surgical debulking is enhanced by adjuvant systemic interferon. Am J Obstet Gynecol 1992; 166:815–820.
35. Wills R, et al. Interferon kinetics and adverse reactions after intravenous, intramuscular, and subcutaneous injection. Clin Pharm Ther 1984; 35:722–727.
36. Bernstein DI, Miller RI, Harrison CJ. Effects of therapy with an immunomodulator (imiquimod, R-837) alone and with acyclovir on genital HSV-2 infection in guinea-pigs when begun after lesion development. Antiviral Res 1993; 20:45–55.
37. Spruance S, et al. Multicenter trial of 5% imiquimod (IQ) cream for treatment of genital and perianal warts. American Society for Microbiology, 33rd ICAAC meeting, New Orleans, Louisiana, 17–20 October 1993; session 131, abstract 1432.
38. Strauss, et al. Placebo-controlled trial of vaccination with recombinant glycoprotein D of herpes simplex type 2 for immunotherapy of genital herpes. Lancet 1994; 343:1460–1463.
39. Wiltz OH, Torregrosa M, Wiltz O. Autogenous vaccine: the best therapy for perianal condyloma acuminata? Dis Colon Rect 1995; 38(8):838–841.
40. Vella S. Update on a proteinase inhibitor. AIDS 1994; 8(suppl 3):S25.
41. Massarl E, et al. Abstracts of the 35th ICAAC, 1995, LB-6.
42. Katz DH, et al. Antiviral activity of 1-docosanol, an inhibitor of lipid-enveloped viruses including herpes simplex. Proc Natl Acad Sci 1991; 88:10825–10829.
43. Katz DH, et al. n-Docosanol: broad spectrum antiviral activity against lipid-enveloped viruses. In: Slow infections of the central nervous system. Ann NY Acad Sci 1994; 724:472–488.
44. Habbema L, et al. 1-Docosanol cream: an effective topical treatment of recurrent cutaneous herpes infection. American Academy of Dermatology annual meeting, San Francisco, California August 1994.
45. Wahren B, Oberg B. Reversible inhibition of cytomegalovirus replication by phosphonoformate. Intervirology 1980; 14:7–15.
46. Shepp DH, Dandlicker PS, Meyers JD. Treatment of varicella-zoster virus infection in severely immunocompromised patients. A randomized comparison of acyclovir and vidarabine. N Engl J Med 1986; 314:208–212.

6
Vinca Alkaloids and Epipodophyllotoxins

Alan B. Weitberg
Roger Williams Medical Center and Brown University School of Medicine, Providence, Rhode Island

I. VINCA ALKALOIDS VINCRISTINE AND VINBLASTINE ARE ALKALOIDS OF THE PERIWINKLE PLANT, VINCA ROSEALINN

A. Chemistry

Vincristine and vinblastine are similar chemically. They are assymetrical dimeric compounds with only minor structural differences resulting in significant differences in toxicity and antineoplastic activity (Figure 1).

B. Mechanism of Action

The vinca alkaloids, cell cycle-specific agents, block mitosis with metaphase arrest by binding to tubulin. Tubulin is a critical component of microtubules (1). Vinca alkaloids disrupt the mitotic apparatus after binding to tubulin resulting in mitotic arrest in metaphase. This effect on the mitotic spindle accounts for the cytotoxicity of these agents, although other cellular functions depend on microtubular integrity as well (CNS function, neuromuscular transmission). These may be affected as well and account for the toxicity observed with the vinca alkaloids.

Cross-resistance does not occur between between vinca alkaloids, but has been observed with several antitumor antibiotics, suggesting a shared transport mechanism for cell entry.

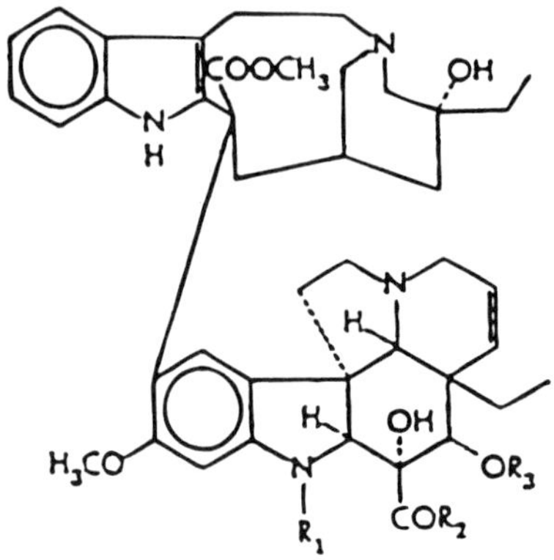

	Vincristine	Vinblastine
R_1:	$-CHO$	$-CH_3$
R_2:	$-OCH_3$	$-OCH_3$
R_3:	$-COCH_3$	$-COCH_3$

Figure 1

C. Pharmacology

Both vincristine and vinblastine are erratically absorbed after oral administration and both bind extensively to plasma proteins and to all of the cellular elements of the blood, but particularly to platelets. The peak concentration of each drug after administration of normal clinical doses is 0.4 μM. After intravenous injection, vincristine and vinblastine have a multiphasic pattern of clearance from the plasma. After distribution, vinblastine disappears from the plasma with half-lives of 1 and 20 h, while the terminal half-life of vincristine is approximately 2.5 h (2,3). Both drugs are metabolized in the liver with vinblastine being metabolized to the biologically active derivative desacetylvinblastine. No biologically active derivatives of vincristine have been identified. For vinblastine, 15% is detected intact in the urine after administration of a standard dose and 10% is recovered in the feces after biliary excretion. The major route of elimination of vincristine is biliary and 70% of an administered dose appears in the feces (4). Greater toxicity is encountered when vincristine is administered to patients with obstructive jaundice and doses should be reduced in patients with biliary obstruction.

D. Clinical Indications

Vincristine is used in combination with other chemotherapeutic agents to treat a variety of solid and hematological malignancies. These include acute lymphoblastic leukemia, Hodgkin's and non-Hodgkin's lymphomas, soft tissue sarcomas,

Wilms' tumor, and neuroblastoma, although its greatest efficacy is recognized in the hematological malignancies. Vinblastine has a similar spectrum of clinical activity, although vincristine is more useful in lymphocytic leukemias, especially the acute variety in children, and vinblastine is more effective in the treatment of metastatic testicular tumors.

E. Adverse Reactions

Neurotoxicity is the most common side effect of therapy with vincristine and is more freqeuntly observed in adults than children (5). It presents initially with peripheral neuropathies manifested by loss of deep tendon reflexes and distal parasthesias. Muscular weakness and sensory impairment may occur with continued administration of the drug, and severe jaw pain has been observed. Autonomic neuropathies also occur and include constipation, abdominal cramping, patalytic ileus, bladder atony, and orthostatic hypotension. Mental status changes, including confusion and coma, have been described as well. Neurotoxicity is dose related, and thus single doses of greater than 2 mg should not be administered. Doses should be reduced when early, mild toxicity occurs, but should be suspended if there is progression of toxicity or if more serious complications occur. Early toxicity is usually reversible, but motor deficits may persist. Because autonomic dysfunction can occur, patients receiving vincristine should be on a regimen of stool softeners and laxatives, and drugs that decrease bowel motility should be avoided. Myelosuppression is rare with vincristine, but a syndrome of dilutional hyponatremia secondary to the inappropriate secretion of antidiuretic hormone has been described (6). Reversible alopecia occurs in approximately 20% of patients treated with vincristine.

Vinblastine causes myelosuppression, particularly leukopenia. The nadir of the leukopenia occurs at 7 d, with recovery completed by 14 d. Gastrointestinal side effects include nausea, vomiting, anorexia, diarrhea, and stomatitis. Hair loss and dermatitis occur infrequently.

II. EPIPODOPHYLLOTOXINS

Teniposide (VM-26) and etoposide (VP-16) are semisynthetic derivatives of podophyllotoxin, an extract of the mandrake plant.

A. Chemistry

The chemical structure of teniposide and etoposide are shown in Figure 2. They are two of many derivatives of podophyllotoxin synthesized over many years.

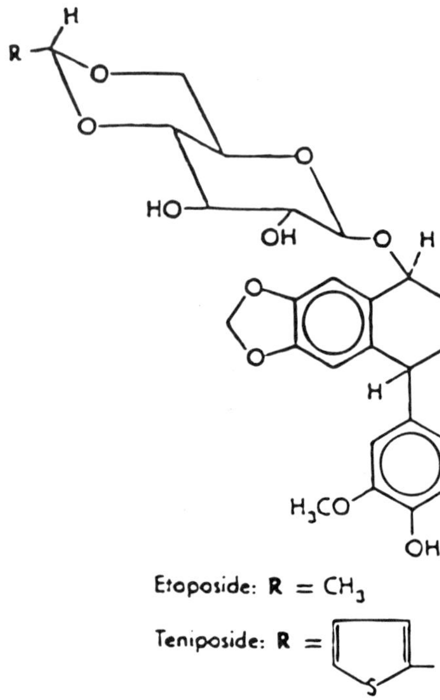

Figure 2

B. Mechanism of Action

The mechanism of the epipodophyllotoxins differs from the parent podophyllotoxin which inhibits microtubule formation. Their lack of microtubule assembly inhibition is due to the glucoside moiety on the C ring of the molecule. These agents are cell cycle specific, arresting cells at the S-G2 interface, and cause single-strand breaks in DNA (7). This effect appears to be due to the inhibition of topoisomerase II, a nuclear enzyme responsible for the breakage and resealing of DNA (8). The epipodophyllotoxins also can inhibit nucleoside transport and impair incorporation of nucleosides into cellular nucleic acids.

C. Pharmacology

Both teniposide and etoposide are highly potein bound. After oral administration, approximately 50% of the drug is absorbed. Following intravenous injection of etoposide, there is a biphasic pattern of clearance with half-lives of 3 h and 12 h (9). Forty-five percent of the dose is excreted in the urine (two-thirds unchanged and one-third as metabolites), and decrease clearance rates have been observed in patients with renal insufficiency requiring dose reductions (10). Fifteen percent is recovered in the feces and less than 10% of the plasma concentration accumulates in the CSF.

Teniposide has a multiphasic pattern of clearance after intravenous injection, which is its most common form of administration. Approximately 45% of the drug is excreted in the urine, but unlike etoposide, most (80%) is recovered as metabolites. Less than 1% of the drug concentrates in the CSF. Teniposide undergoes some biliary elimination after conjugation with glucuronide or sulfate derivatives.

D. Clinical Indications

Teniposide has not been extensively used clinically but has been shown to be effective in the treatment of small cell carcinome of the lung. Activity also is noted in acute lymphoblastic lymphoma, neuroblastoma, and the lymphomas.

Etoposide clearly is effective in the treatment of small cell lung cancer and is useful as part of combination chemotherapy for testicular carcinoma, Hodgkin's and non-Hodgkin's lymphoma, and acute and chronic leukemias. It is also used in platinum-based combinations for the treatment of non-small cell carcinoma of the lung (11).

E. Adverse Reactions

The clinical toxicity of etoposide and teniposide are similar. Myelosuppression is the major dose-limiting toxicity of both, with leukopenia and neutropenia occurring most frequently. Nadirs are observed at 10–14 d with complete recovery noted by 3 wk. Thrombocytopenia occurs less frequently and usually is mild. Nausea, vomiting, and diarrhea occur in 10–15% of patients, while most patients develop complete, though reversible, alopecia. Hypersensitivity reactions occur, but are uncommon, although hypotension has been reported after rapid infusions of etoposide.

REFERENCES

1. Krauhs E, Little M, Kempf T, et al. Complete amino acid sequence of beta-tubulin from porcine brain. Proc Natl Acad Sci USA 1981; 78:4156.
2. Owellen RJ, Hartke CA, Hains OF. Pharmacokinetics and metabolism of vinblastine in humans. Cancer Res 1977; 37:2597.
3. Bender RA, Castle MC, Margileth DA, Oliverio VT. The pharmacokinetics of [3H]-vincristine in man. Clin Pharm Ther 1977; 22:430.

4. Jackson DV, Castle MC, Bender RA. Biliary excretion of vincristine. Clin Pharm Ther 1978; 24:101.
5. Miller BR. Neurotoxicity and vincristine. JAMA 1985; 253:2045.
6. Robertson GL, Bhoopalam N, Zelkowitz LJ. Vincristine neurotoxicity and abnormal secretion of antidiuretic hormone. Arch Intern Med 1973; 132:717.
7. Derwinko B, Barlogie B. Survival and cycle-progression delay of human lymphoma cells in vitro exposed to VP 16–213. Cancer Treat Rep 1976; 60:1295.
8. Ross W, Rowe T, Glisson B, et al. Role of topoisomerase II in mediating epipodophyllotoxin-induced DNA cleavage. Cancer Res 1984; 44:5857.
9. Allen LM, Creaven PJ. Comparison of the human pharmacokinetics of VM-26 and VP-16, two antineoplastic epipodophyllotoxin glucopyranoside derivatives. Eur J Cancer 1975; 11:697.
10. D'Incalci M, Rossi C, Zucchetti M, et al. Pharmacokinetics of etoposide in patients with abnormal renal and hepatic function. Cancer Res 1986; 46:2566.
11. O'Dwyer PJ, Leyland-Jones B, Alonso MT, et al. Etoposide (VP 16–213): current status of an active anticancer drug. N Engl J Med 1985; 323:378.

7
Bleomycin

Charles J. McDonald
Brown University, Providence, Rhode Island

Antibiotics used as chemotherapeutic agents are very complex substances that are usually derived from primary cultures of a variety of microorganisms. A substantial number of agents obtained in this manner have demonstrated antineoplastic activity. Antitumor antibiotics are among the most active compounds in clinical use for treating cancer and include the anthracycline derivatives doxorubicin, daunorubicin, and idarubicin, all products of the fungus *Streptomyces peucetus* var. *caesius,* and bleomycin which is a fermentation product derived from a strain of *Streptomyces verticalis.* In dermatology, the bleomycins are the most commonly used antineoplastic antibiotics.

I. CHEMISTRY

Bleomycin is a water-soluble complex mixture of small molecular-weight, closely related, copper-chelating glycopeptides. Chemically the various bleomycin species are structurally similar and differ from each other in very minor ways, principally in the substitution of complex peptide and inorganic substances in the terminal amine moieties (1) (Figure 1). The substituted terminal amine moieties are apparently not essential for bleomycin clinical activity. However, in order to become active antitumor agents, the copper component must be replaced by ferrous ions (Fe^{2+}).

Crude bleomycin mixtures can be purified by chromatography into several components: bleomycins A_{1-6}, B_{1-4}. Bleomycin A_2 and B_2 at 70% and 25%, respectively, make up the bulk of bleomycins found in commercial preparations.

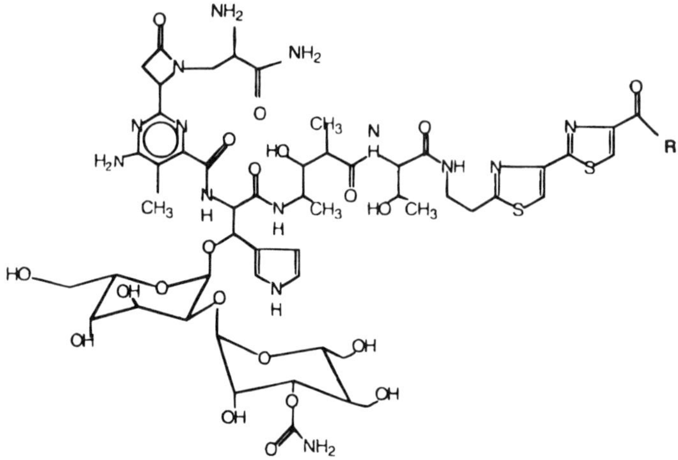

Bleomycin A_2 : **R** = $NHCH_2CH_2CH_2-\overset{+}{S}(CH_3)_2$

Figure 1 Chemical structure of bleomycin.

II. MECHANISM OF ACTION

The bleomycins bind with both double- and single-strand cellular DNA, producing site-specific and nonspecific single- and double-strand scissions and progressive fragmentation of the DNA chain. DNA is cleaved preferentially at guanine-cytosine and guanine-thymine sequences. Cleavage occurs after ferrous ions are chelated to nitrogen-containing groups, such as the pyrimidine ring, and the imidazole of C-histidine on the bleomycin molecule. As bleomycin intercalates with DNA, the complexed iron is brought into close proximity to a deoxyribose moiety. The ferrous ion is then spontaneously oxidized to the ferric state. Oxidation is associated with the generation of free oxygen radicals as the superoxide or hydroxyl radical; strand breakage then occurs.

Additional effects of bleomycin on DNA include alteration of the activity of DNA-dependent DNA polymerase and inhibition of DNA ligase. Thus, in the presence of bleomycin, cells are rendered incapable of repairing DNA damage secondary to the chemical effect of bleomycin.

Additionally, bleomycin may form noncovalent intermolecular cross-links with DNA. Bleomycin has no activity against RNA. Cells in the S1G1 and G2 phases of the cell cycle are sensitive to bleomycin, however, cells in mitosis are most sensitive. Bleomycin can produce partial synchrony in vitro by blocking progression of the cell through the S-G2 boundary and causing accumulation of cells in the G2 phase (2).

The bleomycins appear to have a special affinity for epithelia tissues, especially those tissues containing low levels of an inactivating enzyme bleomycin aminohydrolase (3). This enzyme hydrolyzes the amide of bleomycin to a weakly active deamido-bleomycin. Particularly low levels of the enzyme are found in skin and lung. Although bleomycin exerts its greatest toxicity in tissues with low levels of bleomycin hydrolase, it has found greatest use in the treatment of squamous cell carcinoma of the skin, head, neck, and lungs, as well as in the treatment of cutaneous T-cell lymphoma and Kaposi's sarcoma.

III. PHARMACOLOGY

Bleomycin is most often administered by parenteral routes. Intravenous or intramuscular administration appear equally effective. Subcutaneous and intracavitary instillation are also acceptable routes of administration. Bleomycin clearance from plasma is biphasic. The serum half-life after intravenous bolus administration is 24 min, and plasma peak concentrations range from 1–10 mμ/ml. The terminal half-life is 2–4 h. After intramuscular administration bleomycin has a half-life of 2–3 h, and peak serum concentrations depend on the dosage of drug given. Bleomycin clearance from plasma is altered with continuous infusions. The half-life increases to 80 min and terminal half-life increases up to 9 h. Steady-state concentration occurs after approximately 12 h of continuous infusions (4).

Bleomycin and its metabolites are primarily excreted in urine. Severe renal failure will prolong the serum half-life, leading to increased drug toxicity. In patients with normal renal function, 50% of an intravenous dose is excreted in the first 4 h, and within 24 h approximately 70% is excreted in urine. Intramuscular administration produces approximately the same clearance values.

The degree of bleomycin accumulation in normal and tumor tissue is inversely proportional to the activity and amount of bleomycin hydrolase. Normal skin and lung are hydrolase-free or deficient tissues (3). Hence, they are tissues where bleomycin sensitivity is most pronounced and toxicity occurs most frequently.

IV. CLINICAL INDICATIONS

When administered alone bleomycin has broad spectrum antitumor activity, as demonstrated in squamous cell cancers of the head and neck, cervix, esophagus, lungs, vulva, and skin.

Efficacy has also been demonstrated when used singly or in combination with other agents in Hodgkin's disease, non-Hodgkin's lymphoma, Kaposi's, sarcoma, and germ cell testicular cancer.

V. ADVERSE REACTIONS

Bleomycin causes very little bone marrow toxicity and thus it has found frequent use in combination chemotherapy regimens. The most commonly encountered adverse reactions occur in those tissue lacking in bleomycin hydrolase, that is, skin and lungs. The most severe and serious toxicity occurs in the lungs. A nonresponsive interstitial pneumonitis followed by severe pulmonary fibrosis occurs in about 10% of treated patients. This entity is to be distinguished from a hypersensitivity reaction in the lungs that does respond to systemic corticosteroid treatment (5,6). Pulmonary toxicity appears to be age and drug dosage dependent. It is observed most often in patients over 70 y of age and in those receiving a dosage of 400 ν or greater. The earliest signs and symptoms of bleomycin pulmonary toxicity include dyspnea, fine pulmonary rales, x-ray findings of diffuse pulmonary opacities, as well as decreased total lung capacity, decreased diffusion capacity, and decreased vital capacity. In an attempt to discover pulmonary toxicity at an early stage, all patients on bleomycin should have frequent chest x-ray examinations and pulmonary function tests. These examinations should also be taken prior to initial drug administration. It has not been clearly established that pulmonary function tests are predictive, sufficient that repeated testing will give ample warning of impending bleomycin pulmonary toxicity, or will provide an adequate index for discontinuation of drug in time to prevent progressive pulmonary involvement.

An idiosyncratic reaction characterized by profound hyperpyrexia, chills, hypotension, and sustained cardiorespiratory collapse has been noted in 1–5% of patients with lymphoma. This reaction does not appear to be related to classic anaphylaxis, but has resulted in a number of deaths. It may occur immediately or be delayed for several hours, and usually occurs with the first or second dosages of drug. A very similar response has been observed by the author in a single patient being treated for Kaposi's sarcoma with bleomycin and vincristine. It has been suggested that in patients with lymphoma small test doses of bleomycin (1–2μ) be given on the first two treatment occasions, each to be followed by a 24 h period of observation. A period of pyrexia alone lasting for 24–48 h may occur in up to 25% of patients treated with bleomycin and should not be confused with the more severe systemic reaction above.

Cutaneous reactions occur in 50% or more patients. These reactions vary from simple erythematous dermatitis to vesiculation followed by ulcerations, hyperkeratoses, and sclerodermoid skin changes, particularly in skin overlying bony prominences (7). Pruritus followed by scratching of the skin causes "feathery" areas of erythema followed by persistent hyperpigmentation. Sclerodermoid skin changes that may occur with drug dosages as low as 100μ can be associated with cutaneous edema, arthralgias, increased serum sedimentation rate, and positive antinuclear factor. Unlike pulmonary fibrosis, some affected patients may respond to the use of systemic corticosteroids or aminobenzoate potassium (POTABA). Other mucocutaneous reactions include alopecia and stomatitis, which often occur within 3–4 w after a cumulative dose of 150–200 units of bleomycin.

REFERENCES

1. Carter SK, Crooke ST, Umezawa H. Recent studies on biochemistry and action of bleomycin. In: Carter SK, Crooke ST, Umezawa H, eds. Bleomycin: current status and new development. New York: Academic Press, 1978: 15–19.
2. Barranco SC. A review of the survival and cell-kinetics effect of bleomycin. In: Carter SK, Crooke ST, Umezawa H, eds. Bleomycin: current status and new developments. New York: Academic Press, 1978: 81–90.
3. Yoshioka O, Noriko A, Takahashi K, Matsuda A, Umezawa H. Intracellulare fate and activity of bleomycin. In: Carter SK, Crooke ST, Umezawa H, eds. Bleomycin: current status and new developments. New York: Academic Press, 1978: 35–56.
4. Crooke ST, Prestayko AW. Clinical pharmacology of bleomycin. In: Carter SK Crooke ST, Umezawa H, eds. Bleomycin: current status and new developments. New York: Academic Press, 1978: 117–130.
5. Hoyle PY, Lunga MA, Mackay B, Bedrosian CW. Bleomycin hypersensitivity pnemonitis. Ann Int Med 1978; 88:47–49.
6. Brown LD, Reimer RR, Ahmed M, Hewlett JS. Successful treatment of bleomycin lung. Clev Clin O 1980; 47:92–96.
7. McDonald CJ, Friedman DA, Muglia JJ. Alopecia and other cutaneous reactions to cancer chemotherapeutic agents. In: Abeloff M, Armitage J, Lichter A, Niederhuber J, eds. Clinical oncology. New York: Churchill Livingstone, 1993.

8
Cytokines

Aditya K. Gupta, Ron Prussick, Gulnar M. Shivji, Daniel N. Sauder
University of Toronto, Sunnybrook Health Science Centre, Toronto, Ontario, Canada

I. INTRODUCTION

Cytokines represent a complex network of soluble mediators of immunological and inflammatory reactions. They play an important role in intercellular communication and signal transduction. Cytokines possess a wide range of biological activities and frequently have overlapping functions. Initially these mediators were thought to be restricted to the immune system, and they were designated as lymphokines, but they are now known to be synthesized and secreted from a wide variety of cell types including keratinocytes. The major subclasses of cytokines are a)interferons (IFNs), b) interleukins (ILs), c) hematopoietic colony stimulating factors (CSFs), d) growth factors and inhibitory factors, and e) tumor necrosis factors (TNFs). Cytokines act in a network with the final response being determined by a repertoire of synergistic and antagonistic signals. These mediators modulate activation, proliferation, and differentiation of immune and nonimmune cells.

In general, cytokines initiate their action by binding with the target cell that bears the specific cytokine receptor. This may initiate a cascade of cellular events including release of other cytokines which may modulate release of the initial cytokine. Although cytokines have heterogeneous properties, they possess common characteristics including a) they are glycoproteins of low molecular weight (usually <70 kD), b) most are synthesized as larger precursor molecules, c) they are potent at relatively low concentrations such as nanomoles or picomoles, d) cytokines often interact with a specific high-affinity cell surface receptor, and e) receptors on target cells may be present in relatively low numbers, for example, less than 10,000 receptors per cell (1). The cytokines synthesized and expressed in skin are summarized in Table 1.

II. INTERFERONS

Interferons are an important and integral part of the cytokine network and were the first cytokines to be used therapeutically (2). Interferon was first identified by Isaacs and Lindenmann in 1957 who demonstrated that a soluble factor prevented influenza-A virus from infecting chick chorioallantoic membranes (3). Interferons were so named because they interfere with viral infection. They have now been found to possess nonspecific viral activity (4).

A. Chemistry

The IFNs are a multigene family. Three major classes of IFNs have been identified: IFN-α, IFN-β, and IFN-γ. The classification was initially based on the cell types producing them (Table 2) (5–7). Interferons have been found to be generally species specific. Thus, IFNs produced by one species may not be active in another species. The production of natural IFN-γ in stimulated leukocyte cultures was described by Wheelock in 1965 (8). The DNA sequence of the human IFN-γ gene was isolated and characterized by Gray and Goddel in 1982 (9). Initially IFNs were produced on a small scale from human cell cultures. The availability of recombinant DNA techniques has enabled large amounts of IFN protein to be produced for use in clinical trials. Typically the recombinant IFN differs from naturally occurring IFN by one amino acid substitution (10). IFN-α-2a and interferon-α-2b differ only in the amino acid residue on position 23, which is arginine and lysine, respectively (11).

Table 1 Cytokines Synthesized and Expressed in Skin

Interleukins (ILs): IL-1, IL-3 (murine only), IL-4, IL-6, IL-7, IL-8, IL-10, IL-11
Colony stimulating factors (CSFs): granulocyte macrophage colony-stimulating factor (GM-CSF), macrophage colony-stimulating factor (M-CSF), granulocyte colony-stimulating factor (G-CSF)
Tumor necrosis factor (TNF): TNF-α
Growth factors: Nerve growth factor, transforming growth factor-α (TGF-α), transforming growth factor-β (TGF-β), parathyroid-like peptide, basic fibroblast growth factor, platelet-derived growth factor (PDGF), epidermal growth factor (EGF)

B. Mechanism of Action

In general, INFs have antiviral, antipoliferative, and immunomodulatory activities. Interferons also have antitumoral properties and may inhibit growth of benign and malignant tumors (12). Interferons exert their cellular activities by binding to specific membrane receptors on the cell surface. The type 1 IFNs (IFN-α and IFN-β) share a common receptor that is distinct from that for IFN-γ. Once the IFN has bound to its receptor a complex sequence of intracellular events is initiated. There may be internalization of the interferon-receptor complex into the cells. Another possibility is that a "second messenger" is generated at the cell surface following activation of a plasma membrane-bound enzyme. Regardless of the exact nature of changes that occur, a signal is transduced to the nucleus, resulting in gene activation and subsequent enzyme production (13–16). Interferons can induce receptors for other cytokines such as a tumor necrosis factors (TNFs) (14). Interferons can also induced or enhance expression of cell surface receptors for the Fc portion of IgG.

Interferons can affect immunological function in several ways (Table 3) (14,17). INF-γ is a more potent immunomodulator that IFN-α and IFN-β and can activate macrophages more efficiently than type 1 IFNs (6).

Interferons augment specific cytotoxicity of lymphocytes for target cells. The activity of cytotoxic effector cells is increased by type 1 IFNs. This includes enhancement of natural killer (NK) cell activity, cytotoxic T lymphocytes and antibody-dependent cellular cytotoxicity (13). Type 1 IFN can activate NK cells quite rapidly, in contrast with IFN-γ which occurs more slowly over 12–18 h. It is possible that type I and type II IFNs activate NK cells by different mechanisms. Interferons, particularly IFN-γ, inhibit T suppressor lymphocytes and induce ICAM-I on keratinocytes which may enhance the delayed hypersensitivity response (17–19). IFN-γ can also induce ICAM-I expression on endothelial cells and melanoma cells (20).

Type I and II IFNs can induce or enhance expression of class I MHC and β_2 microglobulin on different cell types, particularly lymphocytes and monocytes (13). In addition, IFN-γ can induce class II MHC antigens on a variety of cell types including monocytes, lymphoid cells, keratinocytes, melanocytes and endothelial cells.

Both type I and II IFNs can have an effect on B cells by enhancing antibody formation. This may, in part, be mediated by indirect effects such as an improvement in antigen presentation by accessory cells. Interferons may also have a direct effect on B-cell maturation.

Type I IFNs are more potent in their inhibition of normal and malignant cell growth compared to type II IFNs (14,21). This may explain the efficacy of IFN-α in the treatment of capillary hemangiomas, warts, and cutaneous carcinoma. Some cells may become arrested in the G1 phase of the cell cycle.

Table 2 Comparison Between the Interferons

	IFN-α	IFN-β	IFN-γ
IFN type	1	1	2
Molecular weight (daltons)	19,000	22,000	45,000(dimer)
Number of species (isotypes)	18–20	2	1
IFN genes	At least 23 different genes, code for 15 functional proteins	1	1 IFN-B
Nucleic acid homology	45% homology between IFN-α and IFN-β	45% homology between IFN-α and β	No homology between IFN-α and IFN-β
Introns	None	None	3
Amount of glycosylation	Some glycosylated	Glycoslylated	Glycosylated
Polypeptide chain length (amino acids)	165/166	180/194	143/146
Tertiary protein structure	Type 1 mature protein contains disulfide bridges	Type 1 mature protein contains disulfide bridges	Mature protein does not contain disulfide bridges
Resistance to heat and acids	Acid stable	Acid stable	Lower resistance to heat and acids compared to type 1 IFN, inactivated at lower pH.
Chromosome location	Multiple gene family 2,5,7, short arm 9 (9p21–p22)	Multiple gene family 2,5,7, short arm 9 (9p21–p22)	Long arm of chromosome 12 (12q 24.1)
Interferon receptor	common between IFN-α and IFN-β; 110–130 kD	Common between IFN-α and IFN-β; 110–130 kD	Separate receptor from IFN-α and IFNβ. 54 kD. No homology with the IFN-α and IFN-β receptor
Inducers	Viruses, bacteria	Viruses, bacteria	Mitogens, lectins, specific antigens
Produced mainly by	Leukocytes. Sometimes by keratinocytes, fibroblasts, endotheliocytes, and mesenchymal cells.	Fibroblasts, leukocytes, epithelial cells	Lymphocytes

Activity	Antiviral. Antiproliferative. Antitumoral MHC I expression/up-regulation. No significant immunomodulative activity.	Antiviral. Antiproliferative. MHC I expression/up-regulation. Stimulation of macrophages, NK cells. Fc receptor expression. Modulation of B-cell activity. Differentiation of certain cell types.	Antiviral. Antiproliferative. MHC 1/II expression/up-regulation. Stimulates macrophage function. Enhances cytotoxic activity of NK cells and neutrophils. Induces expression of adhesion molecules. Induces differentiation of NK and cyrotoxic T cells. Induces synthesis of IgG 2α by activated B cells. Causes antagonism of some IL-4 actions.
Immunomodulating activity	Less potent immunomodulator than Type II IFNs.	Less potent immunomodulator than type II IFNs.	More potent immunomodulator than type I IFNs.

Table 3 Effect of Interferons on Immunologic Function (14,17)

	IFN-α	IFN-β	IFN-γ
Antiviral activity	+	+	+
Cytostatic activity	+	+	+
Activation of macrophages	+[a]	+[a]	+
T-cell proliferation	−		0
Induction of ICAM 1			+
Stimulation of NK cells	+[b]	+[b]	+
Stimulation of LAK cells	−	−	+
MHC Class I expression	+	+	+
MHC Class II expression	+/0	+/0	+/0
Isotype selection			+
B-cell activation			−
B-cell proliferation	+	+	+
Collagen synthesis by human dermal fibroblasts	−	−	−
Antitumor activity in vivo	+	+	+
Induce fever	+	+	+

[a] Higher doses of type I IFN required compared to type II IFN.
[b] The activation of NK cells by type I IFN is a rapid effect; this activation occurs more slowly with IFN-γ.

Key:
+ Stimulation
0 No effect
− Inhibitory

Interferons can inhibit transcription of genes such as the proto-oncogene *c-myc* as well as other genes such as those involved in mitogenic response (21).

C. Adverse Reactions

The nature and severity of side effects of INFs (Table 4) (22–36) is generally dependent upon the dosage administered, route of administration, and the disorder being treated. However, patient sensitivity varies. Most reactions are mild to moderate in severity. In many cases the adverse effects are transient and diminish with ongoing therapy. The adverse effects are generally reversible, although in some cases it may take several weeks for symptoms to resolve. If the IFN is given regularly, for example on a daily basis, some degree of tolerance occurs.

The most common adverse effect is a "flulike" syndrome. This occurs in nearly all patients to one degree or another. Some tolerance develops within 7–10 d of therapy. Some of the symptoms may be diminished by taking doses at bedtime. For symptomatic relief use of acetaminophen and nonsteroidal antiinflammatory

Table 4 Adverse Reactions Following Interferon Therapy (22–36)

Flu-like symptoms:
more common: fever, fatigue, chills, myalgia, headache, general feeling of discomfort
less common: joint/back pain

Gastrointestinal symptoms:
more common: anorexia, nausea, vomiting, diarrhea, dry mouth, thirst, change in taste or metallic taste
less common: abdominal pain, dyspepsia, constipation, loose stools, weight loss, cold sores or stomatitis, gingivitis

Symptoms related to the nervous system:
more common: dizziness, tiredness
less common: depression, irritability, confusion, impaired concentration, paresthesia, hypoesthesia, amnesia, anxiety, nervousness, somnolence

Respiratory symptoms:
less common: dyspnea, sinusitis, coughing, nasal congestion, rhinitis, rhinorrhea, pharyngitis, bronchospasm, wheezing, sneezing, pneumonia, pleural pain, cyanosis

Dermatological symptoms:
more common: erythematous eruption with inflammation
less common: pruritus, dry skin, reaction at injection site (such as inflammation, pain, burning, bleeding, necrosis, erythema), purpura, alopecia (diffuse thinning, acceleration of male pattern baldness, telogen effluvium), abnormal hair texture, increased hair growth, moniliasis, edema/facial edema, photosensitivity, lichenoid dermatitis, acne, furunculosis, urticaria, melanosis, skin depigmentation, induction of cutaneous malignancy (basal and squamous cell carcinomas, dermatofibroma sarcoma protruberans, sebaceous carcinoma), atrophic plaques, exacerbation/induction/improvement of psoriasis.

Cardiovascular:
less common: arrhythmias, chest pain, hypotension

Endocrine:
less common: hyperthyroidism or hypothyroidism, aggravation of diabetes mellitus, gynecomastia, virilism, loss of libido

Special senses:
less common: blurred vision, conjunctivitis, diplopia, periorbital edema, photophobia

Miscellaneous:
less common: increased sweating, malaise

Laboratory test abnormalities:
more common: anemia (usually asymptomatic), leukopenia (usually asymptomatic), thrombocytopenia (usually asymptomatic)
less common: hepatotoxicity (usually asymptomatic); symptomatic-anemia, granulocytopenia, leukopenia, thrombocytopenia

drugs (NSAIDs) to prevent or reduce fever and headaches may be of benefit (37–41). Patients should be well hydrated, especially during the early stages of therapy, to reduce the risk of hypotension associated with fluid depletion. At higher doses of systemic therapy, hematological toxicity and hepatotoxicity may become manifest. At ever higher doses the frequency of cardiovascular and neurological toxicity increases.

Interferon should be administered with adherence to the appropriate monitoring guidelines. Since photosensitivity can sometimes occur, sun protection measures should be taken. Interferons may interact with cytochrome P-450 giving rise to the potential for interactions with medications known to affect the P-450 system, for example, reduced clearance of aminophylline when given with IFN-α-2b (42–45).

In some cases IFN therapy may result in the development of antibodies that may neutralize the effects of IFN. The significance of such antibodies is not certain.

D. Clinical Indications

Interferons are not completely effective as antiviral agents (46). The efficacy of IFN as an antiviral agent does not increase linearly as the dosage is increased (23,47). Condyloma acuminata may be treated by IFN-α by various routes such as parenterally, intramuscularly, subcutaneously, topically, and intralesionally but appears to be more effective when given intralesionally. A recommended regimen is administering 1 million IU/lesion three times a week intralesionally for 3 wk. Maximum benefit should occur within 4–8 wk following injections; if results are not satisfactory at 12–16 wk as second course of therapy may be required. The intralesional route allows for localized administration of drug with a reduction in the severity of side effects (10). One limitation of intralesional administration is that areas with subclinical infection that appear clinically uninfected may not receive treatment. Although IFN-α is effective in clearing condyloma acuminata, it has not proved to have clear-cut superiority over conventional therapies (48,49).

Several reports have suggested the use of IFN-α in the treatment of cutaneous T-cell lymphoma (CTCL) (50). Various treatment regimens have been tried, with the response being dependent upon the stage of the disease and the general condition of the patient. Interferon-γ may not be as effective as IFN-α in CTCL (51). When high-dose recombinant IFN-α is used as monotherapy (up to 5×10^7 IU/m^2 three times a week) for a prolonged period of time a 50% complete response rate has been reported (52). In some cases side effects have necessitated a dosage reduction. In CTCL (stages Ia to IVa), when recombinant IFN-α was given at a dose of 3–36 $\times$ 10^6 UI/day for 10 wk an objective response was noted in 64% of patients (28). Some patients developed severe side effects during treatment. In many cases IFN-α is used as adjunctive therapy with other modalities

(53). A combination of recombinant IFN-α and etretinate may be effective in the treatment of CTCL, especially in early stage disease (31,54–57). A combination of recombinant IFN-α and PUVA (psoralen plus ultraviolet-A light) also appears to be effective in the treatment of CTCL, particularly early stage disease (58).

Surgical treatment of basal cell carcinomas (BCCs) and squamous cell carcinomas (SCCs) usually results in cure rates exceeding 95%. Although the response rate with IFN-α therapy is generally inferior, it may provide a suitable alternative in patients who are not surgical candidates, those who prefer nonsurgical treatment or possibly as adjuvant therapy (6,59–62). In many protocols recombinant IFN-α has to be injected three times a week for 3 wk. For example, in one study superficial BCCs were treated with IFN-α-2b at a dose of 1.5×10^6 IU three times weekly for 3 wk injected directly into the skin cancer. At follow-up, after 16–20 wk, histological examination revealed remission in 86% of patients. When reexamined 1 y after therapy 81% of patients were tumor free (63). Similar results have been obtained in patients with SCCs (64,65).

The effect of an intralesional sustained-release formulation of recombinant IFN-α-2b on BCCs has been studied. The IFN-α-2b was packaged as a protamine zinc chelated formulation (10 million IU/injection) (60). Thirty-three patients received a single injection and 32 patients were administered one injection per week for 3 wk. After 16 wk of therapy 80% of evaluable tumors treated with three injections and 52% treated with one injection were found to be cured histologically.

IFN-α has also been used as an adjunctive therapy with retinoids with enhancement of efficacy. A combination of recombinant IFN-α-2a (3 million units/d) with 13-*cis* retinoic acid (1 mg/kg/d) given for at least 2 mo to patients with advanced inoperable SCC resulted in a response rate of 93% (66).

Interferons may have antitumor effects against malignant melanoma. In a review of the experience with recombinant IFN-α-2a in the treatment of metastatic melanoma, an overall response rate of 12.6% was noted in 189 evaluable patients from a total of 196 entered patients (67–73). In another review, 46 of 309 evaluable patients demonstrated a response, giving an overall response rate of 15% (74). Trials utilizing interrupted (intermittent) schedules were less effective than studies where IFN was administered regularly (for example, daily or three times a week). When IFN-α-2b was used to treat metastatic melanoma there was a response of 22.6% in 106 evaluable patients (75–78). With recombinant IFN-γ, in 69 evaluable patients with metastatic melanoma there was a response in 5 patients (7%) (79–81).

In order to improve response rates IFN therapy has been combined with other cytotoxic and biological agents. These include interleukin-2 (IL-2), TNF-α, cimetidine, indomethacin, vinblastine, α-difluoromethylornithine (DFMO), dimethyltriazenoimidazole, carboxamide (DTIC), and *cis*-platinum (CDPP) (82–

87). Further experience needs to be obtained to determine the most efficacious combination and its dosage profile.

IFN-γ has shown some benefit in atopic dermatitis. IFN-γ is known to affect the balance between subsets of T-helper cells. T-helper (Th) cells can by subdivided into two subsets that produce different lymphokines. Following activation by antigens or mitogenic lectins Th1 T-cell clones produce IL-2 and IFN-γ, whereas Th2 cell clones secrete IL-4 and IL-5 (88). In atopic dermatitis there is defective regulation of IgE production, with elevated IgE levels being present (89). Human IgE production is regulated by several factors including the balance between Th1 cytokines, such as IFN-γ, and Th2 cytokines, such as IL-4. Interferon-γ inhibits production of IgE, whereas IL-4 promotes it. Lymphocytes from patients with atopic dermatitis have a diminished ability to secrete IFN-γ (90–92). The reduced IFN-γ may enhance IgE secretion in patients with atopic dermatitis and contribute to the pathogenesis of the cutaneous condition.

Various studies have found IFN-γ therapy to be effective in atopic dermatitis. In one such study 100 μg of recombinant IFN-γ was administered subcutaneously on 5 d of the first week and then three times a week for a further 3 wk (93). This resulted in an improvement of skin lesions and pruritus with decreased serum IgE production.

The use of IFN in the management of keloids has been investigated. Interferon-γ inhibits type I and III collagen synthesis by dermal and synovial fibroblasts, and type II collagen synthesis by chondrocytes in a dose-dependent manner (94). However, other studies have demonstrated that IFN-γ does not significantly decrease collagen synthesis of keloid fibroblasts *in vitro*. Some clinical reports have shown that recombinant IFN-γ injected into progressively enlarging keloids may be of some benefit (95,96). It is possible that intralesional IFN-α may be more effective for the treatment of keloids (53).

III. INTERLEUKINS

Cytokines were initially named according to their biological activities. Since cytokines possess multiple overlapping activities a new nomenclature system was devised. At one time it was thought that cytokines were synthesized primarily by leukocytes and that most of their actions were on other leukocytes, thus the term interleukin ("between leukocytes") was proposed in 1981 (97–99).

At the sixth International Congress of Immunology in 1986, it was decided that a new lymphokine/cytokine would initially be named according to its biological properties. Following establishment of the amino acid sequence of the human form, it would be assigned an interleukin number (100). For example, B-cell

Table 5 Nomenclature of Interleukins

Interleukin	Other Names
IL-1	Edogenous pyrogen, leukocytic pyrogen, lymphocyte activating factor, leukocyte endogenous mediator, epidermal thymocyte activity factor, proteolysis inducing factor, synovial factor, fibroblast proliferating factor, osteoclast activating factor, catabolin
IL-2	T-cell growth factor
IL-3	Multicolony stimulating factor
IL-4	B-cell growth factor-1, B-cell stimulating factor
IL-5	B-cell growth factor-2, eosinophil differentiating factor
IL-6	B-cell hepatocyte stimulating factor, B-cell stimulating factor-2
IL-7	Pre-B-cell growth factor
IL-8	Neutrophilic chemotactic factor, leukocyte adhesion inhibitor
IL-9	T-cell-derived growth factor
IL-10	Cytokine synthesis inhibitory factor
IL-11	Adipogenesis inhibitory factor
IL-12	Natural killer cell stimulating factor
IL-13	P-600

growth factor-1 is now termed interleukin-4 (IL-4) (Table 5) (100). It should be noted that many cytokines continue to be referred to by their original names, for example, the interferons and the colony stimulating factors. There are 13 known interleukins (Table 5). This review will focus mainly on the interleukins that are currently used therapeutically and those that play a prominent role in the pathogenesis of certain skin diseases. For more detailed reviews the reader is referred to other texts (97–113).

A. Interleukin-1

Interleukin-1 (IL-1) is produced by almost every nucleated cell in the body including keratinocytes, Langerhans cells, endothelial cells, fibroblasts, natural killer cells, kidney mesangial cells, glial cells and astrocytes in the nervous system, corneal epithelium, and dendritic cells (Table 6) (101,114–118). Both *in vivo* and *in vitro* human keratinocytes express the IL-1 gene, IL-1 mRNA, and protein (119–123). A large proportion of the IL-1 is found in an intracellular location although a portion is membrane associated (124).

1. Chemistry

Two forms of IL-1 (IL-1α and IL-1β) have been cloned (123,125). Both IL-1α and IL-1β genes are synthesized as precursors of weight 31–33 kD and subsequently

Table 6 Actions of IL-1 (97,99,101)

T lymphocytes	1. Lymphokine production
	2. IL-2 receptor expression
	3. IL-2 production
	4. Chemotaxis
B lymphocytes	1. Chemotaxis
	2. Proliferation
	3. Augmented antibody production
Macrophages/monocytes	1. Stimulate PGE-2 synthesis
	2. Tumor necrosis factor synthesis
	3. Cytotoxic activity
	4. Chemotaxis
Neutrophils	1. Enzyme release
	2. Degranulation
	3. Oxidative metabolism
	4. Chemotaxis
	5. Collagenase production
Epithelial cells	1. Proliferation
	2. Type IV collagen synthesis
Keratinocytes	1. Proliferation
	2. Induction of GM-CSF
Skeletal muscle	1. Proteolysis
Hepatocytes	1. Synthesis of acute phase proteins
	2. Hypoferremia
	3. Hypozincemia
Osteoclasts	1. Bone resorption
	2. Collagenase synthesis
Bone marrow	1. Neutrophil production
Synovial cells	1. Collagenase synthesis
Cartilage/chondrocytes	1. Collagenase and plasminogen activator synthesis
Fibroblasts	1. Collagenase synthesis
Endothelial cells	1. Procoagulant activity
	2. Increased macrophage and neutrophil adhesion
Brain	1. Hypothalamus pyrexia
	2. Somnolence
	3. Anorexia
	4. Cerebral cortex slow-wave sleep

proteolytically cleaved to active molecules which are 15–17 kD proteins (126). Cleavage of the intracellular precursor results in removal of the N-terminal segment of the molecule, with bioactivity residing in the carboxy terminal portion of the molecule (127). The 17 kD peptide can be further fragmented into 4 kD and 2 kD species with retention of some biological activity (128). IL-1α and IL-β both lack the hydrophobic sequences of amino acids that are typically present in secretory proteins (114,126,129). It is possible that IL-1 remains within the cells and that its release occurs following cell damage (126).

2. Mechanism of Action

T-cell Activation. Macrophages or other antigen-presenting cells bearing the class II major histocompatibility complex (MHC) react with the processed antigen in association with the T-cell receptor on helper T cells (114,126,130). Helper T cells produce interleukin-2 (IL-2) following activation by the processed antigen in conjunction with IL-1 secreted by activated macrophages. Activated T cells respond to IL-2 by differentiating into effector lymphocytes including cytotoxic T cells. These activated helper T cells produce cytokines such as IL-2, IL-3, IL-4, IL-5, and IL-6 (114). IL-1 may augment IL-2 function both at the level of IL-2 production and IL-2 action, and may be required for the expression of the IL-2 receptor (IL-2R) (114,126,131–133).

Effects of Interleukin-1 on Monocytes. IL-1 can mediate cytotoxicity of monocytes via TNFs (tumor necrosis factors) (114). It should be noted that many of the properties of IL-1 overlap with those TNF-α and TNF-β (Table 7) (97,125,126,134).

Effects of Interleukin-1 on B Cells. IL-1 may be involved in the maturation of pre-B cells into a mature B cell and may also have an effect on sensitive B cells during the phase of clonal expansion following antigenic stimulation. IL-1 acts synergistically with other cytokines in promoting B-cell proliferation and differentiation. These include, IL-2, IL-4, IL-5, and IFN-γ (114,134,135).

3. Clinical Applications

Pharmacological doses of recombinant IL-1 have been used in clinical trials as a bone marrow protective agent in an attempt to reduce the toxicity of high-dose chemotherapy (136). Clinical trials are under way in chemoprotection during cancer chemotherapy. IL-1 plays an important role in wound healing and acts as a mitogen for fibroblasts resulting in collagen production (112,123,137). This suggests that recombinant IL-1 may be beneficial in wound healing, with IL-1 antagonists having a possible role in the prevention of keloid formation.

Table 7 Comparison of Biological Activities of Interleukin-1 (IL-1) and Tumor Necrosis Factor (TNF) (adapted from 97,125)

	IL-1	TNF
Activation of T cells	+	±
Cytotoxicity	±	+
Activation of neutrophils	+	+
Activation of macrophages	+	+
Induction of B-cell growth factors	+	−
Activation of eosinophils for parasite killing	−	+
Increased adhesion of leukocytes or tumor cells to endothelium	+	+
Induction of procoagulant activity on endothelial cells	+	+
Mitogenic action of fibroblasts	+	+
Induction of IL-1 synthesis	+	+
Induction of TNF synthesis	+	+
Induction of GM-CSF	+	+
Induction of EGF-receptor	NK	+
Inhibition of IFN-β-2	+	+
Induction of synovial collagenase and PGE-2 synthesis	+	+
Induction of hypothalamic PGE-2	+	+
Induction of pyrexia, slow-wave sleep, and anorexia	+	+
Inhibition of lipoprotein lipase	+	+
Induction of acute phase proteins	+	+
Inhibition of lipoprotein lipase	+	+
Decreased hepatic albumin synthesis	+	+

Key: NK - not known.

B. Interleukin-2

1. Chemistry

Interleukin-2 (T-cell growth factor) is a pleiotropic protein that exerts its action on a variety of cells in the immune system (138–144). As with all cytokines IL-2 binds to specific receptors. The IL-2 receptor may exist as a low-affinity, intermediate-affinity, or high-affinity receptor. The low-affinity receptor is an α chain (MW = 55 kD, or p55 subunit). The intermediate-affinity receptor is a combination of a β chain (MW = 75 kD, or p75) and a γ chain (MW = 64 kD, or p64) (145). The high-affinity receptor is a combination of the low- and intermediate-affinity receptors. Cells that express the α chain (p55 chain) on their cell surface are designated Tac$^+$ cells and are recognized by the CD25 (anti-TAC) monoclonal antibody. Activated T and B cells express high-affinity receptors for IL-2. The β chain (p75 subunit) is expressed on large granular lymphocytes and mediates the induction of LAK (lymphokine-activated killer) cell activity (146–148). During signal transduction IL-2 first associates with the α chain (low-affinity receptor, p55 chain). The subsequent internalization of IL-2 and the signal to induce cellular proliferation are correlated with IL-2 binding to the β chain (p75 chain) (149,150).

2. Mechanism of Action

IL-2 can stimulate T-helper, cytotoxic, suppressor cell activity, macrophages, natural killer cells, and B cells (151). IL-2 can also induce the production of other cytokines such as interferons, other interleukins, and tumor necrosis factors (145,152).

T cells are activated by binding specific antigens to the cell surface in the presence of IL-1 or IL-6 (145). Activated T cells produce IL-2 and simultaneously upregulate high-affinity IL-2 receptors (97,153). In vitro it has been found that upon removal of the antigen, the T-cell surface receptors for IL-2 become down-regulated (97). IL-2 can augment natural killer cell activity in vitro with enhanced tumoricidal activity in vivo (97). In 1980 Rosenberg and colleagues described the characteristics of LAK cells (140,154). LAK cells are often non-T, non-B, "null" lymphocytes. The LAK cells were able to lyse most fresh, noncultured cells in animal and human systems as well as NK-resistant tumor cells (140). No antigenic stimulus was required and there was no MHC restriction (145). Later it was demonstrated in animal models that tumors responded best when treated with a combination of IL-2 and LAK (140,155).

More recently attention has turned to adoptive immunotherapy with tumor-infiltrating lymphocytes (TILs). Biopsy specimens of the original tumor mass, such as a melanoma, provide material from which the TILs can be grown. Suspensions of the original tumor are cultured with IL-2. There is an expansion of TILs with destruction of the tumor cells (145). The TIL cells demonstrate increased specific activity in lysing autologous tumor cells, with less IL-2 being required compared to LAK activity. Some comparisons between LAK and TIL immunotherapy are given in Table 8 (145,156,157).

3. Clinical Indications

IL-2 is approved for the treatment of metastatic renal cell carcinoma in adults; however, it is being used in a variety of solid tumors including metastatic melanoma, Kaposi's sarcoma, colorectal carcinoma, and non-Hodgkin's lymphoma.

Rosenberg and colleagues have reported on their experience in treating 652 patients with high-dose recombinant IL-2 (158). The majority had metastatic cancer where standard therapy had failed or the carcinoma had no standard effective therapy. The patients received either recombinant IL-2 alone or in combination with other therapies. When recombinant IL-2 was given as monother-

Table 8 Comparison Between Lymphokine Activated Killer (LAK) Cells and Tumor Infiltrating Lymphocytes (TIL) (145,156,157)

	LAK	TIL
History	Used prior to TIL therapy	
IL-2 requirement for activity		Amount of IL-2 required for TIL activity less compared to LAK
Cell origin	Blood	Autologous tumor site
Phenotype	CD3 phenotype	Generally CD3 phenotype
Composition	Some T cells, natural killer cells; no significant diversity	T cells, B cells, natural killer cells; composition varies depending on the autologous tumor
Processing	Plasmapheresis	Requires original tumor which is more difficult to obtain and culture
Effectiveness		TIL considered more effective than LAK therapy
MHC-dependent activity	Not MHC restricted	May show specific MHC-restricted killing

apy it was administered intravenously in bolus doses every 8 h (144,158). In most cases the dose was 100,000 U/kg given for 5 d. This was followed by a 7–10 d rest period and treatment for a subsequent 5 d. In the protocol for IL-2 plus LAK cells, IL-2 was administered for up to 5 d followed by 4–5 d of leukapheresis to obtain peripheral lymphocytes (158–161). The LAK cells were generated in culture and then reinfused along with concomitant administration of IL-2 during the second treatment cycle, as in the protocol with IL-2 alone.

The results of immunotherapy as of March 1989 revealed that in 130 evaluable patients with advanced cancer treated with IL-2 alone, there was complete response in 4 patients and a partial response in 18 patients (17% complete or partial response rate) (158). In comparison, there were 177 evaluable patients treated with IL-2 plus LAK therapy, with complete response in 14 patients and a partial response in 30 patients (25% complete or partial response rate). There were 42 evaluable patients with melanoma treated with IL-2 alone. In these there was no patient who experienced a complete response. There were 10 partial responses (24% response rate). There were 48 evaluable melanoma patients treated with IL-2 plus LAK. In these there were 4 complete and 6 partial responses (complete and partial response rate of 21%). Rosenberg and his group have also reported on a prospective randomized trial of 181 patients who were randomized to receive either IL-2 alone or a combination of IL-2 plus LAK cell therapy

(158). The overall response rate was similar in the two groups, although the incidence of complete responses was greater in the group of patients receiving IL-2 plus LAK therapy ($p = 0.04$).

Adoptive immunotherapy using TIL (Table 8) for patients with advanced cancer has also been tried. The in vitro activity to TIL suggests that some patients with cancer are able to exhibit an immune response to their malignancy. In murine models adoptive transfer of TIL was found to be 50–100 times more potent than therapy with LAK in mediating regression of established cancer in several murine tumor models (162–165).

In therapy with TIL the lymphocytes are extracted from freshly resected melanomas and then expanded in vitro. These can mediate specific lysis of autologous tumor cells but not of autologous normal cells or allogenic tumor (162). Prior to therapy with TIL, the tumor bearing host was pretreated with cyclophosphamide 25 mg/kg. Thirty-six hours later the TIL were administered intravenously. Patients received a total of one to seven infusions of TIL over 1 or 2 d. Following the first infusion of TIL, patients received recombinant IL-2 (100,000 units/kg given intravenously every 8 hr) (162). The IL-2 was administered until there was dose-limiting toxicity. The median IL-2 treatment time was 5 d (25th percentile, 4 d; and 75th percentile, 6 d), compared to 15 d required for a course of treatment with LAK cells plus IL-2 (162). In the 20 patients with metastatic melanoma treated in this manner, objective regression of cancer occurred in 9 of 15 patients (60%) who had not been previously treated with IL-2 and in 2 of 5 patients (40%) in whom previous IL-2 therapy had failed. Although this treatment can produce higher response rates, sufficiently long follow-up has not been performed to determine whether survival is affected (162).

The value of constant infusion of recombinant IL-2 in adoptive immunotherapy has been confirmed, with increased safety and comfort of patients (166,167). Furthermore, with bolus administration of recombinant IL-2 the greater fluctuation in serum levels, with transiently high values compared to that seen following constant infusion, is more likely to result in toxic side effects.

In other immunotherapies IL-2 has been combined with tumor necrosis factor (TNF) or IFN-α (158,168–170). Studies are ongoing using antitumor therapy with other lymphokines either as monotherapy or as combination therapy.

4. Adverse Reactions

Adverse reactions with IL-2 therapy are frequent, and can be serious and sometimes fatal (Table 9) (171–188). The frequency and severity of adverse reactions appears to be related to the dose and/or schedule of administration (145,171,172,174,175). When IL-2 is combined with LAK therapy, most of the side effects are related to IL-2. Infusion of LAK cells alone is generally associated with few side effects, such as transient fever and chills (154,189–191). Although

Table 9 Adverse Reactions with Recombinant Interleukin (IL-2R) Therapy (171–188)

General symptoms

more common: fever/chills, pain (abomdinal, chest, back), fatigue/weakness/malaise, edema

less common: infection, weight gain (> 10%), headache, weight loss (> 10%), conjunctivitis, nasal congestion injection site reactions, allergic reactions

Cardiovascular complications

more common: hypotension requiring pressors, sinus tachycardia, arrhythmias (atrial, supraventricular, junctional, ventricular)

less common; bradycardia, premature ventricular/atrial contractions, myocardial ischemia, myocardial infarction, angina, congestive heart failure, myocarditis/endocarditis, stroke, gangrene, pericardial effusion, thrombosis

Pulmonary complications

more common: dyspnea at rest, pulmonary congestion, pulmonary edema

less common: respiratory failure, tachypnea, pleural effusion, wheezing, apnea, pneumothorax, hemoptysis

Gastrointestinal symptoms

more common: nausea, vomiting, diarrhea, stomatitis, anorexia

less common: gastrointestinal bleeding requiring surgery, jaundice, dyspepsia, constipation, intestinal perforation/ileus, pancreatitis, ascites, hepatomegaly

Neuropsychiatric complications

more common: mental status or behavioral changes (for example, confusion, disorientation, somnolence), cognitive impairment, dizziness, sensory dysfunction

less common: special sensory disorders (vision, speech, taste), syncope, motor dysfunction, coma, seizure, severe depression, malignant hyperthermia

Renal complications

more common: oliguria/anuria, proteinuria, elevated creatinine (> 5–10 fold-limit of normal)

less common: hematuria, dysuria, urinary retention, urinary frequency, allergic interstitial nephritis

Hematological abnormalities

more common: anemia, thrombocytopenia <50,000/μL, eosinophilia > 2000/μL, anemia requiring blood transfusion, leucopenia, coagulation disorders

less common: leucocytosis

Dermatological findings

more common: pruritus, erythema, erythroderma, dry skin, exfoliative dermatitis, edema

less common: purpura/petechiae, urticaria, angioedema, alopecia, edema, delayed reaction to intravenous control media, bullous drug eruption, induction or exacerbation of cutaneous condition (psoriasis, pemphigus vulgaris, linear IgA disease), erythema nodosum

Table 9 Continued

Musculoskeletal complications
less common: arthralgias, myalgias, arthritis (acute arthritis de novo or exacerbation of pre-existing disease), muscle spasm
Laboratory findings
more common: hematologic—anemia, thrombocytopenia < 50,000/μL, eosinophilia > 2000/μl; renal—elevated creatinine, elevated BUN; hepatic—bilirubin↑, transaminase↑, alkaline phosphatase↑; electrolytes—hypomagnesemia, hypocalcemia, hypophosphatemia, acidosis
less common: hypokalemia, hyperuricemia, hypoalbuminemia, hypoproteinemia, hyponatremia, hyperkalemia, alkalosis, hypoglycaemia, hyperglycemia, hypocholesterolemia, hypercalcemia, hypernatremia, hyperphosphatemia
Endocrine complications
less common: thyroid dysfunction (hyperthyroidism or hypothyroidism), adrenal hemorrhage

IL-2 may directly cause some of the side-effects, it is also possible that IL-2 stimulates T helper cells to secrete cytokines, for example, IFN-γ that may be responsible for some of the side effects (154,192). Upon discontinuation of IL-2 therapy, the side effects are generally, but not always, reversible within a few days. Generalized symptoms such as fever, myalgia, and fatigue occur in the vast majority (> 85%) of patients following IL-2 administration (Table 9). These are usually mild and may occur within a few hours of IL-2.

The most frequent and adverse effect of IL-2 is probably the result of the capillary or vascular leak syndrome, characterized by damage to endothelial cells. This results in extravasation of plasma proteins and fluid from capillaries into the extravascular space (145,172). This syndrome is not unique to IL-2 and has been reported with GM-CSF administration (193). The clinical manifestations of this syndrome include hypotension, generalized nonpitting edema, and weight gain. Other cardiopulmonary complications include dyspnea, respiratory distress, and pulmonary congestion with interstitial infiltrates on chest x-ray. The reduced central arterial pressure may decrease renal perfusion resulting in oliguria, elevated serum BUN, and creatinine (145,172). Cardiovascular complications such as myocardial toxicity, arrhythmias, and cardiomyopathy may also be a consequence of the capillary leak syndrome. The pathogenesis of this syndrome is not certain. Activated T cells produce tumor necrosis factor, which can induce neutrophil activation and perhaps initiate the capillary leak syndrome (145). IL-2 activates T cells which may bind and activate complement (194,195). Complement products are known to potentially increase vascular permeability. Furthermore, IL-2 may suppress secretion of endothelin-1 by endothelial cells, which may have an effect on their permeability and function (196).

The spectrum of dermatological side effects is shown in Table 9. In the majority of patients receiving high-dose IL-2, and in many on intermediate doses of IL-2, an eruption characterized by macular erythema, burning, and cutaneous pruritus will develop 2–3 day after IL-2 infusion (197). In patients without preexisting skin disease the eruption will usually begin on the face and neck. In subjects receiving IL-2 plus LAK a more rapid onset may occur. Within 48–72 h of discontinuing IL-2 the eruption usually resolves, often with desquamation. The eruption is dose dependent in most instances (198).

Infrequently reported cutaneous side effects include exacerbation of preexisting psoriasis, angioneurotic edema and urticaria, erythema nodosum, and life-threatening bullous skin lesions (145,199–202). Recombinant IL-2 may induce a recurrence of pemphigus vulgaris. Since IL-2 stimulates the immune system it should be used cautiously in patients with a history of autoimmune disease (188). When IL-2 is administered subcutaneously transient inflammation at the injection site may occur (203). Nodular lesions similar to subcutaneous lipomas have developed at the injection sites and resolved over the following 6 mo.

C. Interleukin-6

Interleukin-6 (IL-6) is a multifunction protein for use by lymphoid and non-lymphoid cells, as well as by normal and transformed cells. The IL-6 precursor protein is 212 amino acids with two potential N-glycosylation sites. The hydrophobic N-terminal 28 amino acid signal peptide is cleaved to produce a mature protein of 184 amino acids with the molecular weight of 21 kD (204–206). Interleukin-6 exerts its activity by binding to a high-affinity receptor complex consisting of two membrane glycoproteins—an 80 kD IL-6 binding receptor protein (IL-6R) and a signal-transducing protein, gp130 (207–209).

IL-6 is a proinflammatory cytokine produced by a variety of cells including keratinocytes. Both primary cytokines IL-1 and TNF-α can induce the expression of IL-6 in keratinocytes (210,211). IL-6 plays a role in the acute phase response as it can up-regulate the production of acute phase proteins and inhibit the secretion of albumin in the acute phase response (212). Increased expression of IL-6 has been demonstrated in contact dermatitis at the patch test site (213). An increase in IL-6 plasma levels in mice following elicitation of allergic contact dermatitis was observed (214). It has been documented that IL-6 can directly and indirectly stimulate T-cell proliferation (215,216). In addition, IL-6 induces B-cell differentiation, immunoglobulin production, and the proliferation of some transformed B-cell lines (217). In psoriatic skin, monocytes and serum IL-6 expression have been shown to be up-regulated (218–220). In contrast, in normal skin, in situ hybridization did not detect IL-6 and its receptor message. However, the message is expressed in perilesional uninvolved skin, in the transitional zone, and in the psoriatic lesion (221). Recently, transgenic mice, which overexpress

IL-6 in the skin, have been employed to get a better picture of the role of IL-6 in psoriasis. This study showed that IL-6 overexpression did not enhance epidermal proliferation or leukocyte infiltration, but did induce a thicker stratum corneum (222).

D. Interleukin-8

Interleukin-8 (IL-8) (Table 6) belongs to the supergene family of proinflammatory and chemotactic cytokines recently renamed chemokines. IL-8 is a potent neutrophil chemotactic and activating factor. The precursor protein consists of 99 amino acids with the putative signal peptide being cleaved to generate the nonglycosylated mature protein of 8 kD. At least four N-terminal variants of IL-8 containing 69, 72, 77, and 79 amino acids have been described (223–225). Both the 72 amino acid (monocyte or leukocyte) form and the 77 amino acid (endothelial) form have similar biological activities (226). IL-8 exerts its biological activity by binding to specific cell surface receptors. There are two distinct but homologous human IL-8 receptors (type 1 or α and type 2 or β). The two receptors share 77% amino acid sequence identity and both are members of the superfamily of G protein-coupled receptors (227–230).

The primary source of IL-8 is monocytes, but a number of other cell types can also produce this chemokine (231–233). Primary cytokines IL-1 and TNF-α have been shown to induce the expression of IL-8 in keratinocytes (233). This cytokine was initially investigated for its chemotactic effect on neutrophils. But now it has also been shown to be a potent T-cell chemotactic. In the presence of monocyte chemotactic activating factor (MCAF), IL-8 can effectively recruit monocytes to the site of inflammation (234,235). Increased levels of IL-8 were detected in "neutrophilic dermatoses" such as psoriasis and palmoplantar pustulosis (236,237). Another study confirmed the up-regulation of IL-8 in psoriatic epidermis and scales (1). And yet another study demonstrated that the neutrophilic chemotactic activity in suction blister fluids of psoriatic skin did not correlate well with that of IL-8 activity (238).

E. Interleukin-10

Interleukin-10 (IL-10) is a multifunctional molecule that is made by a number of cells including macrophages, B lymphocytes, mast cells, and keratinocytes (239–243). IL-10 was originally described as a Th2 cell-derived cytokine with the ability to inhibit Th1 cell function by down-regulating IFN-γ, IL-2, and the production of other cytokines (244–246). These Th1 cells are involved in successful induction of the delayed type of hypersensitivity response (247). IL-10 has been shown to down-regulate class II MHC expression on monocytes and thus antigen-specific T-cell proliferation (248). It has also been demonstrated that IL-

10 inhibits the expression of the costimulator B7 on murine macrophages which is vital for T-cell activation (241,249). IL-10 can also inhibit the antigen-presenting function of Langerhans cells (250). In an *in vivo* study, IL-10 was shown to inhibit the effector phase of contact hypersensitivity (251). In a recent study, IL-10 was implicated in playing an important role in the "natural regulation" of contact hypersensitivity *in vivo* (252).

IV. HEMATOPOIETIC GROWTH FACTORS

The hematopoietic growth factors include erythropoietin, granulocyte-macrophage colony-stimulating factor (GM-CSF), granulocyte colony-stimulating factor (G-CSF), macrophage colony-stimulating factor (M-CSF), and interleukin-3 (IL-3). In 1906 Carnot and Deflandre were able to induce erythrocytosis in normal rabbits by infusing them with plasma from anemic animals (253,254). It thus became recognized that circulating factors may regulate red cell production. Subsequently culture systems capable of growing bone marrow progenitor cells *in vitro* were developed (255,256). These factors were originally termed CSFs since they stimulated the production of cell colonies from individual bone marrow progenitors. In the cascade of cell differentiation from the multipotent progenitor to the circulating mature cell there is an interaction with hematopoietic growth factors at various levels. The hematopoietic growth factors regulate the proliferation and differentiation of hematopoietic progenitor cells and enhance the functioning and survival of mature blood cells (253). The hematopoietic growth factors may be divided into two groups: those that stimulate the proliferation and differentiation of pluripotent stem cells and progenitor cells (GM-CSF, IL-3, IL-6), and those that stimulate the development of mature progenitor cells to specific cell lineages (G-CSF, M-CSF, and erythropoietin) (257).

A. Chemistry

Human GM-CSF has an effect mainly, but not exclusively, on myeloid cells (258–261). The precursor protein for GM-CSF is 144 amino acids long (262). The mature protein is 127 amino acids with 17 amino acids being cleaved from the NH_2 terminal. The human gene is composed of four exons with three intervening sequences (263). Each growth factor is coded for by a single gene (264–268). The genes for GM-CSF, M-CSF, and IL-3 are located on the long arm of chromosome 5 (269–271). In contrast the gene for G-CSF is found on chromosome 17 (272). The GM-CSF and G-CSF glycoproteins that are produced exhibit different amounts of glycosylation; however, it appears that glycosylation is not a requirement for *in vitro* or *in vivo* activity (273). On the other hand, the extent of glycosylation may determine the antigenicity of the protein (274,275).

B. Mechanism of Action

Hematopoietic growth factors can provide intercellular communication signals that can activate or prime effector cells such as neutrophils and macrophages. Furthermore, the effect on eosinophils may be to enhance their effectiveness as cytotoxic cells (276). The direct effects of CSFs include membrane changes, modulation of receptor expression, and inhibition of migration. Their indirect effects can be regarded as "priming" effects requiring the presence of an additional stimulus. This includes enhanced chemotaxis, phagocytosis, oxidative metabolism, enhanced cytotoxicity, arachidonic acid release, leukotriene B_4 synthesis, and potentiation of antigen processing (276). The hematopoietic growth factors GM-CSF and G-CSF are critical to the normal development of granulocytes (277). These factors play an important role in the regeneration of bone marrow and replacement of leukocytes. The effects of GM-CSF on mature granulocytes and monocytes include promoting adherence of neutrophils to blood vessels *in vivo,* potentiation of superoxide production, and enhancing the uptake and killing of parasitic organisms by neutrophils (278–280). Furthermore, macrophages are stimulated to destroy tumor cells and intracellular parasites. GM-CSF is able to induce maturation of Langerhans cells and enhance antigen presenting cell function activity (281,282). The effects of the hematopoietic growth factors are mediated by factors binding to receptors on the surface of target cells (283,284).

C. Pharmacokinetics of GM-CSF

Following intravenous boluses of nonglycosylated GM-CSF (0.3–3 μg/kg) the terminal-phase elimination half-life was 0.2–1.2 h (275,285). When the boluses were administered intravenously over 20–30 min at the higher dose of 3–30 μg/kg the half-life was 0.6–9.1 h (285). Following bolus doses the distribution half-life was 5 min (275). Following both intravenous infusion and subcutaneous injection the peak level was dose related.

D. Pharmacokinetics of G-CSF

When nonglycosylated G-CSF 3–60 μg/kg was administered intravenously over 20–30 min the terminal-phase elimination half-life was 1.3–7.2 h (275). The peak levels were dose related and were as high as 600 ng/ml.

E. Clinical Indications

The growth factors GM-CSF and G-CSF have been used in various clinical stimulations where there is some degree of hematopoietic failure (253,277). Hematopoietic growth factors such as GM-CSF and G-CSF may allow the physician to counteract the myelotoxic effects of chemotherapy. There have been phase I and II clinical trials looking at the efficacy of GM-CSF and G-CSF in the treatment of various conditions including a) bladder cancer: G-CSF, b) small cell lung cancer: G-CSF, c) some advanced neoplasms: G-CSF, d) Hodgkin's lymphoma with autologous bone marrow transplantation: G-CSF, e) inoperable metastatic cancers: GM-CSF, f) lymphoid leukemia and Hodgkin's and non-Hodgkin's lymphoma: GM-CSF, and g) breast cancer and melanoma with autologous bone marrow transplantation: GM-CSF (277). The administration of these growth factors can act as myelostimulating agents, enhancing myeloid recovery and reducing the duration and degree of neutropenia induced by chemotherapy. The accelerated recovery of leukocytes (granulocytes and monocytes) following drug-induced myelosuppression can also help reduce the frequency of infection and duration of hospitalization in many cases (277).

Phase I and II clinical trials have also been carried out looking at the efficacy of GM-CSF and G-CSF in the treatment of myelodysplastic disorders such as preleukemia and refractory acute nonlymphoblastic leukemia (277). The growth factor G-CSF may help induce differentiation of leukemic cells. Although GM-CSF enhanced recovery of granulocytes, monocytes, and reticulocyte, many patients also had elevated blast counts (277). Thus GM-CSF may need to be combined with cytotoxic or differentiation-inducing drugs. The rationale is that the GM-CSF would activate resting leukemic cells into a phase so that they could be destroyed by cycle-specific chemotherapy (273).

Both GM-CSF and G-CSF has been used to treat congenital and idiopathic neutropenias (277). In cyclic and idiopathic neutropenias G-CSF may help induce normal neutrophil and monocyte counts. The cycling seen in cyclic neutropenia may be terminated or the periodicity of cycling lengthened. Therapy with G-CSF may also help reduce the frequency and severity of recurrent infections, ulcers, mucositis, and periodontal disease seen in these patients.

In some patients with mild to moderate aplastic anemia GM-CSF has produced temporary improvement in granulopoiesis. The poor response of GM-CSF and G-CSF in some cases may be explained by the lack of effect of these growth factors at the level of early pluripotential stem cell differentiation, which is where the defect might lie in aplastic anemia (277).

In AIDS the main objective of administering GM-CSF is to stimulate hematopoiesis. When intravenous GM-CSF is administered to leukopenic patients with AIDS there is a dose-dependent increase in neutrophils and eosinophils with a slight elevation in the monocyte count (286). Following discontinuation of therapy the counts returned to pretherapy values (253). The efficacy of GM-CSF therapy may be increased if it is given concurrently with retroviral agents such as zidovudine (287,288).

F. Adverse Effects of GM-CSF

As is seen with G-CSF, administration of GM-CSF also causes an elevation of neutrophil counts, although not to the same extent. With GM-CSF the circulating neutrophil half-life is prolonged; in G-CSF therapy the half-life of neutrophils is not altered (275). Unlike G-CSF, GM-CSF increases the production rate of eosinophils and the proportion of eosinophil precursors. Therapy with GM-CSF is able to increase the number of progenitor cells of all lineages in the peripheral blood. This occurs to a greater extent at the higher doses of GM-CSF; unfortunately, at such doses the side effects may be dose limiting. However, initially upon administration of GM-CSF there is a transient leukopenia resulting from the disappearance of circulating neutrophils, eosinophils, and monocytes (275,289). Furthermore, neutrophils may also undergo pulmonary sequestration (290).

GM-CSF given at doses of 0.3–10 μg/kg/d may result in anorexia, weight change, lethargy, flushing, myalgia, bone pain, and cutaneous lesions (275,289,291). These include raised, elevated lesions at sites of subcutaneous injections (291). However, the side effects are generally well tolerated. Following the first dose of GM-CSF, particularly when given intravenously rather than by the subcutaneous route, and at a dose of ≥1 μg/kg, a reaction consisting of transient flushing, nausea, vomiting, tachycardia, hypotension, musculoskeletal pain, and dyspnea may be observed (275,290). When GM-CSF is given at doses ≥3 μg/kg fevers and chills may occur (292). At even higher doses (≥20 μg/kg/d) the side effects may in fact be dose limiting, and include weight gain with fluid retention, pleuritis, pericarditis, effusions, and venous thrombosis (275,284,289,291). This may be the manifestation of a capillary-leak syndrome. Some of the side effects could be explained by GM-CSF-induced cytokine production (275). These include TNF and IL-1 (293).

Localized cutaneous adverse effects seen with GM-CSF therapy include reactions at the injection site such as phlebitis, irritation (294,295), a pustular eruption (296), erythematous plaques and purpuric lesions (297). Facial flushing may also occur (276). Mehregan et al. have reviewed cutaneous reactions in 26 patients who received GM-CSF as part of a chemotherapeutic protocol (298). In 14 of these patients an immediate localized angioedematous reaction was observed at the site of the subcutaneous GM-CSF injection. In 21 patients there was a generalized cutaneous reaction. Horn et al. have reported confluent erythematous macules and papules developing within 1–2 d of administration of recombinant GM-CSF (259). At the conclusion of therapy desquamation of skin was observed. In the upper dermis the inflammatory infiltrate consisted of neutrophils and mononuclear cells with an increase in the number and size of macrophages. The differential diagnosis of the eruption would include hypersensitivity to other concomitant medications, cutaneous eruption due to infectious causes, and the eruption of lymphocyte recovery (259,299).

Treatment with hematopoietic growth factors such as GM-CSF may worsen a preexisting inflammatory condition or vasculitis, particularly where eosinophils play an important role in the etiology (300–302). Bullous pyoderma gangrenosum has been reported to develop at the site of previous eczema; the pyoderma gangrenosum subsided when the GM-CSF was discontinued (300). In a patient with myelodysplasia GM-CSF therapy led to the flare-up of preexisting psoriasis (294,303). Rarely, the development or worsening of leukocytoclastic vasculitis has been reported in association with GM-CSF (304–308). In another patient recurrent painful pustular lesions on the face, arms, and upper trunk developed with 24 h of a GM-CSF injection and would last 1–2 wk. A positive rechallenge to GM-CSF was elicited on several occasions (304). Treatment with GM-CSF is often accompanied by an eosinophilia (275). In a case of epidermolysis bullosa acquisita induced by GM-CSF the eosinophils may have mediated blister formation (309).

In certain situations GM-CSF should either be given cautiously or even withheld. GM-CSF may reactivate idiopathic thrombocytopenic purpura and should perhaps not be given to such patients (291). Furthermore, GM-CSF and G-CSF should be considered cautiously in patients who have a history of chronic inflammatory or autoimmune disease, since these conditions (for example, rheumatoid arthritis, thyroiditis, and hemolysis) may become reactivated (294,310–314).

G. Adverse Effects of G-CSF

G-CSF has been given intravenously and subcutaneously in both normal subjects and those with cancer (275,315–317). Generally the G-CSF is well tolerated (253). When G-CSF is given there is an initial transient decrease in leukocyte counts. The trough in leukocyte counts occurs 30–60 min after subcutaneous injection and at 5–15 min when given by the intravenous route (275). The initial fall in the circulating neutrophil and monocyte count is later followed by a dose-dependent increase in circulating neutrophils (317). The neutrophilia is a left shift toward more immature cell types such as myelocytes and promyelocytes. At higher G-CSF doses ($\geq$10 μg/kg/d) an elevation in lymphocyte and monocyte levels is also seen. Furthermore, G-CSF (10–60 μg/kg/d) given over 10 d may result in a decrease in the platelet count of up to 25% (317). Neutrophil counts fall to pretherapy levels within 4–7 d of stopping therapy. Other laboratory abnormalities that have been reported include elevated leukocyte alkaline phosphatase levels and an increase in lactate dehydrogenase (286,318–320).

The most frequently reported symptom is bone pain (316,321). It may occur in 20% of cases (275,322). Usually the pain is dull and transient; it is controlled in most instances with analgesics. Localized cutaneous adverse reactions include the development of erythematous plaques, vesicles, and papules at injection sites (323). It is also possible that recombinant G-CSF may induce an inflammatory process de novo, particularly one where neutrophils play an important role. The development of Sweet's syndrome in a patient following G-CSF therapy may possibly be due to increased production of, or an enhanced sensitivity to, G-CSF (294). Rarely reported side effects of G-CSF include development of vasculitis (263,322), bullous pyoderma gangrenosum (323), folliculitis (304), and an anaphylactoid reaction (incidence $< 0.01\%$) (324,325). Recombinant G-CSF therapy may also exacerbate preexisting cutaneous conditions such as leukocytoclastic vasculitis (307) and psoriasis (303).

V. GROWTH FACTORS

The term *growth factors* is used to denote a group of low molecular weight, locally acting peptides that have the ability to affect cellular differentiation and/or proliferation. Growth factors are also characterized by their specific high-affinity cell surface receptors (326). They were originally distinguished from the "cytokine" group of peptides by their lesser immunoregulatory effects. Recent evidence reveals overlapping functions between the so-called growth factors and cytokines, leading to the realization that these two groups of peptides are less distinct than originally thought. While their names reflect the biological activities initially described, their functional spectrum continues to expand as a result of ongoing research. Each growth factor actually represents a family of related peptides with homologous amino acid sequences with similar, but sometimes distinct, functions (326).

A. Growth Factors in Wound Healing

The release of platelet derived growth factor (PDGF) and transforming growth factor-β (TGF-β) from platelets is an important initial process in acute wounds. These are among the most significant factors in the chemoattraction of neutrophils and macrophages. Neutrophils produce PDGF-like peptides and other growth factors that allow further chemoattraction of cells, debridement, and matrix accumulation. Macrophages are seen later, at about 48 h, and release TGF-β, TNF-α, IL-1, PDGF-like peptides, and other growth factors. These are involved in all aspects of wound repair such as fibroblast proliferation, angiogenesis, and matrix production. Reepithelialization is a consequence of the action of chemotactic factors such as epidermal growth factor (EGF), TGF-α, and fibroblast growth factor (FGF) on keratinocytes (327).

Several clinical studies have examined the clinical efficacy of topical growth factors in both acute and chronic wounds. Brown et al. studied rates of reepithelization at skin graft donor sites with silver sulfadiazine cream, as compared to silver sulfadiazine cream containing EGF (10 mg/ml) (328). Treatment with EGF significantly decreased the average length of time of healing. Robson et al. reported that topical recombinant PDGF-BB at 100 μg/ml resulted in a statistically significant healing response when compared to a placebo for chronic pressure ulcers (329). Knighton et al. studied healing in chronic leg ulcers using a platelet-derived wound healing formula (PDWHF) (330). This topical agent is known to contain at least five locally acting growth factors: platelet-derived growth factor (PDGF); platelet-derived angiogenesis factors (PDAF); platelet-derived epidermal growth factor (PDEGF); transforming growth factor-β (TGF-β); and platelet factor 4 (PF4). In the treatment group 81% had reepithelialization after 8 wk, as compared to only 15% in the control group. After crossover to treatment with PDWHF all of the patients in the control group achieved reepithelization in an average of 7.1 wk. This study suggested that various combinations of growth factor peptides may be more effective than monotherapy with single agents.

B. Growth Factors in Pathological Disease

It is believed the TGF-β and PDGF are involved in keloid formation. TGF-β increases collagen formation when injected in vivo (331). In experimental studies on animal wounds the use of TFG-β antibodies decreases scar formation (332). It has been hypothesized that decorin, a proteoglycan that binds TFG-β, or the injection of soluble TGF-β receptors to competitively inhibit the active molecule, may decrease scar or keloid formation (327). Alternatively, topical application of PDGF (333), TGF-β in a slow-release vehicle (334), and basic FGF injections (335) all have been shown to increase wound tensile strength, which may be useful under some clinical circumstances.

The role of growth factors has also been studied in hyperproliferation diseases such as psoriasis and cutaneous neoplasms. Fibroblasts in affected psoriasis skin are more responsive to PDGF stimulation (336). There is increased EGF binding (337) and TFG-α expression (338) in psoriasis keratinocytes. Squamous cell carcinomas show an increased number of EGF receptors, and TFG-α may be important (339) in the pathogenesis of keratoacanthomas, and possibly squamous cell carcinomas (340).

Although more studies are needed to confirm the clinical usefulness of topical growth factors in wound healing or the reduction of keloid formation, this approach appears promising. Future studies should focus on demonstrated important variables, such as mode of application, optimization of vehicles, and dosages. As well, the use of various combinations of peptides may be found to be more effective than single agents alone. Understanding the role of growth factors in the various hyperproliferative diseases may lead to alternative treatment options in the future.

VI. TUMOR NECROSIS FACTORS

A. History

TNF-α (cachectin) and TNF-β (lymphotoxin) are cytokines with pleiotropic actions. TNF-α and TNF-β function by binding to TNF receptors (55 and 75 kb) expressed on cells in a variety of tissues. William Coley, in the 19th century was the first to examine the role of TNF-α in infectious disease, and other potential therapeutic uses such as inducing hemorrhagic necrosis of tumors (341–344). Once human TNF-α protein was isolated then molecular cloning (cDNA) and cloning of TNF locus followed shortly thereafter (345–348). This was an exciting period in history, and TNF was believed to be a powerful weapon in combating cancer. In contrast, lymphotoxin/TNF-β was discovered independently and was believed to play a role in delayed-type hypersensitivity response (349–351). TNF-α and TNF-β share common features including similar amino acid identity and their high affinity to bind to the same TNF receptors (352–355).

B. Chemistry

Human TNF-α and TNF-β are functionally related with similar primary structures. TNF-α is synthesized as a 25 kD precursor protein and cleaved to 17 kD trimer prior to secretion. This precursor protein is stored in microsomal compartments and upon stimulation (with lipopolysaccharide) is transported to the cell surface, processed, and secreted (345,346). As for TNF-β, a 20 kD and 24 kD secreted protein have been reported (356).

C. Mechanism of Action

A major cellular source of TNF is from activated mononuclear cells, followed by mast cells and also keratinocytes (357–359). TNF-α, a primary cytokine, is known for its pleiotropic effects on cells within the skin and influences the normal homeostasis. This cytokine has been implicated to play a cardinal role in the inflammatory cascade and thus in the pathogenesis of cutaneous diseases. Evidence to support this hypothesis points to the ability of TNF-α to induce its own production (autocrine) as well as induce the release of other cytokines and inflammatory mediators such as IL-1, IL-6, GM-CSF, PDGF, neutrophil chemotactic factors [IL-8, monocyte activating factor (MCAF)], and prostaglandins (360–365). Another property of TNF-α that supports its role in the cutaneous inflammatory disease process includes the up-regulation of intercellular adhesion molecule-1 (ICAM-1), vascular cell adhesion molecule-1 (VCAM-1), and endothelial leukocyte adhesion molecule-1 (ELAM-1) expression on endothelial cells (366–368). These effects may result in an increase in vascular permeability, up-regulation of dermal endothelial cell adhesion molecule expression, and induction of neutrophil chemotactic factors that influence cutaneous recruitment of inflammatory cells.

D. Role of TNF-α in Contact Dermatitis

Langerhans cell, the major antigen-presenting cell in the epidermis, is believed to play an important role in the initiation of allergic contact dermatitis (ACD) (369–372). These dendritic cells have been reported to be effective antigen presenters in the presence of the class II major histocompatibility complex (Ia) to naive T lymphocytes in the draining lymph node (373–375). TNF-α can sustain cellular integrity, maintain viability of murine Langerhans cells *in vitro,* and also stimulate the migration of Langerhans cells to the draining lymph node for antigen presentation (376,377). Piguet et al. demonstrated total abrogation of allergic and irritant contact dermatitis in animals injected with anti-TNF-α antibody prior to challenge (378). TNF-α has also been implicated to participate in UVB impaired allergic contact dermatitis (379,380). A human study employing sodium lauryl sulfate-induced contact dermatitis reported an increase in TNF-α levels in the local lymph node samples shortly after exposure (378,381). Another study with nickel sulfate did not demonstrate any significant increase in keratinocyte expression of TNF-α (213). Other investigators have shown that humans treated with poison ivy–poison oak extract experience an up-regulation of TNF-α and adhesion molecules on keratinocytes (382). These conflicting results may be explained by the unique properties of each hapten in a review that highlights TNF-α having a beneficial or deleterious effect depending on timing, target cells, and the intensity of the inflammatory reaction (383).

E. Role of TNF-α in Psoriasis

TNF-α has been implicated in the pathogenesis of psoriasis, although results are conflicting. Increased epidermal hyperproliferation and inflammation is observed in psoriasis. Psoriatic plaques display excessive keratinocyte growth and cellular infiltration consisting primarily of leukocytes. This inflammatory process may represent an early event that precedes abnormal keratinocyte proliferation and differentiation (384). Neutrophils and mononuclear cells may be the earliest cell in the psoriatic lesion (385,386). There is also evidence supporting the presence of mast cells early and in increasing numbers in the psoriatic dermis (387,388). Macrophages containing TNF-α are also present in psoriatic lesion (389). TNF-α is able to induce the release of secondary cytokines such as IL-6 and IL-8 (in keratinocytes) which are observed in psoriatic lesions (220). In addition, TNF-α is capable of up-regulating adhesion molecules in the epidermis, endothelial cells, and keratinocytes (368). This step is necessary for successful leukocyte recruitment into the site of inflammation.

In a clinical trial, several patients with severe refractory psoriasis vulgaris were treated with TNF-α for 5 d at 3 wk intervals (dose range 90–225 μ/m²/d) (391). Two patients had complete clearing and three other patients had substantial clearing. In a report by the same group they showed that two patients with severe psoriasis responded well to TNF-α systemic treatment while one patient with more localized psoriasis did not improve following TNF-α treatment (392). TNF-α levels in blister fluids, serum, and horny tissue from psoriasis patients were not elevated significantly compared to normal skin (393,394). In one study TNF-α message was not detected in epidermis or dermis of psoriatic skin (395). Yet, in another study, using *in situ* hybridization the investigators were able to demonstrate TNF-α message in normal skin (396,397). It has also recently been reported that in both normal and psoriatic skin, epidermal cells express the 55 kD TNF-α receptor and not the 75 kD receptor (397). The precise role of TNF-α in the pathogenesis of psoriasis remains unclear.

REFERENCES

1. Sauder DN. The role of epidermal cytokines in inflammatory skin diseases. J Invest Dermatol 1990; 95:27S–28S.
2. Interferon nomenclature. Nature 1980; 286:110.
3. Isaacs A, Lindenmann J. Virus interference: I. The interferon. Proc R Soc Lond 1957; 147:258–267.
4. Bocci V. The physiological interferon response. Immunol Today 1985; 6:7–9.
5. Stadler R, Mayer-da-Silva A, Bratzke B, et al. Interferons in dermatology. J Am Acad Dermat 1989; 20:650–656.
6. Stadler R, Ruszczak Z. Interferons: new additions and indications for use. Dermat Clin 1993; 11:187–199.
7. Adolf GR. Structure and effects of interferon-gamma. Oncology 1985; 42:33–40.
8. Wheelock EF. Interferon-like virus-inhibitor induced in human leukocytes by phytohemagglutinin. Science 1965; 149:310–311.
9. Gray PW, Goddel DV. Structure of the human immune interferon gene. Nature 1982; 298:859–863.
10. Higgins PJ. Interferons. J Clin Pathol 1984; 37:109–116.
11. Thomson DB. Interferon-α as cancer therapy. Med J Aust 1988; 149:290–292.
12. Strander H. Interferon treatment of human neoplasia. Adv Cancer Res 1986; 46:1–265.
13. Tovey MG. Interferon and cyclic nucleotides. Gresser Interferon 1982; 4:23–47.
14. Balwill FR. Peptide regulatory factors: interferons. Lancet 1989; :1060–1063.
15. Dani C, Mechti N, Piechaczyk M, et al. Increased rate of degradation of c-myc mRNA in interferon-treated Daudi cells. Proc Natl Acad Sci USA 1985; 82:4896–4899.
16. Friedman RL, Manly SP, McMahon M, et al. Transcriptional and postranscriptional regulation of interferon-induced gene expression in human cells. Cell Immunol 1984; 38:745–755.

17. Knop J. Immunologic effects of interferon. J Invest Dermat 1990; 95:72S–74S.
18. Barker JNWN, Allen MH, McDonald DM. The effect of in vivo interferon-gamma on the distribution of LFA-1 and ICAM-1 in normal human skin. J Invest Dermat 1989; 93:439–442.
19. Nickoloff BJ, Griffiths CEM. T-lymphocytes and monocytes bind to keratinocytes in frozen sections of biopsy specimens of normal skin treated with gamma interferon. J Am Acad Dermat 1989; 20:736–743.
20. Garbe C, Schröder K, Krasagakis K, et al. Presence of ICAM-1 on melanoma cells in vitro and enhancement of its expression by interferons. J Invest Dermat 1989; 93:550.
21. Kimchi A. Autocrine interferon and the suppression of the c-myc nuclear oncogene. Interferon 1987; 8:86–110.
22. United States Pharmacopeial Convention. Interferons. In: Drug information for the health care professional. Taunton, Mass. Rand McNally, 1994:1583–1593.
23. Drug facts and comparisons. Biologicals. St. Louis, Mo.: Facts and Comparisons, 1994:2149–2226.
24. Prussick R, Knowles S, Shear NH. Cutaneous drug reactions. Curr Probl Dermat 1994; 6:81–124.
25. Luger TA, Schwarz T. Epidermal cell derived secretory regulins. In: Schuler G, ed. Epidermal langerhans cells. Boca Raton: Fla. CRC Press, 1991:219–251.
26. Cnudde F, Gharakhanian S, Luboinski J, et al. Cutaneous local necrosis following interferon injections. Int J Dermat 1991; 30:147.
27. Detman U, Agathos M, Nerl C. Allergy of delayed type to recombinant interferon alpha-2C. Contact Dermat 1989; 20:149–150.
28. Olsen EA, Rosen ST, Vollmer RT, et al. Interferon alfa-2a in the treatment of cutaneous T cell lymphoma. J Am Acad Dermat 1989; 20:395–407.
29. Wagner RF, Sanchez RL. Presenation of sebaceous carcinoma and dermatofibrosarcoma protuberans subsequent to intralesional interferal alfa-2b for the treatment of in situ squamous cell carcinoma. Arch Dermat 1991; 127:127–272.
30. Tosti A, Misciali C, Bardazzi F, et al. Telogen effluvium due to recombinant interferon α-2b. Dermatology 1992; 184:124–125.
31. Quesado JR, Gutterman JH. Psoriasis and alpha-interferon. Lancet 1986; 2:1466.
32. Shiohara T, Abe K, Nagashima M. Psoriasis occurring predominantly on warts: possible involvment of interferons alfa. Arch Dermat 1988; 124:1816–1821.
33. Jacgla A, Marcoval J, Curco N, et al. Psoriasis with articular involvment induced by interferon alfa. Arch Dermat 1991; 127:910–911.
34. Funk J, Langeland T, Schrumpf E, et al. Psoriasis induced by interferon-α. Br J Dermat 1991; 125:463–465.
35. Morhenn VB, Pregerson-Rodan K, Mull RH, et al. Use of recombinant interferon gamma administered intramuscularly for the treatment of psoriasis. Arch Dermat 1987; 123:1633–1637.
36. Fierlbeck G, Rassner G, Müller C. Psoriasis induced at the injection site of recombinant interferon gamma. Arch Dermat 1990; 126:351–355.
37. McManus Balmer C. The new alpha interferons. DICP 1985; 19:887–893.

38. Gutterman JU, Fine S, Quesada J, et al. Recombinant leukocyte A interferon: pharmacokinetics, single-dose tolerance, and biologic effects in cancer patients. Ann Intern Med 1982; 96:549–556.
39. Muss HB, Kempf RA, Matino S, et al. A phase II study of recombinant alpha interferon in patients with recurrent or metastatic breast cancer. J Clin Oncol 1984; 2:1012–1016.
40. Wagstaff J, Chadwick G, Howell A, et al. A phase I toxicity study of human rDNA interferon in patients with solid tumors. Cancer Chemother Pharm 1984; 2:1012–1016.
41. Mora JS, Ko-Pei K, Munsat TL. Indomethacin reduces the side effects of intrathecal interferon [letter]. N Eng J Med 1984; 310:126–127.
42. Stiehm ER, Kronenberg LH, Rosenblatt HM, et al. Interferon: immunobiology and clinical significance. Ann Intern Med 1982; 96:80–93.
43. Levine M, Jones MW. Interferon and drug metabolism [letter]. Clin Pharm 1983; 2:210–211.
44. Bauman JH, Fuentes JH. Interferon and drug metabolism [letter]. Clin Pharm 1983; 2:211.
45. Parkinson A, Lasker J, Kramer MJ, et al. Effects of three recombinant human leukocyte interferons on drug metabolism in mice. Drug Metab Dispos 1982; 10:579–585.
46. Ho M. Interferon as an agent against herpes simplex virus. J Invest Dermat 1990; 95:158S–161S.
47. Ho M. Kinetic considerations of the inhibitory action of an interferon appearing in chick cell cultures infected with Sindbis virus. Virology 1962; 17:265–275.
48. Edwards L. Interferon: promises, disappointments, and tempered optimism. Arch Dermat 1987; 123:743–744.
49. Naples SP, Brodell RT. Verrucae vulgaris: treatment with natural interferon alfa using a needleless injector. Arch Dermat 1993; 129:698–700.
50. Zachariae H, Thestrup-Pedersen K. Interferon alpha and etretinate combination treatment of cutaneous T-cell lymphomas. J Invest Dermat 1990; 95:206S–209S.
51. Mahrle G, Schulze H-J. Recombinant interferon-gamma (rIFN-gamma) in dermatology. J Invest Dermat 1990; 95:132S–136S.
52. Bunn PA Jr, Ihde DC, Foon KA. Recombinant interferon alfa-2a, an active agent in advanced cutaneous T-cell lymphomas. Cancer Res 1987; 40:9–13.
53. Stadler R, Luger T. Interferon-combined therapies in cutaneous T-cell lymphoma and miscellaneous skin diseases—European experience. In: Burgdorf WHC, Katz SI, eds. Dermatology: progress & perspectives. New York: Parthenon, 1992:329–334.
54. Bunn PA, Norris DA. The therapeutic role of interferons and monoclonal antibodies in cutaneous T-cell lymphomas. J Invest Dermat 1990; 95:209S–212S.
55. Testrup-Pedersen K, Kaltoft K, et al. Treatment of mycosis fungoides with recombinant interferon-2a alone and in combination with etretinate. Br J Dermat 1988; 118:811.

56. Dréno B, Claudy A, Meynadier J, et al. The treatment of 45 patients with cutaneous T-cell lymphoma with low doses of interferon alpha 2a and etretinate. Br J Dermat 1991; 125:456–459.
57. Thestrup-Pedersen K, Hammer R, Kaltoft K, et al. Treatment of mycosis fungoides with recombinant interferon-α2a alone and in combination with etretinate. Br J Dermat 1988; 118:811–818.
58. Roegnigk HH, Kuzel TM, Skoutelis AP, et al. Photochemotherapy alone or combined with interferon alpha-2a in the treatment of cutaneous T-cell lymphoma. J Invest Dermat 1990; 95:198S–206S.
59. Greenway HT, Cornell RC, Tanner DJ, et al. Treatment of basal cell carcinoma with intralesional interferon. J Am Acad Dermat 1986; 15:437.
60. Edwards L, Tucker SB, Perednia D, et al. The effect of an intralesional sustained-release formulation of interferon alfa-2b on basal cell carcinomas. Arch Dermat 1990; 126:1029–1032.
61. Smalley RB, Borden EC. Interferons: current status and future directions of this prototypic biological. Springer Semin Immunopathol 1986; 9:73–83.
62. Pestka S. Interferon: a decade of accomplishments, foundations of the future in research and therapy. Semin Hematol 1986; 23:27–37.
63. Grob JJ, Collet AM, Munoz MH, et al. Treatment of large basal-cell carcinoma with intralesional interferon alpha 2a. Lancet 1988; 1:232.
64. Ikic D, Padovan I, Pipic N, et al. Treatment of squamous cell carcinoma with interferon. Int J Dermat 1988; 30:58.
65. Wickramasinghe L, Hindson TC, Wacks H. Treatment of neoplastic skin lesions with intralesional interferon. J Am Acad Dermat 1989; 20:71–74.
66. Lippmann SM, Parkinson DR, Iri LM, et al. 13-cis retinoic acid and interferon alpha 2a: effective combination therapy for advanced squamous cell carcinoma of the skin. J Natl Cancer Inst 1992; 84:235–341.
67. Kirkwood JM, Ernstoff MS. Role of interferons in the therapy of melanoma. J Invest Dermat 1990; 95:180S–185S.
68. Creagan ET, Ahmann DL, Green SJ, et al. Phase II study of low-dose recombinant leukocyte A interferon in disseminated malignant melanoma. J Clin Oncol 1984; 2:1002–1005.
69. Creagan ET, Ahmann DL, Green SJ, et al. Phase II study of recombinant leukocyte A interferon (rIFN-A) in disseminated malignant melanoma. Cancer Res 1984; 54:2844–2849.
70. Coates A, Rallings M, Hersey P, et al. Phase-II study of recombinant α_2-interferon in advanced malignant melanoma. J Interferon Res 1986; 6:1–4.
71. Hersy P, Hasie E, MacDonald M, et al. Effects of recombinant leukocyte interferon (rIFN-alpha A) on tumor growth and immune responses in patients with metastatic melanoma. Br J Cancer 1985; 51:815–826.
72. Legha SS, Papadopoulos NE, Plager C, et al. Clinical evaluation of recombinant interferon alfa-2a (Roferon-a) in metastatic melanoma using two different schedules. J Clin Oncol 1987; 5:1858E.
73. Steiner A, Wolf C, Pehamberger H. Comparison of the effects of three different treatment regimens of recombinant interferons (r-IFN alpha, r-IFN gamma, and r-

IFN alpha + Cimetidine) in disseminated malignant melanoma. J Cancer Res Clin Oncol 1987; 113:459–465.

74. Legha SS. Interferons in the treatment of malignant melanoma: a review of recent trials. Cancer Res 1986; 57:1675–1677.
75. Robinson WA, Mughal TI, Thomas MR, et al. Treatment of metastatic malignant melanoma with recombinant interferon alpha-2. Immunobiology 1986; 172:275–282.
76. Kirkwood JM, Ernstoff MS, Davis CA, et al. Comparison of intramuscular and intravenous recombinant alpha-2 interferon in melanoma and other cancers. Ann Intern Med 1985; 103:32–36.
77. Dorval T, Palangie T, Jouve M, et al. Clinical phase II trial of recombinant DNA interferon (interferon alfa 2b) in patients with metastatic malignant melanoma. Cancer Res 1986; 58:215–218.
78. Sertoli MR, Bernengo MG, Ardizzoni A, et al. Phase II trial of recombinant alpha-2b interferon in the treatment of metastatic skin melanoma. Oncology 1989; 46:96–98.
79. Ernstoff MS, Trautman T, Davis CA, et al. A randomized phase I/II study of continuous versus intermittent intravenous interferon gamma in patients with metastatic melanoma. J Clin Oncol 1987; 5:1804–1810.
80. Creagan ET, Ahmann DL, Long HJ, et al. Phase II study of recombinant interferon-gamma in patients with disseminated malignant melanoma. Cancer Treat Rep 1987; 71:843–844.
81. Perez R, Lipton A, Harvey HA, et al. A phase I trial of recombinant human gamma interferon (IFN-g4A) in patients with advanced malignancy. J Biol Respon Modif 1988; 7:309–317.
82. Ruocco V, Satriano RA, Castello G. Malignant melanoma: biotherapeutic strategies for management with the interferons. Clin Dermat 1991; 9:505–510.
83. Castello G, Ruocco V, Satriano RA, et al. Role of interferons in the therapy of melanoma. Melanoma Res 1992; 1:311–325.
84. Taguchi T, Abe S, Nakano K, et al. Synergistic enhancement of the antitumor activity of recombinant human TNF-alpha by recombinant human IFN-gamma. Cancer Detect Prevent 1988; 12:105–114.
85. Krigel RL, Padavic-Shaller KA, Rudolph AR, et al. A phase I study of recombinant interleukin-2 plus recombinant beta-interferon. Cancer Res 1988; 48:3875–3881.
86. Cameron RB, McKintosh JK, Rosenberg SA. Synergistic antitumor effects of combination immunotherapy with recombinant interleukin-2 and a recombinant hybrid α-interferon in the treatment of established murine hepatic metastases. Cancer Res 1988; 48:5810–5817.
87. Iigo M, Sakurai M, Tamura T, et al. Invivo antitumor activity of multiple injection of recombinant interleukin-2, alone and in combination with three different types of recombinant interferon, on various syngeneic murine tumors. Cancer Res 1988; 49:260–264.
88. de Waal Malefyt R, Yssel H, Roncarolo M-G, et al. Interleukin-10. Curr Opin Immunol 1992; 4:314–320.
89. Reinhold U, Kukel S, Brzoska J, et al. Systemic interferon gamma treatment in severe atopic dermatitis. J Am Acad Dermat 1993; 29:58–63.

90. Reinhold U, Pawelec G, Wehrmann W, et al. Immunoglobulin E and immunoglobulin G subclass distribution in vivo and relationship to in vitro generation of interferon-gamma and neopterin in patients with severe atopic dermatitis. Int Arch Allergy Appl Immunol 1988; 87:120–126.
91. Reinhold U, Wehrmann W, Kukel S, et al. Evidence that defective interferon-gamma production in atopic dermatitis patients is due to intrinsic abnormalities. Clin Exp Immunol 1990; 79:374–379.
92. Rousset F, Robert J, Andary M, et al. Shifts in interleukin-4 and interferon-gamma production by T cells of patients with elevated serum IgE levels and the modulatory effects of these lymphokines on spontaneous IgE synthesis. J Allergy Clin Immunol 1991; 86:444–448.
93. MacKie RM. Interferon-α for atopic dermatitis. Lancet 1990; 335:1282–1283.
94. Granstein RD, Rook A, Flotte TJ, et al. A controlled trial of intralesional recombinant interferon-γ in the treatment of keloidal scarring. Arch Dermat 1990; 126:1295–1302.
95. Safai B, Bason M, Friedman-Birnbaum R, et al. Interferon in the treatment of AIDS-associated Kaposi's sarcoma: the American experience. J Invest Dermat 1990; 95:166S.
96. Ruszczak ZV, Detmar M, Imcke E, et al. Effects of rIFN alpha, beta and gamma on the morphology, proliferation and cell surface antigen expression of human dermal microvascular endothelial cells *in vivo.* J Invest Dermat 1990; 95:693.
97. Sauder DN. Interleukins. Progress Dermat 1988; 22:1–8.
98. Cohen SC. Physiologic and pathologic manifestations of lymphokine action. Human Pathol 1986; 17:112–121.
99. Feldmann M. Cell cooperation in the antibody response. In: Roitt I, Brostoff J, Male D, eds. Immunology. St. Louis: Mosby, 1993:7.1–7.16.
100. Dinarello CA, Mier JW. Medical intelligence: current concepts lymphokines. N Eng J Med 1987; 317:940–945.
101. Male D, Champion B, Cooke A, et al. Cytokines. In: Male D, Champion B, Cooke A, et al., eds. Advanced immunology. New York: Raven Press, 1991:11.1–11.16.
102. Yoshizaki K, Kishimoto T. Interleukin 6. In: Luger TA, Schwarz T, eds. Epidermal growth factors and cytokines. New York: Marcel Dekker, 1994:49–62.
103. Schröder J-M, Sticherlin M, Smid P, et al. Interleukin 8 and structurally related cytokines. In: Luger TA, Schwarz T, eds. Epidermal growth factors and cytokines. New York: Marcel Dekker, 1994:89–112.
104. Enk AH. Interleukin 10. In: Luger TA, Schwarz T, eds. Epidermal growth factors and cytokines. New York: Marcel Dekker, 1994:113–130.
105. Dinarello CA. Interleukin-1 and its biologically related cytokines. In: Cohen S, ed. Lymphokines and the immune response. Boca Raton, Fla.: CRC Press, 1990:145–180.
106. Balkwill FR. The other interleukins. In: Balkwill FR, ed. Cytokines in cancer therapy. Oxford: Oxford University Press, 1989:150–181.
107. Gery I, Gershon RK, Waksman BH. Potentiation of the T-lymphocyte response to mitogens: I. The responding cell. J Exp Med 1972; 136:128.

108. Kampschmidt RF, Upchurch HF, Worthington ML. Further comparisons of endogenous pyrogen and leukocytic endogenous mediators. Infect Immun 1983; 41:6–10.

109. Aarden LA, Brunner KT, Cerottini JC. Revised nomenclature for antigen-nonspecific T cell proliferation and helper factors. Mol Immunol 1980; 17:641–643.

110. Dinarello CA, Cannon JG, Mier JW, et al. Multiple biological activities of human recombinant interleukin-1. J Clin Invest 1986; 71:1734–1739.

111. Dinarello CA, Marnoy SO, Rossenwasser LJ. Role of arachidonate metabolism in the immunoregulatory function of human leukocytic pyrogen/lymphocyte-activating factor-interleukin-1. J Immunol 1983; 130:890–895.

112. Durum SK, Schmidt JA, Oppenheim JJ. Interleukin-1: an immunological perspective. Annu Rev Immunol 1985; 3:263–287.

113. Durum SK, Gershon RK. Interleukin-1 can replace the requirement for I-A positive cells in the proliferation of antigen-primed T cells. Proc Natl Acad Sci USA 1982; 79:4747–4750.

114. Caussy D, Sauder DN. The role of interleukin-1 in the immunological response. Transfus Med Rev 1989; 3:194–205.

115. Oppenheim JJ, Kovacs EJ, Matsushima K, et al. There is more than one interleukin-1. Immunol Today 1986; 7:45–56.

116. Sauder DN, Dinarello CA, Morheun VS. Langerhans cell production of interleukin-1. J Invest Dermat 1984; 82:605–607.

117. Sauder DM, Carter CA, Katz SI, et al. Epidermal cell production of thymocyte activation factor (ETAF). J Invest Dermat 1982; 79:34–39.

118. Sauder DN. Biologic properties of epidermal cell thymocyte-activating factor (ETAF). J Invest Dermat 1985; 85:176S–179S.

119. Kupper TS, Ballard D, Chua AO, et al. Human keratinocytes contain mRNA indistinguishable from monocyte interleukin 1 and mRNA: keratinocyte epidermal cell-derived thymocyte activating factor is identical to interleukin 1. J Exp Med 1986; 164:2095.

120. Schmitt A, Hauser C, Jaunin F, et al. Normal epidermis contains high amounts of natural tissue IL-1: biochemical analysis by HPLC identifies a MW approximately 17 kD form with a pl 5.7 and a MW approximately 30 kD form. Lympokine Res 1986; 5:105–118.

121. Kupper TS, Chua AO, Flood P, et al. Interleukin 1 gene expression in cultured human keratinocytes is augmented by ultraviolet irradiation. J Clin Invest 1987; 80:430–436.

122. Hauser C, Dayer JM, Jaunin F, et al. Intracellular epidermal interleukin 1 like factors in the human epidermoid carcinoma cell line A431. Cell Immunol 1986; 100:89.

123. Kupper TS. Interleukin 1 and other human keratinocyte cytokines: molecular and functional characterization. Adv Dermat 1988; 3:293–308.

124. Goldminz D, Kupper TS, McGuire. Keratinocyte membrane associated epidermal cell derived thymocyte activating factor (ETAF). J Invest Dermat 1987; 88:97.

125. Sauder DN, Arsenault TV, Stetsko D. Isolation and partial characterization of a putative cDNA clone (k-IL-1a): ETAF is distinct from IL-1α or Il-1β. Clin Res 1987; 35:714A.

126. Le J, Vilcek J. Biology of disease: tumor necrosis factor and interleukin 1: cytokines with multiple overlapping biological activities. Lab Invest 1987; 56:234–248.
127. March CJ, Mosley B, Larsen A, et al. Cloning, sequence and expression of two distinct human interleukin-1 complementary DNAs. Nature 1985; 315:641.
128. Dinarello CA. An update on human interleukin-1: from molecular biology to clinical relevance. J Clin Immunol 1985; 5:287.
129. Lomedico PT, Gubler U, Hellmann CP, et al. Cloning and expression of murine interleukin-1 cDNA in *escherichia coli.* Nature 1984; 312:458–462.
130. Kaye J, Janeway CA Jr. Induction of receptors for interleukin-2 requires T cell Ag:In receptor crosslinking and interleukin 1. Lymphokine Res 1984; 3:175–182.
131. Williams JM, Delovia D, Hansen J, et al. The events of primary T cell activation can be staged by use of Sepharose-bound anti-T3 (64.1) monoclonal antibody and purified interleukin-1. J Immunol 1985; 135:2249–2255.
132. Kaye J, Gillis S, Mizel SB, et al. Growth of a cloned helper T cell line induced by a monoclonal antibody specific for the antigen receptor: interleukin-1 is required for the expression of receptors for interleukin-2. J Immunol 1984; 133:1339–1345.
133. Lowenthal JW, Cerotini JC, MacDonald HR. Interleukin-1 dependent induction of both interleukin-2 secretion and interleukin-2 receptor expansion by thymoma cells. J Immunol 1986; 137:1226–1231.
134. Ruddle NH. Tumour necrosis factor and related cytokines. Immunol Today 1987; 8:129–136.
135. Hoffmann MK. Macrophages and T cells control distinct phases of B cell differentiation in the humoral immune response in vitro. J Immunol 1980; 125:2076–2081.
136. Futami H, Jansen R, MacPhee MJ. Chemoprotective effect of recombinant human interleukin-1α in cyclophosphamide treated tumor bearing mice. J Immunol 1990; 145:21–30.
137. Dinarello CA. Interleukin. Rev Infect Dis 1984; 6:51.
138. Gillis S, Conlon PJ, Cosman D, et al. Lymphokines: from conjecture to the clinic. Semin Oncol 1986; 13:218–227.
139. Gillis S, Baker PE, Ruscetti FW, et al. Long-term culture of human antigen-specific cytotoxic T-cell lines. J Exp Med 1978; 148:1093.
140. Fisher RI, Coltman CA Jr, Doroshow JH, et al. Metastatic renal cancer treated with interleukin-2 and lymphokine-activated killer cells. Ann Intern Med 1988; 108:518–523.
141. Morgan DA, Ruscetti FW, Gallo RC. Selective in vitro growth of T lymphocytes from normal human bone marrows. Science 1976; 193:1007–1008.
142. Mier JW, Gallo RC. Purification and some characteristics of human T-cell growth factor from phytohemagglutinin-stimulated lymphocyte-conditioned media. Proc Natl Acad Sci USA 1980; 77:6134–6138.
143. Taniguchi T, Matsui H, Fujita T, et al. Structure and expression of a cloned cDNA for human interleukin-2. Nature 1983; 302:305.
144. Rosenberg SA, Grimm EA, McGrogan M, et al. Biological activity of recombinant human interleukin-2 produced in *escherichia coli.* Science 1984; 223:1412–1414.
145. Whittington R, Faulds D. Interleukin-2: a review of its pharmacological properties and therapeutic use in patients with cancer. Drugs 1993; 46:446–514.

146. Khan IU, Shear NH. Cytokines in anticancer therapy. Clin Dermat 1992; 9:523–533.
147. Tsudo M, Goldman CK, Bongiovanni KF, et al. The p75 peptide is the receptor for interleukin-2 expressed on large granular lymphocytes and is responsible for the interleukin-2 activation of these cells. Proc Natl Acad Sci USA 1987; 84:5394–5398.
148. Minami Y, Konok T, Yamada K, et al. The interleukin-2 receptors: insights into a complex signalling mechanism. Biochim Biophys Acta 1992; 1114:163–177.
149. Robb RJ, Greene WC. Internalization of interleukin 2 is mediated by the β chain of high-affinity interleukin 2 receptor. J Exp Med 1987; 165:1201–1206.
150. Wang H-M, Smith KA. The interleukin 2 receptor: functional consequences of its bimolecular structure. J Exp Med 1987; 166:1055–1069.
151. Stewart AM, Tweardy DJ, McCarthy SA, et al. GM-CSF augmentation of IL-2 induced LAK activity: enhancement does not appear to be mediated through either IL-1 of IFN-y. J Immunother 1992; 11:146.
152. Xia X, Lee H-K, Clark SC, et al. Recombinant interleukin (IL) 2-induced human B cell differentiation is mediated by autocrine IL 6. Eur J Immunol 1989; 19:2275–2281.
153. Raulet DH. Expression and function of interleukin-2 receptors on immature thymocytes. Nature 1985; 314:101–103.
154. Rosenberg SA, Lotze MT, Muul LM, et al. Observations on the systemic administration of autologous lymphokine-activated killer cells and recombinant interleukin-2 to patients with metastatic cancer. N Eng J Med 1985; 313:1485–1492.
155. Lafreniere R, Rosenberg SA. Successful immunotherapy of murine experimental hepatic metastases with lymphokine-activated killer cells and recombinant interleukin 2. Cancer Res 1985; 45:3735–3741.
156. Itoh K. Tumour-infiltrating lymphocytes in human metastatic melanoma. Cancer Bull 1991; 43:109–116.
157. Baars JW, Fonk JCM, Scheper RJ, et al. Treatment with tumour infiltrating lymphocytes and interleukin-2 in patients with metastatic melanoma: a pilot study. Biotherapy 1992; 4:289–297.
158. Rosenberg SA, Lotze MT, Yang JC, et al. Experience with the use of high-dose interleukin-2 in the treatment of 652 cancer patients. Ann Surg 1989; 210:474–485.
159. Rosenberg SA, Lotze MT, Muul LM, et al. Observations on the systemic administration of autologous lymphokine-activated killer cells and recombinant interleukin-2 to patients with metastatic cancer. N Eng J Med 1985; 313:1485–1492.
160. Rosenberg SA, Lotze MT, Muul LM, et al. A progress report on the treatment of 157 patients with advanced cancer using lymphokine activated killer cells and interleukin-2 or high dose interleukin-2 alone. N Eng J Med 1987; 316:889–905.
161. Muul LM, Nason-Burchenal K, Carter CS, et al. Development of an automated closed system for generation of human lymphokine activated killer (LAK) cells for use in adoptive immunotherapy. J Immunol Meth 1987; 101:171–181.
162. Rosenberg SA, Packard BS, Aebersold PM, et al. Use of tumor-infiltrating lymphocytes and interleukin-2 in the immunotherapy of patients with metastatic melanoma. N Eng J Med 1988; 319:1676–1680.
163. Rosenberg SA, Spiess P, Lafreniere R. A new approach to the adoptive immunotherapy of cancer with tumor-infiltrating lymphocytes. Science 1986; 233:1318–1321.

164. Spiess PJ, Yang JC, Rosenberg SA. In vivo antitumor activity of tumor-infiltrating lymphocytes expanded in recombinant interleukin-2. J Natl Cancer Inst 1987; 79:1067–1075.
165. Rosenberg SA, Packard BS, Aebersold PM, et al. Use of tumor infiltrating lymphocytes and interleukin-2 in the immunotherapy of patients with metastatic melanoma: a preliminary report. N Eng J Med 1988; 319:1676–1680.
166. West WH, Tauer KW, Yannelli JR, et al. Constant-infusion recombinant interleukin-2 in adoptive immunotherapy of advanced cancer. N Eng J Med 1987; 316:898–905.
167. Ettinghausen SE, Rosenberg SA. Immunotherapy of murine sarcomas using lymphokine activated killer cells: optimization of the schedule and route of administration of recombinant interleukin-2. Cancer Res 1986; 46:2784–2792.
168. Cameron RB, McIntosh JK, Rosenberg SA. Synergistic antitumor effects of combination immunotherapy with recombinant interleukin-2 and a recombinant hybrid interferon-alpha in the treatment of established murine hepatic metastases. Cancer Res 1988; 48:5810–5817.
169. McIntosh JF, Mule JJ, Merino MJ, et al. Synergistic antitumor effects of immunotherapy with recombinant interleukin-2 and recombinant tumor necrosis factor-α. Cancer Res 1988; 48:4011–4017.
170. Brouckaert PGG, Larous-Roels GG, Guisez Y, et al. In vivo anti-tumour activity of recombinant human and murine TNF, alone and in combination with murine IFN-γ, on a syngeneic murine melanoma. Int J Cancer 1986; 38:763–769.
171. Antineoplastic agents. In: Drug facts and comparisons. St. Louis, Mo.: Facts and Comparisons, 1994:2593–2800.
172. Vial T, Descotes J. Clinical toxicity of interleukin-2. Drug Safe 1992; 7:417–433.
173. Scheibenbogen C, Keilholz U, Pezzutto A, et al. Rheumatic disease following immunotherapy. Ann Rheum Dis 1993; 52:165.
174. Interleukin-2. In: The United States Pharmacopediaol Convention, ed. Drug information for the health care professional. Taunton, Mass.: Rand McNally, 1994:2881–2886.
175. Siegel JP, Puri RK. Interleukin-2 toxicity. J Clin Oncol 1991; 9:694–704.
176. Hesketh P, Caguioa P, Koh H, et al. Clinical activity of a cytotoxic fusion protein in the treatment of cutaneous T-cell lymphoma. J Clin Oncol 1993; 11:1682–1690.
177. Zukinski AA, David CL, Coan J, et al. Increased incidence of hypersensitivity to iodine-containing radiographic contrast media after interleukin-2 administration. Cancer 1190; 65:1520–1530.
178. Abi-aad A, Figlin R, Belldegrunk A, et al. Metastatic renal cell cancer: interleukin-2. J Am Acad Dermat 1992; 26:567–574.
179. Shulman KL, Thompson JA, Benyunes MC, et al. Adverse reactions to intravenous contrast media in patients treated with interleukin-2. J Immunother 1993; 13:208–212.
180. Choyke PL, Miller DL, Lotze MT, et al. Delayed reactions to contrast media after interleukin-2 immunotherapy. Radiology 1992; 183:111–114.
181. Oldham RK, Brogley J, Braud G. Contrast medium "recalls": interleukin-2 toxicity. J Clin Oncol 1990; 8:942–943.

182. Wolkenstein P, Chosidow O, Wechsler J, et al. Cutaneous side-effects associated with interleukin 2 administration for metastatic melanoma. J Am Acad Dermat 1993; 28:66–70.
183. St. Georgiev V. Immunomodulating drugs: major advances in research and development. Ann NY Acad Sci 1993; 685:1–10.
184. Denicoff KD, Rubinow DR, Papa MZ, Simpson C, Seipp CA, Lotze MT, Change AE, Rosenstein D, Rosenberg SA. The neuropsychiatric effects of treatment with interleukin-2 and lymphokine-activated killer cells. Ann Intern Med 1987; 107:293–300.
185. Lee RE, Gaspari AA, Lotze MT, et al. Interleukin 2 and psoriasis. Arch Dermat 1988; 124:1811–1815.
186. Ramseur WL, Richards F II, Duggan DB. A case of fatal pemphigus vulgaris in association with beta interferon and interleukin-2 therapy. Cancer Res 1989; 63:2005–2007.
187. Guilleume JC, Escudier B, Espagne E, et al. Dermatose bulleuse avec depots lineaires d'IgA le long de la membrane basale au coufs d'un traitement par l'interferon gamma et l'interleukine-2. Ann Dermat Venereol 1990; 117:899–902.
188. Prussick R, Plott TR, Stanley JR. Recurrence of pemphigus vulgaris associated with interleukin-2 therapy. Arch Dermat (in press).
189. Rosenberg SA. Immunotherapy of cancer by systemic administration of lymphoid cells plus interleukin-2. J Biol Respon Modif 1984; 3:501–511.
190. Mazumder A, Eberlein TJ, Grimm EA, et al. Phase I study of the adoptive immunotherapy of human cancer with lectin activated autologous mononuclear cells. Cancer 1984; 53:896–905.
191. Cochat P, Floret D, Bouffet E, et al. Renal effects of continuous infusion of recombinant interleukin-2 in children. Ped Nephrol 1991; 5:33–37.
192. Lotze MT, Frana LW, Sharrow SO, et al. In vivo administration of purified human interleukin 2. I. Half-life and immunologic effects of the Jurkat cell line-deriveau interleukin 2. J Immunol 1985; 134:157–166.
193. Emminger W, Emminger-Schmidmeier W, Peters C, et al. Capillary leak syndrome during low dose granulocyte-macrophage colony-stimulating factor (rhGM-CSF) treatment of a patient in a continuous febrile state. Blut 1990; 61:219–221.
194. Wagstaff J, Vermorken JB, Schwartsmann G, et al. A progress report of a phase I study of interferon-gamma and interleukin-2 and some comments on the mechanism of toxicity due to interleukin-2. Cancer Treat Rev 1989; 16:105–109.
195. Moore FD Jr, Schoof DD, Rodrick M, et al. The systemic complement activation caused by interleukin-2/lymphokine-activated killer-cell therapy of cancer causes minimal systemic neutrophil activation. Int J Cancer 1991; 49:504–508.
196. Taniguchi K, Morimoto S, Fukuo K, et al. Interleukin-2 suppresses endothelin-1 secretion of cultured endothelial cells. Hyperten Res 1993; 15:171–175.
197. Gaspari AA, Lotze MT, Rosenberg SA, et al. Dermatologic changes associated with interleukin 2 administration. JAMA 1987; 258:1624–1629.
198. Dummer R, Miller K, Eilles C, et al. The skin: an immunoreactive target organ during interleukin-2 administration? Dermatologica 1991; 183:95–99.

199. Baars JW, Wagstaff J, Hack CE, et al. Angioneurotic oedema and urticaria during therapy with interleukin-2 (IL-2). Ann Oncol 1992; 3:243–244.
200. Weinstein A, Bujak D, Mittelman A, et al. Erythema nodosum in a patient with renal cell carcinoma treated with interleukin 2 and lymphokine-activated killer cells. JAMA 1987; 258:3120–3121.
201. Staunton MR, Scully MC, LeBoit PE, et al. Life-threatening bullous skin eruptions during interleukin-2 therapy. J Natl Cancer Inst 1991; 1991:56–57.
202. Wiener JS, Tucker JA Jr, Walther PJ. Interleukin-2-induced dermatotoxicity resembling toxic epidermal necrolysis. South Med J 1992; 85:656–659.
203. Sleijfer D, Janssen RAJ, Buter J, et al. Phase II study of subcutaneous interleukin-2 in unselected patients with advanced renal cell cancer on an out-patient basis. J Clin Oncol 1992; 10:1119–1123.
204. Novick D, Engelmann H, Wallach D, et al. Soluble cytokine receptors are present in normal human urine. J Exp Med 1989; 170:1409.
205. Honda M, Yamamoto S, Cheng M, et al. Human soluble IL-6 receptor: its detection and enhanced release by HIV infection. J Immunol 1992; 148:2175–2180.
206. Ehlers MRW, Riordan JF. Membrane proteins with soluble counterparts: role of proteolysis in the release of transmembrane proteins. Biochemistry 1991; 30:10065–10074.
207. Yasukawa K, Saito T, Funkunaga T, et al. Purification and characterization of soluble human IL-6 receptor expressed in CHO cells. J Biochem 1990; 108:673–676.
208. Suzuki H, Yasukawa K, Saito T, et al. Serum soluble interleukin-6 receptor in MRL/lpr mice is elevated with age and mediates the interluekin-γ signal. Eur J Immunol 1993; 23:1078–1082.
209. Narazaki M, Yasukawa K, Saito T, et al. Soluble forms of the interleukin-6 signal-transducing receptor component gp130 in human serum possessing a potential to inhibit signals through membrane-anchored gp130. Blood 1993; 82:1120.
210. Barker JNWN, Mitra RS, Griffiths CEM, et al. Keratinocytes as initiators of inflammation. Lancet 1991; 337:211–214.
211. Hettmannsperger U, Detmar M, Owsianowki M, et al. Cytokine-stimulated human dermal microvascular endothelial cells produce interleukin-6 inhibition by hydrocortisone, dexamethasone and calcitriol. J Invest Dermat 1992; 99:531–536.
212. Heinrich PC, Castell JV, Andus T. Interleukin-6 and the acute phase response. Biochem J 1990; 265:621–636.
213. Oxholm A, Oxholm P, Avnstorp C, et al. Keratinocyte expression of interleukin 6 but not tumor necrosis factor alpha is increased in allergic and in the irritant patch test reaction. Acta Derm Venereol (Stockh) 1991; 7:93–98.
214. Kimber I, Cumberbath M, Humphries M, et al. Contact hypersensitivity induces plasma interleukin 6. Int Arch Allerg Appl Immunol 1990; 92:97–99.
215. Helle M, Boeije L, Aarden LA. Interleukin 6 is an intermediate in interleukin 1 induced thymocyte proliferation. J Immunol 1989; 142:4335–4338.
216. Tosato B, Pike SE. Interferon beta 2/interleukin 6 is a costimulator for human T lymphocytes. J Immunol 1988; 141:1556–1662.
217. Wong GG, Clark SC. Multiple actions of interleukin 6 within a cytokine network. Immunol Today 1988; 9:137–139.

218. Grossman RM, Krueger J, Yourish D, et al. Interleukin 6 is expressed in high levels in psoriatic skin and stimulates proliferation of cultured human keratinocytes. Proc Natl Acad Sci USA 1989; 86:6367–6371.
219. Neuner P, Urbanski A, Trautinger F, et al. Increased IL-6 production by monocytes and keratinocytes in patients with psoriasis. J Invest Dermat 1991; 97:27–33.
220. Krueger JG, Krane JF, Carter DM, et al. Role of growth factors, cytokines and their receptors in the pathogenesis of psoriasis. J Invest Dermat 1990; 94:135S–140S.
221. Ohta Y, Katayama I, Funato T, et al. In situ expression of messenger RNA of interleukin-1 and interleukin-6 in psoriasis: interleukin-6 involved in formation of psoriatic lesions. Arch Dermat Res 1991; 283:351–356.
222. Turksen K, Kupper T, Degenstein L, et al. Interleukin-1 receptor antagonist in normal and psoriatic epidermis. J Clin Invest 1992; 90:571–583.
223. Yoshimura T, Robinson E, Appella E, et al. Three forms of monocyte-derived neutrophil chemotactic factor (MDNCF) distinguished by different lengths of the amino-terminal sequence. Mol Immunol 1989; 26:87–93.
224. SchrÖder J-M, Sticherling M, Henneicke HH, et al. IL-α or tumor necrosis factor-α stimulate release of three nap-1/il-8-related neutrophil chemotactic proteins in human dermal fibroblasts. J Immunol 1990; 144:2223–2232.
225. Gimbrone MA Jr, Obin MS, Brock AF, et al. Endothelial interleukin-8: a novel inhibitor of leukocyte-endothelial interactions. Science 1989; 246:1601–1603.
226. Hebert CA, Luscinskas FW, Kielry JM, et al. Endothelial and leukocyte form of IL-8. Conversion by thrombin and interactions with neutrophils. J Immunol 1990; 145:3303–3340.
227. Thomas KM, Taylor L, Navarro J. The interleukin-8 receptor is encoded by a neutrophil-specific cDNA clone, F3R. J Biol Chem 1991; 266:14839–14841.
228. Murphy PM, Tiffany HL. Cloning of complementary DNA encoding a functional human interleukin-8 receptor. Science 1991; 253:1280–1283.
229. Holmes WE, Lee J, Kuang W-J, et al. Structure and functional expression of a human interleukin-8 receptor. Science 1991; 253:1278–1280.
230. LaRosa GJ, Thomas KM, Kaufmann ME, et al. Amino terminus of the interleukin-8 receptor is a major determinant of receptor subtype specificity. J Biol Chem 1992; 267:25402–25406.
231. Colditz I, Zwahlen R, Dewald B, et al. In vivo inflammatory activity of neutrophil-activating factor, a novel chemotactic peptide derived from human monocytes. Am J Pathol 1989; 134:755–760.
232. Matsushima K, Oppenheim JJ. Interleukin 8 and MCAF: novel inflammatory cytokines inducible by IL-1 and TNF. Cytokine 1989; 1:2–13.
233. Larsen CG, Anderson AO, Oppenheim JJ, et al. Production of interleukin-8 by human dermal fibroblast and keratinocytes in response to interleukin-1 or tumour necrosis factor. Immunol Allerg Clin N Am 1989; 68:31–36.
234. Larsen CG, Anderson AO, Appella E, et al. The neutrophil activating protein (NAP-1) is also chemotactic for T lymphocytes. Science 1989; 243:1464–1466.
235. Robinson EA, Yoshimura T, Leonard EJ, et al. Complete amino acid sequence of a human monocyte chemoattractant, a putative mediator of cellular immune reactions. Proc Natl Acad Sci USA 1989; 86:1850–1854.

236. Schroder JM. Chemotactic cytokines in the epidermis. Exp Dermat 1992; 1:12–19.
237. Nickoloff BJ. The cytokine newtork in psoriasis. Arch Dermat 1991; 127:871–884.
238. Takematsu H, Tagami H. Quantification of chemotactic peptides (c5a anaphilatoxin and IL-8) in psoriatic lesional skin. Arch Dermat 1993; 129:74–80.
239. Howard M, O'Garra A. Biological properties of interleukin 10. Immunol Today 1992; 13:198–200.
240. Go NF, Castle BE, Barrett R, et al. Interleukin 10, a novel B cell stimulatory factor: unresponsiveness of X chromosome-linked immunodeficiency B cells. J Exp Med 1990; 172:1625–1631.
241. Ding L, Linsley PS, Huang LY, et al. IL-10 inhibits macrophage costimulatory activity by selectively inhibiting the up-regulation of B7 expression. J Immunol 1993; 151:1225–1234.
242. Thompsin-Snipes L, Dhar V, Bond MW, et al. Interleukin 10: a novel stimulatory factor for mast cells and their progenitors. J Exp Med 1991; 173:507–510.
243. Enk A, Katz. Identification and induction of keratinocyte-derived IL-10. J Immunol 1992; 149:92–95.
244. Fiorentino DF, Bond MW, Mosmann TR. Two types of mouse T helper cell. IV. Th2 clones secrete a factor that inhibits cytokine production by Th1 clones. J Exp Med 1989; 170:2081–2095.
245. De Waal Malefyt R, Abrams J, Bennett J, et al. Interleukin 10 (IL-10) inhibits cytokine synthesis by human monocytes: an autoregulatory role of IL-10 production by monocytes. J Exp Med 1991; 174:1209–1220.
246. Fiorentino DF, Zlotnik A, Mosmann TR, et al. IL-10 inhibits cytokine production by activated macrophages. J Immunol 1991; 147:3815–3822.
247. Fiorentino DF, Zlotnid A, Vieira P, et al. IL-10 acts on the antigen presenting cell to inhibit cytokine production by Th1 cells. J Immunol 1991; 146:3444–3451.
248. de wall Malefyt R, Haanen J, Spits H, et al. Interleukin 10 (IL-10) and viral IL-10 strongly reduce antigen-specific human T cell proliferation by diminishing the antigen-presenting capacity of monocytes via downregulation of class II major histocompatibility complex expression. J Exp Med 1991; 174:915–924.
249. Reiser H, Freeman GJ, Razi-Wolf CD, et al. Murine B7 antigen provides an efficient costimulatory signal for activation of murine T lymphocytes via the T-cell receptor/Cd3 complex. Proc Natl Acad Sci USA 1992; 89:271–275.
250. Enk AH, Angeloni VL, Udey MC, et al. Inhibition of Langerhans cell antigen-presenting function by IL-10. J Immunol 1993; 151:2390–2398.
251. Scwarz A, Grabbe S, Simon M, et al. Interleukin 10 inhibits the effector phase of contact hypersensitivity. J Invest Dermat 1993; 100:521A.
252. Ferguson TA, Dube P, Griffith TS. Regulation of contact hypersensitivity by interleukin 10. J Exp Med 1994; 179:1597–1604.
253. Groopman JE, Molina J-M, Scadden DT. Medical progress: hematopoietic growth factors. N Eng J Med 1989; 321:1449–1459.
254. Carnot P, Deflandre C. Sur l'activité hémopoiétique des différents organes au cours de la régénération du sang. CR Hebd Acad Sci 1906; 143:432–435.
255. Pluznik DH, Sachs L. The cloning of normal "mast" cells in tissue culture. J Cell Comp Physiol 1965; 66:319–324.

256. Bradley TR, Metcalf D. The growth of mouse bone marrow cells in vitro. Aust J Exp Biol Med Sci 1966; 66:319–324.
257. Ruef C, Coleman DL. Granulocyte-macrophage colony-stimulating factor: pleiotropic cytokine with potential clinical usefulness. Rev Infect Dis 1990; 12:41–62.
258. Gasson JC, Weisbart RH, Kaufman SE, et al. Purified human granulocyte-macrophage colony-stimulating factor: direct action on neutrophils. Science 1984; 226:1339–1342.
259. Horn TD, Burke PJ, Karp JE, et al. Intravenous administration of recombinant human granulocyte-macrophage colony-stimulating factor causes a cutaneous eruption. Arch Dermat 1991; 127:49–52.
260. Kupper TS, Lee F, Coleman D, et al. Keratinocyte derived T-cell growth factor (KTGF) is identical to granulocyte macrophage colony stimulating factor (GM-CSF). J Invest Dermat 1988; 91:185–188.
261. Kupper TS, Lee F, Birchall N, et al. Interleukin-1 binds to specific receptors on human keratinocytes and induces granulocyte/macrophage colony stimulating factor MRNA and protein: a potential autocrine role for interleukin-1 in epidermis. J Clin Invest 1988; 82:1787–1792.
262. Sieff CA. Hematopoietic growth factors. J Clin Invest 1987; 79:1549–1557.
263. Miyatake S, Otsuka T, Yokota T, et al. Structure of the chromosomal gene for granulocyte-macrophage colony stimulating factor: comparison of the mouse and human genes. EMBO J 1985; 4:2561–2568.
264. Lieschke GJ, Burgess AW. Granulocyte colony-stimulating factor and granulocyte-macrophage colony-stimulating factor. N Eng J Med 1992; 327:99–106.
265. Gough NM, Gough J, Metcalf D, et al. Molecular cloning of cDNA encoding a murine haematopoietic growth regulator, granulocyte-macrophage colony stimulating factor. Nature 1984; 309:736–767.
266. Cantrell MA, Anderson D, Cerretti DP, et al. Cloning, sequence, and expression of a human granulocyte/macrophage colony-stimulating factor. Proc Natl Acad Sci USA 1985; 82:6250–6254.
267. Zsebo KM, Cohen AM, Murdock DC, et al. Recombinant human granulocyte colony stimulating factor: molecular and biological characterization. Immunobiology 1986; 172:175–184.
268. Kitamura T, Tojo A, Kuwaki T, et al. Identification and analysis of human erythropoietin receptor on a factor-dependent cell line, TF-1. Blood 1989; 73:375–380.
269. Wong GG, Witek JS, Temple PA, et al. Human GM-CSF: molecular cloning of the complementary DNA and purification of the natural and recombinant proteins. Science 1985; 228:810–815.
270. Pettanti MJ, Le Beau MM, Lemons RS, et al. Assignment of CSF-1 to their involvement in the deletion of the long arm of chromosome 5 in myeloid disorders. Proc Natl Acad Sci USA 1987; 84:2970–2974.
271. Yang YC, Kovacic S, Kriz R, et al. The human genes for GM-CSF and IL-3 are closely linked in tandem on chromosome 5. Blood 1988; 71:958–961.
272. Simmers RN, Webber LM, Shannon MF, et al. Localization of the G-CSF gene on chromosome 17 proximal to the breakpoint in the t(15:17) in acute promyelocytic leukemia. Blood 1987; 70:330–332.

273. Souza LM, Boone TC, Gabrilove J, et al. Recombinant human granulocyte colony-stimulating factor: effects on normal and leukemic myeloid cells. Science 1986; 232:61–65.
274. Moonen P, Mermod JJ, Ernst JF, et al. Increased biological activity of deglycosylated recombinant human granulocyte/macrophage colony-stimulating factor produced by yeast or animal cells. Proc Natl Sci USA 1987; 84:4428–4431.
275. Lieschke GJ, Burgess AW. Granulocyte colony-stimulating factor and granulocyte-macrophage colony-stimulating factor. N Eng J Med 1992; 327:99–106.
276. Weisbart RH, Gasson JC, Golde DW. Colony-stimulating factors and host defense. Ann Intern Med 1989; 110:297–303.
277. Moore MAS. Hematopoietic growth factors in cancer. Cancer Res 1990; 65:836–844.
278. Schiro JA, Kupper TS. Cutaneous eruptions during GM-CSF Infusion. Arch Dermat 1991; 127:110–112.
279. Clark SC, Kamen R. The human hematopoietic colony-stimulating factors. Science 1987; 236:1229–1237.
280. Kupper TS. Immune and inflammatory processes in cutaneous tissues: mechanisms and speculations. J Clin Invest 1990; 86:1783–1789.
281. Witmer-Pack M, Oliver W, Valinsky J, et al. Granulocyte/macrophage colony stimulating factor is essential for the viability and function of cultured murine epidermal langerhans cells. J Exp Med 1987; 166:1484–1498.
282. Koch F, Heufler C, Kampgen E, et al. Tumor necrosis factor alpha maintains the viability of murine epidermal Langerhans cells in culture, but, in contrast to granulocyte/macrophage colony stimulating factor, does not induce their functional maturation. J Exp Med 1990; 171:159–171.
283. Park LS, Friend D, Gillis S, et al. Characterization of the cell surface receptor for human granulocyte/macrophage colony-stimulating factor. J Exp Med 1986; 164:251–262.
284. DiPersio J, Billing P, Kaufman S, et al. Characterization of the human granulocyte-macrophage colony-stimulating factor receptor. J Biol Chem 1988; 263:1834–1841.
285. Cebon J, Dempsey P, Fox R, et al. Pharmacokinetics of human granulocyte-macrophage colony-stimulating factor using a sensitive immunoassay. Blood 1988; 72:1340–1347.
286. Groopman JE, Mitsuyasu RT, DeLeo MJ, et al. Effect of recombinant human granulocyte-macrophage colony-stimulating factor on myelopoiesis in the acquired immunodeficiency syndrome. N Eng J Med 1987; 317:593–598.
287. Miles S, Glaspy J, Chung Y, et al. Recombinant granulocyte colony stimulating factor (r-met HuG-CSF) increases neutrophil number and function, but does not alter HIV expression in patients with AIDS. In: V International Conference on AIDS, Montreal, Quebec, Canada, 4–9 June 1989. Ottawa, Ont.: International Development Research Center, 1989:558 [abstract].
288. Koyanagi Y, O'Brien WA, Zhao JQ, et al. Cytokines alter production of HIV-1 from primary phagocytes. Science 1988; 241:1673–1675.
289. Lieschke GJ, Maher D, O'Connor M, et al. Phase I study of intravenously administered bacterially synthesized granulocyte-macrophage colony-stimulating factor and comparison with subcutaneous administration. Cancer Res 1990; 50:606–614.

290. Lieschke GJ, Cebon J, Morstyn G. Characterization of the clinical effects after the first dose of bacterially synthesized recombinant human granulocyte-macrophage colony-stimulating factor. Blood 1989; 74:2634–2643.

291. Lieschke GJ, Maher D, Cebon J, et al. Effects of bacterially synthesized recombinant human granulocyte-macrophage colony-stimulating factor in patients with advanced malignancy. Ann Intern Med 1989; 110:357–364.

292. Peters WP, Shogan J, Shpall EJ, et al. Recombinant human granulocyte-macrophage colony-stimulating factor produces fever. Lancet 1988; 1:950.

293. Wing EJ, Magee DM, Whiteside TL, et al. Recombinant human granulocyte/macrophage colony-stimulating factor enhances monocyte cytotoxicity and secretion of tumor necrosis factor α and interferon in cancer patients. Blood 1989; 73:643–646.

294. Parkm JW, Mehrotra B, Barnett BO, et al. The sweet syndrome during therapy with granulocyte colony-stimulating factor. Ann Intern Med 1992; 116:996–998.

295. Wakefield PE, James WD, Samlaska CP, et al. Colony-stimulating factors. J Am Acad Dermat 1990; 23:903–912.

296. Passweg J, Buser U, Tichelli A, et al. Pustular eruption at the site of subcutaneous injection of recombinant human granulocyte-macrophage colony-stimulating factor. Ann Hematol 1991; 63:326–327.

297. Farmer KL, Kurzrock R, Gutterman JU. Necrotizing vasculitis at granulocyte-macrophage colony-stimulating factor injection sites. Arch Dermat 1990; 126:1243–1244.

298. Mehregan DR, Fransway AF, Edmonson JH, et al. Cutaneous reactions to granulocyte-monocyte colony-stimulating factor. Arch Dermat 1992; 128:1055–1059.

299. Horn TD, Redd JV, Karp JE, et al. Cutaneous eruptions of lymphocyte recovery. Arch Dermat 1989; 125:1512–1517.

300. Ross HJ, Moy LA, Kaplan R, et al. Bullous pyoderma gangrenosum after granulocyte colony-stimulating factor treatment. Cancer Res 1991; 68:441–443.

301. Glaspy JA, Baldwin GC, Robertson PA, et al. Therapy for neutropenia in hairy cell leukemia with recombinant human granulocyte colony-stimulating factor. Ann Intern Med 1988; 109:789–795.

302. Dreicer R, Schiller J. Granulocyte-macrophage colony-stimulating factor and vasculitis [letter]. Ann Intern Med 1989; 111:91–92.

303. Negrin RS, Haenber DH, Nagler A, et al. Treatment of myelodysplastic syndromes with recombinant human granulocyte colony-stimulating factor. Ann Intern Med 1989; 110:976–984.

304. Ostlere LS, Harris D, Prentice HG, et al. Widespread folliculitis induced by human granulocyte colony-stimulating factor therapy. Br J Dermat 1992; 127:193–194.

305. Welte K, Zeidler C, Reiter A, et al. Differential effects of granulocyte-macrophage colony-stimulating factory and granulocyte colony-stimulating factor in children with severe congenital neutropenia. Blood 1990; 75:1056–1063.

306. Wodzinski MA, Hampton KK, Reilly JT. Differential effect of G-CSF and GM-CSF in acquired chronic neutropenia. Br J Haematol 1991; 77:249–250.

307. Glaspy JA, Baldwin GC, Robertson PA, et al. Therapy for neutropenia in hairy cell leukemia with recombinant human granulocyte colony-stimulating factor. Ann Intern Med 1988; 109:789–795.

308. Kluin-Nelemans JC, Hollander AAMJ, Fibbe WE, et al. Leucocytoclastic vasculitis during GM-CSF therapy. Br J Dermat 1989; 73:419.
309. Ward JC, Gitlin JB, Garry DJ, et al. Epidermolysis bullosa acquisita induced by GM-CSF: a role for eosinophils in treatment-related toxicity. Br J Haematol 1992; 81:27–32.
310. Hazenberg BPC, van Leeuwen MA, van Rijswijk MH, et al. Correction of granulocytopenia in Felty's syndrome by granulocyte-macrophage colony-stimulating factor: simultaneous induction of interleukin-6 release and flare-up of the arthritis. Blood 1989; 74:2769–2770.
311. de Vries EGE, Willemse PHB, Biemsa B, et al. Flare-up of rheumatoid arthritis during GM-CSF treatment after chemotherapy. Lancet 1991; 338:517–518.
312. Hoekman K, vonBlomber-van der Flier BME, Wagstaff J, et al. Reversible thyroid dysfunction during treatment with GM-CSF. Lancet 1991; 338:541–542.
313. Logothetis CJ, Dexeus FH, Sella A, et al. Escalated therapy for refractory urothelial tumors; methotrexate-vinblastine-doxorubicin-cisplatin plus unglycosylated recombinant human granulocyte-macrophage colony-stimulating factor. J Natl Cancer Inst 1990; 82:667–672.
314. Nathan FE, Besa EC. GM-CSF and accelerated hemolysis. N Eng J Med 1992; 326:417.
315. Bronchud MH, Scarffe JH, Thatcher N, et al. Phase I/II study of recombinant human granulocyte colony-stimulating factor in patients receiving intensive chemotherapy for small cell lung cancer. Br J Cancer 1987; 56:809–813.
316. Gabrilove JL, Jakubowski A, Scher H, et al. Effect of granulocyte colony-stimulating factor on neutropenia and associated morbidity due to chemotherapy for transitional-cell carcinoma of the urothelium. N Eng J Med 1988; 318:1414–1422.
317. Lindemann A, Herrmann F, Oster W, et al. Hematologic effects of recombinant human granulocyte colony-stimulating factor in patients with malignancy. Blood 1989; 74:2644–2651.
318. Mitsuyasu R, Levine J, Miles SA, et al. Effects of long term subcutaneous (SC) administration of recombinant human granulocyte-macrophage colony-stimulating factor (GM-CSF) in patients with HIV-related leukopenia. Blood 1988; 72:356.
319. Antman KS, Griffin JD, Elias A, et al. Effects of recombinant human granulocyte-macrophage colony-stimulating factor on chemotherapy induced myelosuppression. N Eng J Med 1988; 319:593–598.
320. Brandt SJ, Peters WP, Atwater SK, et al. Effect of recombinant human granulocyte-macrophage colony-stimulating factor on hematopoietic reconstitution after high-dose chemotherapy and autologous bone marrow transplantation. N Eng J Med 1988; 318:869–876.
321. Gabrilove JL, Jakubowski A, Fain K, et al. Phase I study of granulocyte colony-stimulating factor in patients with transitional cell carcinoma of the urothelium. J Clin Invest 1988; 82:1454–1461.
322. Crawford J, Ozer H, Stoller R, et al. Reduction by granulocyte colony-stimulating factor of fever and neutropenia induced by chemotherapy in patients with small-cell lung cancer. N Eng J Med 1991; 325:164–170.

323. Samlaska CP, Noyes DK. Localized cutaneous reactions to granulocyte-colony-stimulating factor. Arch Dermat 1993; 129:645–646.
324. Jaiyesimi I, Giralt SS, Wood J. Subcutaneous granulocyte colony-stimulating factor and acute anaphylaxis. N Eng J Med 1991; 325:587.
325. Brown SL, Hill E. Subcutaneous granulocyte colony-stimulating factor and acute anaphylaxis. N Eng J Med 1991; 325:587.
326. Green AR. Peptide regulatory factors. Lancet 1989; 1:705–707.
327. Falanga V. Growth factors and wound healing. J Dermat Surg Oncol 1993; 19:711–714.
328. Brown GL, Nanney LB, Griffin J, et al. Enhancement wound healing by topical treatment with epidermal growth factor. N 1989; 321:76–79.
329. Robson MC, Phillips LG, Thomason A, et al. Platelet-derived growth factor BB for the treatment of chronic pressure ulcers. Lancet 1992; 339:23–25.
330. Knighton DR, Ciresi K, Fiegel VA, et al. Stimulation of repair in chronic, non-healing, cutaneous ulcers using platelet-derived wound healing formula. Surg Gyneco Obstet 1990; 170:56–60.
331. Roberts AB, et al. Rapid induction of fibrosis and angiogenesis in vivo and stimulation of collagen formation in vitro. Proc Natl Acad Sci USA 1986; 83:4167–4171.
332. Shah M, Foreman DM, Ferguson MWJ. Control of scarring in adult wounds by neutralising antibody to transforming growth factor-beta. Lancet 1992; 339:213–214.
333. Pierce GF, Mustoe TA, Senior RM, et al. In vivo incisional wound healing augmented by platelet-derived growth factor and recombinant c-sis gene homodimeric proteins. J Exp Med 1988; 167:974–987.
334. Mustoe TA, Pierce GF, Thomason A, et al. Accelerated healing of incisional wounds in rats induced by transforming growth factor-beta. Science 1987; 237:1333–1336.
335. McGee GS, Davidson JM, Buckley A, et al. Recombinant basic fibroblast growth factor accelerates wound healing. J Surg Res 1988; 45:145–153.
336. Gu XF, Raynaud F, Evain-Brion D. Increased chemotactic and mitogenic response of psoriatic fibroblasts to platelet-derived growth factor. J Invest Dermat 1988; 91:599–602.
337. Nanney LB, Ellis D, Dale B, et al. Epidermal growth factor receptors (EGF-R) in idiopathic and virally induced hyperproliferative skin diseases. J Invest Dermat 1988; 91:592A.
338. Elder JT, Fischer GJ, Lindquist PB, et al. Overexpression of transforming growth factor alpha in psoriatic epidermis. Science 1989; 243:811–814.
339. Bauknecht T, Gross G, Hagedorn M. Epidermal growth factor receptors in different skin tumors. Dermatologica 1985; 171:16–20.
340. Prussick R, Knowles S, Shear NH. Cutaneous drug reactions. Curr Probl Dermat 1994; 6:81–124.
341. Coley WB. The treatment of malignant tumors by repeated inoculations of erysipelas; with a report of ten original cases. Am J Med Sci 1893; 105:487–511.
342. Coley WB. Treatment of inoperable malignant tumors with toxins of erysipelas and the bacillus prodigiosus. Trans Am Surg Assoc 1894; 12:183–212.

343. Coley WB. The therapeutic value of the mixed toxins of the streptococcus of erysipelas in the treatment of inoperable malignant tumors, with a report of 100 cases. Am J Med Sci 1896; 112:251–281.
344. Coley WB. Further observations upon the treatment of malignant tumors with the mixed toxins of erysipelas and Bacillus prodigiosus with a report of 160 cases. Bull Johns Hopkins Hosp 1896; 65:157–162.
345. Hung M-C, Macatee S, Leroux ME, et al. Initial characterization of transmembrane domain and cleavage sites of human pro-TNF. Tumor Necros Facto Relat Cytokin 1990; 3:138.
346. Aggarwal BB, Khor WJ, Hass PE, et al. Human tumor necrosis factor. J Biol Chem 1985; 260:2345–2354.
347. Kriegler M, Perez C, DeFay K, et al. A novel form of TNF/cachectin is a cell surface cytotoxic transmembrane protein: ramifications for the complex physiology of TNF. Cell Immunol 1988; 53:45–53.
348. Liu CC, Detmers PA, Jiang S, et al. Identification and characterization of a membrane bound cytotoxin of murine cytolytic lymphocytes that is related to tumor necrosis factor/cachectin. Proc Natl Acad Sci USA. J Biol Chem 1988; 264:3573–3576.
349. Ruddle NH, Waksman BH. Cytotoxic effect of lymphocyte-antigen interaction in delayed hypersensitivity. Science 1967; 157:1060–1062.
350. Ruddle NH, Waksman BH. Cytotoxicity mediated by soluble antigen and lymphocytes in delayed hypersensitivity. I. Characterization of the phenomenon. J Exp Med 1968; 128:1237–1254.
351. Ruddle NH, Waksman BH. Cytotoxicity mediated by soluble antigen and lymphocytes in delayed sensitivity. II. Correlation of the in vitro response with skin reactivity. J Exp Med 1968; 128:1255–1265.
352. Aggarwal BB, Moffat B, Harkins RN. Human lymphotoxin: production by a lymphoblastoid cell line, purification and initial characterization. J Biol Chem 1984; 259:686–691.
353. Muller U, Jongeneel CV, Nedospasov SA, et al. Tumor necrosis factor and lymphotoxin gene map close to h = 2d in the mouse major histocompatibility complex. Nature 1987; 325:265–267.
354. Aggarwal BB, Eessalu TE, Hass PE. Characterization of receptors for human necrosis factor and their regulation by gamma-interferon. Nature 1985; 318:665–667.
355. Stauber GB, Aggarwal BB. Characterization and affinity cross-linking of receptors for human recombinant lymphotoxin (tumor necrosis factor bata) on a human histocytic lymphoma cell line, U-937. J Biol Chem 1988; 264:3573–3576.
356. Aggarwal BB, Henzel WJ, Moffat B, et al. Primary structure of human lymphotoxin derived from 1788 lymphoblastoid cell line. J Biol Chem 1985; 260:2334–2344.
357. Djeu JY, Serbousek D, Blanchard DK. Release of tumor necrosis factor by human polymorphonuclear leucocytes. Blood 1990; 76:1405–1409.
358. Gordon JR, Galli SJ. Mast cells as a source of both preformed and immunologically inducible TNF-alpha/cachetin. Nature 1990; 346:274–276.

359. Kock A, Schwartz T, Krinbaumer R, et al. Human keratinocytes are a source for tumor necrosis factor alpha: evidence for synthesis and release upon stimulation with endotoxin or ultraviolet light. J Exp Med 1990; 172:1609–1614.
360. Philip R, Epstein LB. Tumor necrosis factor as immunomodulator and mediator of monocyte cytotoxicity induced by itself, interferon gamma and interleukin. Nature 1986; 323:86–89.
361. Seelentag WK, Mermod JJ, Montesano R, et al. Addictive effects of interleukin-1 and tumor necrosis factor-alpha on the accumulation of three granulocyte and macrophage colony stimulating factor mRNA in human endothelial cells. EMBO J 1987; 6:2261–2265.
362. Hajjar KA, Hajjar DP, Silverstein RL, et al. Tumor necrosis factor mediated release of platelet derived growth factor from cultured endothelial cells. J Exp Med 1987; 166:235–245.
363. Le JM, Vileck J. Interleukin-6 a multifunctional cytokine regulating immune reactions and the acute phase protein response. Lab Invest 1989; 61:588–602.
364. Strieter RM, Kunkel SL, Showell HJ, et al. Endothelial cell gene expression of a neutrophil chemotactic factor by TNF-alfa, LPS, and IL-1-beta. Science 1989; 243:1467–1469.
365. Dayer JM, Beutler B, Cerami A. Cahectin/tumor necrosis factor stimulates colagenase and prostaglandin E2 production by human synovial cells and dermal fibroblasts. J Exp Med 1985; 162:2163–2168.
366. Kishimoto TK, Larson RS, Corbi AL, et al. The leukocytes integrins. Adv Immunol 1989; 46:149–182.
367. Pober JS, Bevilacqua MP, Mendrick DL, et al. Two distinct monokines, interleukin 1 and tumor necrosis factor, each independently induce the biosynthesis and transient expression of the same antigen on the surface of cultured human vascular endothelial cells. J Immunol 1986; 136:1680–1687.
368. Griffiths CEM, Voorhees JJ, Nickoloff BJ. Characterization of intercellular adhesion molecule-1 and HLA-DR expression in normal and inflamed skin: modulation by recombinant gamma interferon and tumor necrosis factor. J Am Acad Dermat 1989; 20:617–629.
369. Inaba K, Steinman RM. Resting and sensitized T lymphocytes exhibits distinct (antigen presenting cell) requirements for growth and lymphokine release. J Exp Med 1984; 160:1717–1735.
370. Wollf K, Stingl G. The Langerhans cell. J Invest Dermat 1983; 80:17–21.
371. Semma M, Sagami S. Induction of suppressor T cells to DNFB contact hypersensitivity by application of sensitizer through Langerhans cell deficient skin. Arch Dermat Res 1981; 271:361–364.
372. Rheins LA, Nordlund JJ. Modulation of the population density of identifiable Langerhans cells associated with enhancement or suppression of cutaneous immune reactivity. J Immunol 1986; 136:867–876.
373. Macatonia SE, Edwards AJ, Knight SC. Dendritic cells and the initiation of contact sensitivity of fluorescein isothiocyanate. Immunol Allerg Clin N Am 1991; 74:139–145.

374. Kinnaird A, Peters SW, Poster JR, et al. Dentritic cells accumulation in the draining lymph nodes during the induction phase of contact allergy in mice. Int Arch Allerg Appl Immunol 1989; 89:202–210.
375. Cumberbatch M, Illingworth I, Kimber I. Antigen bearing dendritic cells in the draining lymph nodes of contact sensitized mice. Immunol Allerg Clin N Am 1991; 74:129–145.
376. Koch F, Heufler C, Kampgen E, et al. Tumor necrosis factor alpha maintains the viability of murine epidermal Langerhans cells in culture, but, in contrast to granulocyte/macrophage colony stimulating factor, does not induce their functional maturation. J Exp Med 1990; 171:159–171.
377. Cumberbatch M, Kimber I. Dermal tumor necrosis factor-alpha induces dendritic cell migration to draining lymph nodes, and possibly provides one stimulus for Langerhans cell migration. Immunol Allerg Clin N Am 1992; 75:257–263.
378. Piguet PF, Grau GE, Hauser C, et al. Tumor necrosis factor is a critical mediator in hapten induced irritant and contact hypersensitivity reactions. J Exp Med 1991; 173:257–263.
379. Kurimoto I, Streilein JW. Cis-urocanic acid suppression of contact hypersensitivity induction is mediated via tumor necrosis factor alpha. J Immunol 1992; 148:3072–3078.
380. Vermeer M, Streilein JW. Ultraviolet B light induced alterations in epidermal Langerhans cells are mediated in part by tumor necrosis factor alpha. Photodermat Photoimmunol Photomed 1990; 7:258–265.
381. Hunziker T, Brand CU, Kapp A, et al. Increased levels of inflammatory cytokines in human skin lymph derived from sodium lauryl sulphate induced contact dermatitis. Br J Dermat 1992; 127:254–257.
382. Griffths CE, Barker JNWN, Kunkel S, et al. Modulation of leukocyte adhesion molecules, a T-cell chemotaxin (IL-8), and regulatory cytokine TNF-α in allergic dermatitis (rhus dermatitis). Br J Dermat 1991; 124:519–526.
383. Jacob CO. Tumor necrosis factor α in autoimmunity: pretty girl or old witch. Immunol Today 1992; 13:122–125.
384. Jablonska S, Chowaniece O, Beut Aciejowska E, et al. Stripping of the stratum corneum in patients with psoriasis. Arch Dermat 1992; 118:652–657.
385. Braun Falco O, Schmoeckel C. The dermal inflammatory reactions in initial psoriatic lesions. Arch Dermat Res 1977; 258:9–16.
386. Ragaz A, Ackerman AB. Evolution, maturation, and regression of lesions of psoriasis: new observations and correlations of clinical and histologic findings. Am J Dermatopathol 1979; 1:199–214.
387. Schubert C, Christophers E. Mast cell and macrophages in early relapsing psoriasis. Arch Dermat Res 1985; 277:352–358.
388. Cox AJ. Mast cells in psoriasis. In: Farber EM, Cox AJ, eds. Psoriasis. New York: Yorke Medical, 1977:36–43.
389. Nickoloff BJ, Karabin GD, Barker JNWN, et al. Cellular localization of interleukin-8 and its inducer, tumor necrosis factor-alpha in psoriasis. Am J Pathol 1991; 138:129–140.

390. Nickoloff BJ, Griffiths C. Lymphocyte trafficking in psoriasis. J Invest Dermat 1990; 95:35S–37S.
391. Takematsu H, Ozawa H, Yoshimura T, et al. Systemic TNF administration in psoriatic patients: a promising therapeutic modality for severe psoriasis. Third Int Conf TNF Relate Cytokin 1990; W4B-6.
392. Takematsu H, Ozawa H, Yoshimura T, et al. Systemic TNF administration in psoriatic patients: a promising therapeutic modality for severe psoriasis. Br J Dermat 1991; 124:209–210.
393. Takematsu H, Tagami H. Absence of tumor necrosis factor-α in suction blister fluids and stratum corneum from patients with psoriasis. Arch Dermat Res 1989; 281:398–400.
394. Gomi T, Shiohara T, Munakata T, et al. Interleukin 1α, tumor necrosis factor α and interferon γ in psoriasis. Arch Dermat 1991; 127:827–830.
395. Baker JN, Karabin GD, Stoof TJ, et al. Detection of interferon-gamma mRNA in psoriatic epidermis by polymerase chain reaction. J Dermat Surg Oncol 1991; 2:106–111.
396. Boehm KD, Yun JK, Elmets CA. Demonstration of IL-1 and TNF-α mRNAs *in situ* in normal skin. J Invest Dermat 1991; 96:611.
397. Kristensen M, Chu CQ, Eedy DJ, et al. Localization of tumor necrosis factor-alpha (TNF-α) and its receptors in normal and psoriatic skin: epidermal cells express the 55-kD but not the 75-kD TNF receptor. Clin Exp Immunol 1993; 94:354–362.

9

Hydroxyurea: Mechanisms of Action and Usage in Dermatology

Jack L. Arbiser
Harvard Medical School, Boston, Massachusetts
Samuel L. Moschella
Lahey-Hitchcock Clinic, Burlington, Massachusetts

Hydroxyurea is an antimetabolite useful in the outpatient therapy of hematological malignancies, such as chronic myelogenous leukemia, and in the management of severe dermatologic problems, including recalcitrant psoriasis and hypereosinophilic syndrome. Hydroxyurea acts primarily through inhibiting the conversion of ribonucleotides to deoxyribonucleotides, thus halting DNA synthesis and cell growth. In addition, hydroxyurea has lesser known effects on cellular growth and gene regulation which may prove useful in the treatment of other dermatological disorders, such as melanoma. The low cost, oral bioavailability, and rapid reversal of most side effects upon discontinuation of the drug make it a rational choice for recalcitrant psoriasis.

I. MECHANISMS OF ACTION

Hydroxyurea is a compound with a molecular weight of less than 100, which has cytostatic, cytocidal, and immunomodulating properties, and regulates genes at transcriptional and posttranscriptional levels (1). This compound was first synthesized by Dressler and Stein in 1869, but its was not known to be biologically active until 1928, when Rosenthal found it to produce a hematological picture similar to that of pernicious anemia, most notably a megaloblastic anemia (2). This effect led investigators to believe that hydroxyurea acted through the inhibition of DNA synthesis (3,4), and this inhibition has been shown to occur at the level of ribonucleotide reductase, which converts ribonucleotides to deoxyribonucleotides, the precursors of DNA (5,6).

Multiple analogs of hydroxyurea have been synthesized as chemotherapy agents, but none of these agents has been clinically evaluated (7).

Ribonucleotide reductase is a highly conserved enzyme consisting of two component proteins, a regulatory and a catalytic subunit (8). This structure is conserved from bacteria through humans, indicating its importance (9–11). The regulatory subunit of ribonucleotide reductase is regulated by the quantity of deoxyribonucleotides (12,13). The catalytic subunit contains a tyrosine-associated free radical that is inactivated by hydroxyurea (13).

Other factors regulate the activity of these genes. The regulatory subunit is expressed at a constant level in actively dividing cells, while the level of catalytic subunit expression varies with position in the cell cycle, and is regulated by other stimuli, such as DNA-damaging agents and cellular second messengers (14–19). The actual mechanisms of this regulation are currently unknown.

A. Ribonucleotide Reductase Inhibition

The inhibition of ribonucleotide reductase by hydroxyurea leads to profound changes in intracellular nucleotide pool concentrations. This enzyme catalyzes the reduction of ribonucleoside diphosphates into the corresponding deoxyribonucleotide diphosphates, which are subsequently converted into triphosphates, the precursors for DNA synthesis. Not all deoxynucleotide precursors are affected equally. Intracellular levels of deoxyadenosine, deoxyguanosine, and deoxycytidine were decreased by hydroxyurea treatment, while deoxythymidine levels were increased (20).

Resistance to hydroxyurea has been observed in mammalian cells (21,22). The clinical significance of this has yet to be established. Amplification of both M1 and M2 subunits has been observed at the level of DNA, RNA, and protein in mammalian cell lines, as well as alteration of the biochemical properties of the subunits (23,24). Posttransciptional mechanisms have also been shown to play a role in increasing levels of hydroxyurea resistance in cultured cells (25). Other genes have been shown to be amplified in addition to the ribonucleotide reductase genes. These genes include ferritin (26), ornithine decarboxylase (27), and a member of the phospholipase C family (28). Whether these genes are amplified as part of an amplicon or contribute to hydroxyurea resistance remains to be determined.

B. Inhibition of DNA Repair and Gene Amplification

Hydroxyurea has other properties that may lead to its increased usefulness in the clinical setting. Hydroxyurea has been demonstrated to inhibit repair of DNA damage induced by ultraviolet and ionizing radiation, and it has found clinical use as a radiation sensitizer (29,30). Incubation of tumor cells in vitro with hydroxyurea has been shown to cause breakage of mature DNA strands; this damage could be partially prevented by addition of all four deoxynucleotides. The addition of fewer than three deoxynucleotides was ineffective in reversing this DNA damage, suggesting that imbalances in DNA precursors may result in DNA damage (31). Hydroxyurea is unique among the antimetabolites in that its effects are rapidly reversible when the drug is withdrawn. Hydroxyurea has been shown to decrease the level of expression of highly amplified genes in tumor cells, such as the c-myc oncogene and the multidrug resistance gene (mdr1), which exports lipophilic chemotherapeutic agents from tumor cells, and has been shown to contribute to chemotherapy resistance (32–34).

Hydroxyurea has also been found to induce fetal hemoglobin expression in patients with sickle cell anemia—in addition to 5-azacytidine and cytosine arabinoside—and since the side effects of hydroxyurea are milder that 5-azacytidine or cytosine arabinoside, hydroxyurea has found a role in the treatment of sickle cell anemia (35–37).

C. Methylation and Other Effects on Gene Expression

The mechanism by which hydroxyurea affects gene expression remains unknown. Hydroxyurea has been shown to cause hypomethylation of the fetal hemoglobin gene (HbF), and hypomethylation of genes is associated with increased transcription. Other examples of genes induced by hydroxyurea include the human chorionic gonadotropin-α and -β subunit genes (40). Mechanistic studies on the mechanism of hydroxyurea induction of these genes suggest that they are induced by mechanisms other than the cyclic AMP second messenger pathway (41). It is possible that the induction of fetal hemoglobin in patients with sickle cell anemia, the normalization of the morphology of psoriatic skin through the induction of differentiation, and the induction of genes in in vitro systems occurs through hypomethylation or other changes in chromatin. At present, the role of ribonucleotide reductase inhibition in these effects has not been established.

In addition to its inhibition of ribonucleotide reductase, hydroxyurea may have other biological activities. Treatment of cells with hydroxyurea has been shown to induce epigenetic changes, such as loss of amplified genes on episomes or double-minute DNA (42). Treatment of B16 melanoma cells with hydroxyurea has been shown to transiently induce an increase in the activity of cellular glutathione reductase and glutathione peroxidase, enzymes important in maintaining levels of glutathione, a cellular antioxidant (43).

Hydroxyurea may interplay with other cellular second messenger signaling pathways. Inhibition of cell cycle in murine Swiss 3T3 fibroblasts with hydroxyurea leads to down-regulation of MARCKS protein and mRNA, the major substrate of protein kinase C, when these cells were fed with serum poor media (44). This protein can be down-regulated by a number of of peptides through pathways that involve and are independent of protein kinase C. The precise function of MARCKS is not known, but it may link cell cycle regulation to second messenger pathways.

Hydroxyurea is an inexpensive and relatively safe antimetabolite used in the treatment of severe psoriasis, eosinophilic cellulitis, the stable phase of chronic myelocytic leukemia, sickle cell anemia, and polycythemia vera. Increased knowledge of its mechanism of action should lead to expanded use as a radiation sensitizer and biochemical modulator of DNA synthesis.

II. PHARMACOLOGY

Hydroxyurea has found wide use in the treatment of neoplastic and nonneoplastic disease because of its biological activity and pharmacological availablitity. It is most commonly administered orally in the usual dose of 20–30 mg/kg. After administration, it is rapidly absorbed, with peak serum concentrations reached at 1–2 h and a serum half-life of 5.5 h (45). Hydroxyurea crosses the blood-brain barrier easily, and peak CSF levels are obtained 3 h after administration (46). The prime method of excretion is renal, with up to 70% of a given dose being excreted unchanged into the urine. A small proportion is metabolized into carbon dioxide, which is expired (45).

III. CLINICAL INDICATIONS

A. Psoriasis

Hydroxyurea was initially used by Yarbro et al., at a dosage of 40 mg/kg/d, with excellent results, in two patients with refractory psoriasis (47). This was followed by a double-blind study by Leavell and Yarbro (48), who noted significant histological and clinical improvement in the hydroxyurea treated group. This trial involved 10 patients who received either 4 wk of placebo or 4 wk of hydroxyurea at a dosage of 500 mg twice daily, and then were crossed over. Histologically there was a decrease in psoriasiform hyperplasia. Rebound was not observed after discontinuation of the drug, and several patients went into long-term remission. No serious side effects were observed and no significant depression in any of the three hematopoietic lines was observed. A larger group of 60 patients was studied by Moschella and Greenwald over a period of 18 mo, with good to excellent results in 63% (49). In this study, intermittent therapy with intervals of 4–12 wk was utilized to maintain response. A small but significant number of patients became refractory to further courses of hydroxyurea over a period of several months. Clinical improvement in this study was defined in terms of lessening pruritus, reduction in scale and erythema, extent of clearing of psoriatic lesions, and reduction of arthritis and arthralgia. Side effects included flu-like syndromes, cutaneous vasculitis, leukopenia, and in one instance, a fixed drug reaction (49). Hydroxyurea has also been found to be of value in pustular and erythrodermic psoriasis (50). In recent years hydroxyurea has not been used regularly for the treatment of psoriasis. Reasons for this include studies that have shown hydroxyurea to be of little benefit and the belief that hydroxyurea is of benefit for a limited time of several months (51).

Topical hydroxyurea has been attempted in the treatment of psoriasis, but has not been found effective, except in a 10% cream and only when used under occlusion. Perhaps changes in vehicle preparation, or the use of more lipophilic analogs may result in more effective topical preparations, but this is not an area of active investigation.

Hydroxyurea may find its place as a component of combination therapy for psoriasis, in combination with methotrexate, which may regulate ribonucleotide reductase activity (52,53), given that part of its activity is cell-cycle dependent, with ultraviolet light, given that hydroxyurea inhibits DNA repair enzymes, and with retinoids.

IV. HYPEREOSINOPHILIC SYNDROME

Hypereosinophilic syndrome is characterized by increased numbers of circulating eosinophilis and organ damage secondary to eosinophilis in the absence of known causes of eosinophilia. These conditions include asthma, connective tissue disease, parasitic infection, neoplasia, and allergic reactions. The organ damage produced by eosinophils includes space occupying eosinophilic infiltration, eosinophil-mediated cytotoxicity, including that mediated by toxic proteins secreted by eosinophils, and thromboembolic phenomena. The organs most commonly involved are the heart, gastrointestinal tract, central nervous system, and bone marrow. Initial therapy of hypereosinophilic syndrome uses high-dose prednisone; but in patients with disease nonresponsive to steroids, hydroxyurea in doses of 0.5–1.5 g daily is useful in controlling the disease. The major cause of death from hypereosinophilia is endomyocardial fibrosis of inflow tracts to both ventricles. The pathogenic role of the eosinophil in this disorder has been suggested by the similar histological findings in hypereosinophilic syndrome and eosinophilic leukemia (54).

Untreated, the prognosis is poor; with treatment, the prognosis is variable. Some cases are characterized by chromosomal abnormalities progressed to myeloid leukemia (54).

V. MALIGNANT MELANOMA

Metastatic melanoma remains a therapeutic challenge, and current therapy is unsatisfactory. Presently, the agents of choice are dimethylaminotriazenecarboxamide (DTIC), sometimes in combination with tamoxifen, and nitrosoureas (55,56). Interleukin-2-based immunotherapy has provided striking responses in a small number of cases (57). In an early trial, hydroxyurea as a single agent has induced short-lived responses in metastatic melanoma (58). Better responses were seen when hydroxyurea was combined with DTIC and bischloroethylnitrosourea (BCNU) (56). Hydroxyurea as a single agent will probably not find much utility in the treatment of melanoma, but given its partial efficacy and relatively benign side-effect profile, it may become a part of combination chemotherapy regimens for melanoma.

VI. MISCELLANEOUS SKIN DISORDERS

Polycythemia vera is not a primary skin disorder, but is often associated with severe pruritus. The etiology of this pruritus is currently not known, but it has been shown to be responsive to hydroxyurea treatment (59). The main criteria for treatment of polycythemia vera are elevated hematocrit and thrombocytosis, which predisposes to embolic phenomena (60). A major concern in the treatment of polycythemia vera is the progression to myeloid leukemia, which occurs spontaneously, but may be hastened by agents used to control the disorder such as radioactive phosphorus and alkylating agents (61). The increase in the incidence of acute leukemia in patients treated with radioactive phosphorus and alkylating agents has led to their disuse in the treatment of polycythemia vera, and the combination of hydroxyurea and phlebotomy is now a standard therapy. Nand et al. has noted an increased incidence of transformation to acute leukemia in a small series of patients treated with hydroxyurea (62). Thus the use of hydroxyurea for the treatment of polycythemia vera-related pruritus must be balanced against the potential risks of transformation to acute leukemia and should be compared with phlebotomy alone, which has a low risk of malignant transformation, but an increased risk of thrombotic complications.

Sweet's syndrome (acute febrile neutrophilic dermatosis) is a disease of unknown etiology that presents as edematous red plaques on multiple skin sites. Histologically these plaques are characterized by neutrophilic infiltration of the dermis (63). Therapy of these lesions has included prednisone and dapsone (63). Osterwalder et al. report a case associated with an unclassified myeloproliferative disorder that appeared to respond to hydroxyurea (64). Further study is necessary to determine whether hydroxyurea is efficacious for the treatment of Sweet's syndrome.

VII. ADVERSE REACTIONS

The most common and dose-limiting side effect of hydroxyurea is bone marrow suppression, which may occur within 48 h of oral administration. Once the drug is removed, leucocytes recover rapidly, but platelet counts may require up to 2 wk for recovery (30).

A variety of cutaneous side effects have been observed. These include lichen planus and dermatomyositis-like reactions, as well as hyperpigmentation and erythema in previously irradiated sites (65–69). Cutaneous side effects rarely necessitate discontinuation of drug.

Hydroxyurea is a teratogen and is absolutely contraindicated in pregnancy or lactation (51). Other uncommon side effects include transient transaminase increases, proteinuria, and increased creatinine and blood urea nitrogen (30,51). No official guidelines have been established for the dermatological use of hydroxyurea, but the recommendations of Boyd and Neldner are extremely reasonable (51). With careful monitoring and appropriate patient selection, hydroxyurea can be used safely and effectively.

VIII. SUMMARY

Hydroxyurea is a chemically simple agent useful in the treatment of hyperproliferative disorders, both benign and malignant. Its primary site of action is the inhibition of ribonucleotide reductase, resulting in nucleotide pool imbalance and subsequent inhibition of DNA synthesis. This inhibition does not fully explain some of the other effects of hydroxyurea, such as potentiation of radiation sensitivity, decreased gene amplification, and augmentation of fetal hemoglobin production, as well as its degree of selectivity to the skin. Hydroxyurea is a useful agent for psoriasis and hypereosinophilic syndrome. Given its multiple properties, benign side-effect profile, and low cost, it will likely be used in combination chemotherapy for a wide variety of malignancies, including melanoma.

REFERENCES

1. Dressler WF, Stein R. Uber den hydroxylharnstoff. Justus Liebigs Ann Chem 1869; 150:242.
2. Rosenthal F, Wislicki L, Koller L. Uber die beziehungen von schwersten blutgiften zu abbauprodukten des eiweisses: ein betrag zum entstehungmechanismus der pernizoisen anemie. Klin Wochensch 1928; 7:972.
3. Yarbro JW, Kennedy BJ, Barnum CP. Hydroxyurea inhibition of DNA synthesis in ascites tumor. Proc Natl Acad Sci USA 1965; 53:1033.

4. Yarbro JW, Niehaus WG, Barnum CP. Effect of hydroxyurea on regenerating rat liver. Biochem Biophys Res Commun 1965; 19:592.
5. Krakoff IH, Brown NC, Reichard P. Inhibition of ribonucleoside diphosphate reductase by hydroxyurea. Cancer Res 1968; 28:1559.
6. Thelander L, Reichard P. Reduction of ribonucleotides. Annu Rev Biochem 1979; 48:133.
7. Timson J. Hydroxyurea. Mutation Res 1975; 32:115.
8. Reichard P, Ehrenberg A. Ribonucleotide reductase: a radical enzyme. Science 1983; 221:514.
9. Fontecave M, Eliasson R, Reichard P. Enzymatic regulation of the radical content of the small subunit of *escherichia coli* ribonucleotide reductase involving reduction of its redox centers. J Biol Chem 1989; 264:9164.
10. Graslund A, Ehrenberg A, Thelander L. Characterization of the free radical of mammalian ribonucleotide reductase. J Biol Chem 1982; 257:5711.
11. Thelander M, Graslund A, Thelander L. Subunit M2 of mammalian ribonucleotide reductase. J Biol Chem 1985; 260:2734.
12. Atkin CL, Thelander L, Reichard P, et al. Iron and free radical in ribonucleotide reductase. Exchange of iron and Mossbauer spectroscopy of the protein B2 subunit of the *Escherichia coli* enzyme J Biol Chem 1973; 248:7464.
13. Lassman G, Liermann B. ESR studies of structure and kinetics of radicals from hydroxyurea, an antitumor drug directed against ribonucleotide reductase. Free Radic Biol Med 1989; 6:241.
14. Elledge SJ, Davis RW. Two genes differentially regulated in the cell cycle and by DNA-damaging agents encode alternative regulatory subunits of ribonucleotide reductase. Genes Dev 1990; 4:740.
15. Wright JA, Chan AK, Choy BK, Hurta RA, McClarty GA, Tagger AY. Regulation and drug resistance mechanisms of mammalian ribonucleotide reductase, and the significance to DNA synthesis. Biochem Cell Biol 1990; 68:1364.
16. McClarty GA, Chan AK, Choy BK, Wright JA, Thelander L. Elevated expression of M1 and M2 components and drug induced post-transcriptional modulation of ribonucleotide reductase in a hydroxyurea-resistant mouse cell line. Biochemistry 1987; 26:8004.
17. Choy BK, McClarty GA, Wright JA. Transient elevation of ribonucleotide reductase activity, M2 mRNA, and M2 protein in Balb/c 3T3 fibroblasts in the presence of 12-O-tetradecanoyl-13-acetate. Biochem Biophys Res Commun 1989; 162:1417.
18. Fornace AJ, Nebert DW, Hollander MC, et al. Mammalian genes coordinately regulated by growth arrest signals and DNA damaging agents. Mol Cell Biol 1989; 9:4196.
19. McClarty GA, Chan AK, Choy BK, Thelander L, Wright JA. Molecular mechanisms responsible for the drug-induced posttranscriptional modulation of ribonucleotide reductase levels in a hydroxyurea-resistant mouse L cell line. Biochemistry 1988; 27:7524.
20. Bianchi V, Pontis E, Reichard P. Changes of deoxyribonucleoside triphosphate pools induced by hydroxyurea and their relation to DNA synthesis. J Biol Chem 1986; 261:16037.

21. Hurta RA, Wright JA. Amplification of the genes for both components of ribonucleotide reductase in hydroxyurea resistant mammalian cells. Biochem Biophys Res Commun 1990; 167:258.
22. Caras IW, Martin DW. Molecular cloning of the cDNA for a mutant mouse ribonucleotide reductase M1 that produces a dominant mutator phenotype in mammalian cells. Mol Cell Biol 1988; 8:2698.
23. Wright JA. Altered mammalian ribonucleoside diphosphate reductase from mutant cell lines. Int Encycl Pharmacol Ther 1989; 128:89.
24. Choy BK, McClarty GA, Chan Ak, et al. Molecular mechanisms of drug resistance involving ribonucleotide reductase: hydroxyurea resistance in a series of clonally related mouse cell lines selected in the presence of increasing drug concentrations. Cancer Res 1988; 48:2029.
25. McClarty GA, Chan AK, Choy BK, Wright JA. Increased ferritin gene expression is associated with increased ribonucleotide reductase gene expression and the establishment of hydroxyurea resistance in mammalian cells. J Biol Chem 1990; 265:7539.
26. Srinivasan PR, Tonin PN, Wensing EJ, Lewis WH. The gene for ornithine decarboxylase is co-amplified in hydroxyurea resistant hamster cells. J Biol Chem 1987; 262:12871.
27. Chaudhuri MM, Tonin PN, Lewis WH, Srinivasan PR. The gene for a novel protein, a member of the protein disulphide isomerase/form 1 phosphoinositide-specific phospholipase C family, is amplified in hydroxyurea resistant cells. Biochem J 1992; 281:645.
29. Francis AA, Blevins RD, Carrier WL, et al. Inhibition of DNA repair in ultraviolet-irradiated human cells by hydroxyurea. Biochem Biophys Acta 1979; 563:385.
30. Donehower RC. An overview of the clinical experience with hydroxyurea. Semin Oncol 1992; 19:11.
31. Li JC, Kaminskas E. Progressive formation of DNA lesions in cultured Ehrlich ascites tumor cells treated with hydroxyurea. Cancer Res 1987; 47:2755.
32. Christen RD, Shalinsky DR, Howell SB. Enhancement of the loss of multiple drug resistance by hydroxyurea. Semin Oncol 19:94.
33. Von Hoff DD, Waddelow T, Forseth B, Davidson K, Scott J, Wahl G. Hydroxyurea accelerates loss of extrachromosomally amplified genes from tumor cells. Cancer Res 1991; 51:6273.
34. Snapka RM, Varshavsky A. Loss of unstably amplified dihydrofolate reductase genes from mouse cells is greatly accelerated by hydroxyurea. Proc Natl Acad Sci USA 1983; 80:7533.
35. Dover GJ, Charache S. Hydroxyurea induction of fetal hemoglobin synthesis in sickle cell disease. Semin Oncol 1992; 19:61.
36. Goldberg MA, Brugnara C, Dover GJ, et al. Treatment of sickle cell anemia with hydroxyurea nad erythropoietin. N Engl J Med 1990; 323:366.
37. Charache S, Dover GJ. Hydroxyurea therapy for sickle cell anemia. Blood 1987; 69:109.
38. Galanello R, Stamatoyannopoulos G, Papayannopoulou T. Mechanism of HbF stimulation by S-stage compounds: in vitro studies with bone marrow cells exposed to 5-azacytidine, ara-C, or hydroxyurea. J Clin Invest 1988; 81:1209.

39. Watson JD, Hopkins NH, Roberts JW, Steitz JA, Weiner A. eds. Molecular biology of the gene. Reading, Mass.: Benjamin/Cummings, 1987.
40. Arbiser JL, Arbiser ZK, Majzoub JA. Regulation of gene expression in choriocarcinoma by methotrexate and hydroxyurea. Endocrinology 1991; 128:972.
41. Arbiser JL, Arbiser ZK, Majzoub JA. Effect of hydroxyurea and cyclic AMP/protein kinase A inhibitors of human chorionic gonadotropin alpha and c-myc expression in choriocarcinoma. J Endocrinol Invest 1993; 16:849–850.
42. Christen RD, Shalinsky DR, Howell SB. Enhancement of the loss of multiple drug resistance by hydroxyurea. Semin Oncol 1992; 19:94.
43. Eskenazi AE, Pinkas J, Whitin JC, et al. Role of antioxidant enzymes in the induction of increased experimental metastasis by hydroxyurea. J Natl Cancer Inst 1993; 9:711.
44. Herget T, Brooks SF, Broad S, Rozengurt E. Expression of the major protein kinase C substrate, the acidic 80-kD myristoylated alanine-rich C kinase substrate, increases sharply when Swiss 3T3 cells move out of cycle and enter G0. Proc Natl Acad Sci USA 1993; 90:2945.
45. Yarbro JW. Mechanism of action of hydroxyurea. Semin Oncol 1992; 19:1.
46. Dorr RT, Fritz WL. Cancer chemotherapy handbook. New York: Elsevier, 1983:468–471.
47. Yarbro JW. Hydroxyurea in psoriasis. Lancet 1969; 2:846.
48. Leavell UW, Yarbro JW. Hydroxyurea: a new treatment for psoriasis. Arch Dermat 1970; 102:144.
49. Moschella SL, Greenwald MA. Psoriasis with hydroxyurea: an 18-month study of 60 patients. Arch Dermat 1973; 107:363.
50. Stein KM, Shelley WB, Weinberg RA. Hydroxyurea in the treatment of pustular psoriasis. Br J Dermat 1971; 85:81.
51. Boyd AS, Neldner KH. Hydroxyurea therapy. J Am Acad Dermat 1991; 25:518.
52. Sauer GC. Combined methotrexate and hydroxyurea therapy for psoriasis. Arch Dermat 1973; 107:369.
53. Schilsky RL, Ratain MJ, Vokes EE, Vogelzank NJ, Anderson J, Peterson BA. Laboratory and clinical studies of biochemical modulation by hydroxyurea. Semin Oncol 1992; 19:84.
54. Fauci AS. The idiopathic hypereosinophilic syndrome. Ann Intern Med 1982; 97:78.
55. Coconni G, Bella M, Calabresi F, et al. Treatment of metastatic melanoma with dacrbazine plus tamoxifen. N Engl J Med 1992; 327:516.
56. Costanzi JJ, Vaitkevicius V, Quagliana JM, Hoogstraten B, Coltman CA, Delaney FC. Combination chemotherapy for disseminated malignant melanoma. Cancer 1975; 35:342.
57. Rosenberg SA, Lotze MT, Muul LM, et al. Observations on the systemic administration of autologous lymphokine-activated killer cells and recombinant interleukin-2 to patients with metastatic cancer. N Engl J Med 1985; 313:1485.
58. Gottlieb JA, Frei E III, Luce K. Dose schedule studies with hydroxyurea in malignant melanoma. Cancer Chemother Rep 1971; 55:277.
59. Sharon R, Tatarsky I, Ben-Arieh Y. Treatment of polycythemia vera with hydroxyurea. Cancer 1986; 57:718.

60. Donovan PB, Kaplan ME, Goldberg JD, et al. Treatment of polycythemia vera with hydroxyurea. Am J Hematol 1984; 17:329.
61. Kaplan ME, Mack K, Goldberg JD, Donovan PB, Berk PD, Wasserman LR. Long-term management of polycythemia vera with hydroxyurea: a progress report. Semin Hematol 1986; 23:167.
62. Nand S, Messmore H, Fisher SG, Bird ML, Schulz W, Fisher RI. Leukemic transformation in polycythemia vera. Am J Hematol 1990; 34:32.
63. Greer KE, Cooper PH. Sweet's syndrome (acute febrile neutrophilic dermatosis). Clin Rheum Dis 1982; 8:427.
64. Osterwalder B, Schmid L, Jungi WF, Flury R, Schmid U, Staub P, Senn HJ. Myeloproliferatives syndrome und akute febrile neutrophile dermatose (Sweet-syndrome)-eine seltene assoziation. Schweiz Med Wschr 1987; 117:1896.
65. Kennedy BJ, Smith LR, Goltz RW. Skin changes secondary to hydroxyurea. Arch Dermat 1975; 111:183.
66. Renfro L, Kamino H, Raphael J, Moy J, Sanchez M. Ulcerative lichen planus like dermatitis associated with hydroxyurea. J Am Acad Dermat 1991; 24:143.
67. Richard M, Truchetet F, Friedel J, et al. Skin lesions simulating chronic dermatomyositis during long-term hydroxyurea therapy. J Am Acad Dermat 1989; 21:797.
68. Sears ME. Erythema in area of prevoius irradiation in patients treated with hydroxyurea. Cancer Chemother Rep 1965; 40:31.
69. DeSpain JD. Dermatologic toxicity of chemotherapy. Semin Oncol 1992; 19:501.

10
Cyclosporine

Charles J. McDonald
Brown University, Providence, Rhode Island

I. CHEMISTRY

Cyclosporine (cyclosporine A, CSA, Sandimmune®) is an 11 amino acid cyclic polypeptide product of the fungi *Tolypocladium inflatum games* and *Cylindrocarpeu lucidum* (Figure 1). The immunosuppressive properties of this agent have been shown to be quite profound, and yet unlike other conventional immunosuppressives, cyclosporine does not appear to be cytotoxic. Cyclosporine appears to exert its most profound effects through its ability to inhibit clonal expansion and maturation of memory and effector T cells. Cyclosporine effect on treated cells is unique because it is nonlethal. Subsequent to treatment with cyclosporine the immune competence of cyclosporine treated cells will return to normal as does the total immune system of the host. Whereas conventional immunosuppressive agents preferentially kill proliferating lymphocyte clones that respond to antigen and prolonged treatment with conventional agents can lead to depletion of immunological memory at the T-cell level. Additionally, cyclosporine does not interfere with generation and maturation of phagocytic cells within bone marrow and it does not appear to have any measurable effect on peripheral phagocytic function. Thus, unlike patients treated with conventional agents, infections are not problematic in patients treated with cyclosporine alone.

Largely because of its reversible effects on the immune system of the treated host, cyclosporine has become the "gold" standard for treatment of a wide variety of autoimmune disorders of the skin and other organ systems, as well as for prophylaxis of graft rejection in organ transplant recipients (1). Cyclosporine has also been widely used in the treatment of psoriasis, a disease heretofore characterized principally by cellular hyperplasia (2–6).

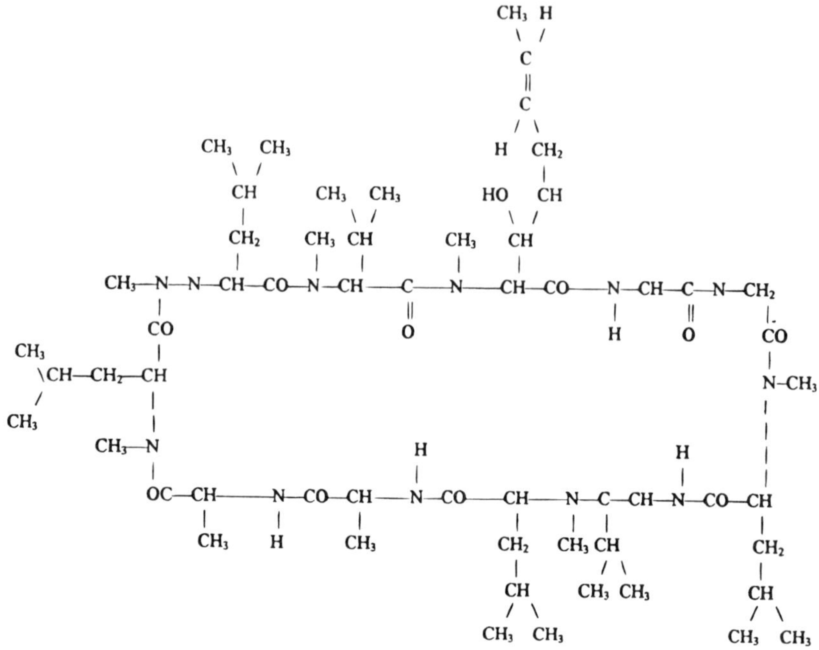

Figure 1 Chemical structure of cyclosporine.

II. MECHANISM OF ACTION

The ability of psoriasis to improve after treatment with cyclosporine has stimulated numerous investigations of cellular immunological mechanisms in this disease. Yet, very much like studies of the immunological mechanisms that enable cyclosporine to prevent graft rejection, results from studies of immunological mechanisms in psoriasis remain controversial. This is especially true of postulates and observations that relate to immunological inhibition and the ultimate effect of such inhibition on cell proliferation. Because of its relevance in understanding cyclosporine's effect in psoriasis, some of the data relative to cyclosporine's effect on immune mechanisms and in vitro cell proliferation will be summarized below (7–11).

It is not difficult to postulate that it is the stimulation of cytokine production within dermis and epidermis that ultimately provokes epidermal cell proliferation in psoriasis. In periods of activity most inflammatory skin diseases including psoriasis, an inflammatory hyperproliferative skin disease, recruit large numbers of immunocompetent cells to the epidermis and dermis. T cells expressing $CD4^+$ and $CD8^+$ molecules, macrophages, and several unique types of antigen-presenting cells may be found in abundance within the epidermis and dermis. In psoriasis the lesional infiltrate is made up predominately of $CD4^+$ and $CD8^+$ T cells and macrophages.

With provocation keratinocytes of the epidermis, at least in culture, are capable of producing a T-cell stimulating factor, principally interleukin-1 (IL-1). They are also capable of producing a variety of other T-cell stimulating cytokines, chemo-attractants, and T-cell inhibitory factors. Among these factors are IL-6, granulocyte macrophage colony-stimulating factor, and IL-8. Even under normal physiological circumstances bone marrow-derived dendritic Langerhans cells that are capable of presenting antigen to T cells and causing T-cell activation and lymphokine release, migrate to and populate the dermis and epidermis.

Although cyclosporine is capable of acting on many cell types in skin with active psoriasis, it probably centers its activity on T-cell function. Cyclosporine blocks the expected increase in lymphokine messenger RNA that normally occurs after the T-cell receptor for antigens has been stimulated (12). It causes a reduction in the density of all T-cell subsets in both dermis and epidermis of active lesions, probably through inhibition of helper T-cell proloferation (13). Cyclosporine inhibits the production of the lymphokines IL-2 and λ-interferon (IFN-λ). There is an early and dramatic effect of cyclosporine on the rapid disappearance of IFN-λ-inducible proteins on the surface of psoriatic keratinocytes (14). Antigen presenting activity in uninvolved and involved psoriatic skin is decreased almost immediately after cyclosporine administration and continues to decline with continuing therapy. Cyclosporine administration causes depletion of Langerhans cells ($CD1^+$, DR^+) and lymph node-based RFD-1^+ interdigitating reticulum cell in lesional dermis of psoriasis (5).

Additionally, it has been proposed that cyclosporine exerts a direct effect on keratinocyte replication that is not mediated through cytokines (8,15). There is considerable controversy surrounding this proposal. Two arguments against are that there is some doubt that intracellular drug concentrations needed to inhibit human keratinocyte proliferation are achievable during standard cyclosporine psoriasis therapy (7); and most data that have been accumulated to date, relative to cyclosporine direct effect on keratinocytes, have been taken from observations in the *in vivo* mouse model and cannot be demonstrated even *in vitro* with keratinocytes from humans. Nonetheless, proponents of a direct cyclosporine effect on keratinocytes give the following data as support: a) the compound (cyclosporine) has been shown to actively inhibit tumor cells *in vitro* (16); and b) the proliferation of human epidermis transplanted to nude mice is inhibited by cyclosporine (17).

Cyclophilin and calmodulin are two binding proteins that have been considered possible mediators of cyclosporine direct effect on keratinocytes. Of the two binding proteins the evidence is best for cyclophilin as a potential mediator. Cyclophilin is widely distributed in human tissue, including epidermis. Although the amount of cyclophilin in abnormal psoriatic epidermal skin does not differ from that in normal skin, its presence is thought to account for the accumulation of cyclosporine within the epidermis. Cyclophilin binds to cyclosporine with a very high affinity, and in the lymphocyte the ability of cyclosporine to bind to cyclophlin correlates well with immunosuppressive activity (18). It has been postulated that cyclosporine's effect on the triggering of T-cell genes in susceptible cells takes advantage of the dependence of lymphokine gene promoters on binding to nuclear factors that require refolding. Cyclophilin is identical structurally to an enzyme peptidyl-prolyl *cis-trans* isomerase that is capable of catalyzing the isomerization of proline, which in turn affects protein folding. Cyclosporine by binding to cyclophilin, a peptidyl-prolyl *cis-trans* isomerase (rotase), blocks peptide bond rotations and folding of proteins activated by T-cell receptors. Because of its ability to regulate protein folding by binding to cyclophilin cyclosporine could adversely affect the exposure of DNA and protein binding sites, thereby disrupting DNA-protein and protein-protein interactions (8).

III. PHARMACOLOGY

Cyclosporine is insoluble in water and for many years was administered to patients in an olive oil vehicle. In recent years a soft gelatin capsule containing corn oil has been developed. Absorption of cyclosporine is incomplete and quite erratic. Absorption is dependent on emulsification of the oil vehicle by bile in the gut. Most data on drug absorption is based on experience using the drug in oil preparation. Approximately 10–50% of an oral dose is absorbed through the small intestine. Once cyclosporine is absorbed through the gut it circulates in blood bound to lipoproteins or dissolved in red blood cell membranes (19). Upon being transported to the liver, bound cyclosporine is transported through large transcellular pores, or fenestrations of endothelial cells, lining sinusoidal spaces. From here the drug enters the hepatic spaces of Disse's. From these spaces drug is actively transported into the hepatocyte or diffuses across hepatic cellular membranes. After the drug is transported into the hepatocyte and endoplasmic reticulum, it is converted by enzymes of the P-450 IIIA family to its major metabolites M1, M17, and M21. M1 and M17 metabolites are produced by hydroxylation of active methyl and ethyl groups and M21 by demethylation. Once cyclosporine is converted to inactive metabolites, some are eliminated from the cell by reentering hepatic sinusoids and then the systemic circulation. However, most drug is transferred from the endoplasmic reticulum of hepatocytes to canalicular membranes and excreted into the bile and then into the stool. Metabolites that are excreted into the systemic circulation circulate bound to protein and blood cells. As a result, cyclosporine blood metabolites are often found in greater abundance than the original compound. About 6% of a given dosage of drug enters the systemic circulation and is excreted throughout the kidneys.

It is important to appreciate that although specific P-450 IIIA enzymes are responsible for metabolic degradation of cyclosporine, each P-450 IIIA enzyme may also exert an effect on multiple agents. Thus, cyclosporine hepatic metabolism is competitive, that is, a large number of drugs compete for P-450 IIIA enzymes, some of which have a greater affinity for the enzyme than does cyclosporine (Table 1). Simultaneous administration of competitive agents can result in the reduced hepatic metabolism of cyclosporine and increased active drug (cyclosporine) circulating in the host. Ketoconazole and erythromycin are examples of competitive inhibitors of P-450 IIIA enzyme activity.

There is also considerable variation among patients in the ability of their P-450 IIIA enzyme to metabolize cyclosporine. It has been proposed that this ability is based primarily on the liver content of P-450 IIIA and that the content may vary tenfold or more among patients (20). This heterogeneity, as these differences are referred to, provides an explanation for the daily dose variation required to attain therapeutic or desirable blood levels in different patients. Other proposed rate-limiting effects are individual variation in absorption, drug delivery through the circulation to the liver, drug uptake by hepatocytes, migration to the endoplasmic reticulum, P-450 IIIA enzymes, and removal of metabolites from the endoplasmic reticulum.

Lastly, cytochrome P-450 enzymes are present to some degree in extrahepatic tissues, such as the intestine. It has been reported that 70% of the total P-450 present in the intestine is P-450 IIIA (21). As a result, it has also been postulated that poor bioavailability of cyclosporine in some individuals is related to metabolism of the drug in the intestine by intestinal P-450 IIIA enzymes (22).

Table 1 Drugs that Affect Cyclosporine Metabolism

Competitive Inhibitors (Increase Levels)	Inducers (Decrease Levels)
Erythromycin	Phenobarbital
Ketoconazole	Phenytoin
Miconazole	Phenylbutazone
Nifedipine	Dexamethasone
Diltiazem	Carbamazepine
Verapamil	
Nicardipine	
Cortisol	
Prednisone	
Prednisolone	
Methylprednisolone	

IV. CLINICAL INDICATIONS

Except for its use in psoriasis, and in transplant medicine, there are few if any uses of cyclosporine that are not experimental. Therefore, its use in dermatological disease should be confined to a) those patients with diseases that have proved unresponsive to standard treatment regimens; b) diseases that have satisfied the first criteria and have a reasonable expectation of responding based on knowledge of the disease, its etiology, and potential response to treatment; c) diseases in which there is no other less toxic or nonstandard treatment; and d) the disease has been evaluated based on the effect that treatment with cyclosporine will have on the patients quality of life.

No one should approach the use of cyclosporine in approved and nonapproved indications without a thorough knowledge of its proposed mechanisms of action, absorption, metabolism, excretion, and its toxicity.

Ho and others have reviewed the use of cyclosporine in nonpsoriatic dermatoses and have categorized diseases into those with excellent responsiveness, moderate responsiveness, variable responsiveness, and minimal responsiveness (Table 2). Although a number of citations on the use of cyclosporine in dermatological disease have been omitted in this survey (23), this should not prevent it from serving as a guide to those contemplating the use of cyclosporine in nonresponsive dermatological disease.

V. ADVERSE REACTION

A variety of organs and organ systems can be adversely affected by cyclosporine. Commonly encountered reactions include hirsutism and acne vulgaris in skin, tremors, headaches and convulsions from the central nervous system, gum hyperplasia, diarrhea, nausea and vomiting, flushing, paresthesias, and leukopenia.

The most common and potentially severe adverse reactions occur as a result of cyclosporine's effect on the kidney. Cyclosporine produces intense renal vasoconstriction rather than acute renal parenchymal cell nephrotoxicity. It is now widely conceded that "some degree of renal vasoconstriction is the price that must be paid by every patient who receives effective cyclosporin therapy" (24). Chronic cyclosporine-induced vasoconstriction ultimately causes occlusion of afferent arterioles and irreversible glomerular and nephron damage secondary to ischemic atrophy. Cyclosporine renal effect is associated with hypertension, decreased glomerular filtration, tubulo-interstitial fibrosis, and renal tubular dysfunction. It appears that this group of adverse reactions are all related to cyclosporine's effect on renal vasculature. Lowering cyclosporine dosage confers only marginal protection against its renovascular effect (25). Although yet to be

Table 2 Dermatoses According to Cyclosporine Responsiveness

A. *Excellent responders*
- Behçet's disease
- Bullous erythema multiforme
- Epidermolysis bullosa acquisita
- Lichen planus
- Psoriasis: erythroderma, pustular

B. *Moderate responders*
- Alopecia areata
- Atopic dermatitis
- Bullous pemphigoid
- Chronic photodermatitis (persistent light reactors, actinic reticuloid)
- Pemphigus vulgaris
- Psoriasis: plaque type, palms and soles

C. *Variable responders*
- Dermatomyositis
- Polymyositis
- Systemic lupus erythematosus
- Systemic Scleroderma

D. *Minimal responders*
- Cutaneous T-cell lymphoma
- Ichthyoses
- Pityriasis rubra pilaris

Modified from Ho, VL. Cyclosporine in non-psoriatic dermatoses [Table 2]. J Am Acad Dermat 1990; 23,1248–1249.

reported in humans, there is some evidence in mice that cyclosporine can also stimulate interstitial fibroblastic proliferation in the kidney (26).

In rare circumstances, cyclosporine has been associated with fulminant acute renal failure and thrombocytopenia. In these patients there is histological evidence of thrombotic microangiopathy and afferent arteriolar thrombosis similar to that seen in the "hemolytic-uremic syndrome" (27).

The severity of cyclosporine renal disease appears to parallel increasing age. The most severe disease being noted in patients over 60 years of age, patients in whom one would expect to find some evidence of preexisting renal disease.

Patients who begin with normal renal function at the start of treatment with cyclosporine can soon show a rapidly reversible reduction in glomerular filtration rate (GFR), even after short-term usage of 6 wk or so. Most patients may not demonstrate renal function abnormalities if standard renal tests such as BUN, creatinine, and creatinine clearance are used to measure function. Gilbert et al. have discussed the insensitivity of standard renal function tests when used to identify cyclosporine caused renal toxicity (28). Chronic or long-term use of cyclosporine for 12 mo or more will cause an irreversible reduction in GFR that may ultimately be associated with histological findings of severe renal disease. Messana et al. recommend frequent use of accurate tests for GFR as the only reliable means of monitoring and preventing cyclosporine renal effect (29). Messana et al. state that if pretherapy and interval GFR determinations are performed and cyclosporine dose is properly adjusted based on GFR findings, significant, irreversible loss of renal function will be uncommon (29). I agree somewhat with this position; however, it is imperative that one be prepared to end the administration of cyclosporine in the presence of a continuing reduction in GFR. It has been demonstrated that after cyclosporine has been discontinued there may be no further evidence of progressive deterioration of the GFR (29). Feutren, for the International Kidney Biopsy Registry of cyclosporine in autoimmune diseases, recommends reducing the risk of nephropathy by limiting the dosage of cyclosporine to 5 mg/kg/d and that the associated increase in serum creatinine be no greater than 30% of pretreatment values (30).

Hypertension is a prime adverse effect of cyclosporine administration. Hypertension is generally a manifestation of cyclosporine renal effect, although increased blood pressure without significant renal effect may be seen in some patients.

Bennett has recommended guidelines for "safe dermatologic use of cyclosporine" (24). These are a) attempt daily cyclosporine dosage of 5 mg/kg or less; b) maintain trough plasma cyclosporine levels at 100 ng/ml or less by radioimmunoassay; c) reduce cyclosporine dose by 25–50% if serum creatinine values increase 30% over baseline; d) with preexisting renal disease or hypertension, monitor (patient) closely; e) avoid over diuresis and concomitant nephrotoxics (i.e., nonsteroidal antiinflammatory drugs).

Fortunately, hypertension secondary to the use of cyclosporine can be managed in the majority of patients with calcium channel antagonists. It is important to remember that calcium channel blockers compete with cyclosporine for hepatic P-450 IIIA enzymes, and as a result, cyclosporine metabolism may be impaired when these two agents are combined (Table 1). Very careful monitoring of cyclosporine blood levels is required in the presence of calcium channel antagonists. The use of diuretics for control of hypertension is discouraged because these agents deplete extracellular fluid volume and can potentially enhance cyclosporine renal effects.

Headaches, hand tremors, paresthesias, and (rarely) seizures may be experienced during cyclosporine administration. Except for seizures, these adverse effects appear to occur secondary to cyclosporine neurological effect rather than secondary to hypertension and renal effects. Headaches tend to occur most often early in the course of treatment, and along with most other CNS effects tend to resolve gradually even during continuing drug treatment.

Hyperbilirubinemia, hyperlipidemia, hypertrichosis, and hypertrophy of the gingiva occur in up to 50% of patients. Hyperuricemia is seen in up to 15% of treated patients. Hyperbilirubinemia is often associated with elevated alkaline phosphatase and serum transaminase. Management in most patients is a reduction in cyclosporine dosage. This is usually sufficient, with all abnormal values returning to normal in a short period of time. Hyperlipidemia, that is elevated total cholesterol, low-density lipoprotein, and triglycerides, are not so easily controlled, and will often test the limits of therapeutics in this disorder. Because cyclosporine has been shown to accelerate atherosclerosis and cardiovascular disease in transplant recipients (31), uncontrolled hyperlipidemia calls for cessation of treatment in patients with most benign skin diseases.

Hypertrichoses, including lanugo and terminal hairs of the face and extremities in both men and women, recedes when cyclosporine use is discontinued. Gingival hypertrophy can be bothersome in a fairly large number of patients. Like gingival hypertrophy occurring with dilantin usage, it is most prevalent in persons with poor dental hygiene. Hyperuricemia secondary to reduced urate clearance is seen most often in renal transplant patients and in elderly men with impaired renal function. Gouty arthritis may occur in some patients secondary to hyperuricemia.

REFERENCES

1. Ho VL, Lui H, McLean DI. Cyclosporine in non-psoriatic dermatoses. J Am Acad Dermat 1990; 23:1245–1259.
2. Mueller W, Herrmann B. Cyclosporine for psoriasis. N Eng J Med 1979; 301:555.
3. Harper JI, Keat AC, Stoughton RC. Cyclosporine for psoriasis. Lancet 1984; 2(8409) 981–982.
4. Marks JM. Cyclosporine a treatment for severe psoriasis. Br J Dermat 1986; 115:745–746.
5. Ellis CH, Gorsulowsky DC, Hamilton TA, et al. Cyclosporine improves psoriasis in a double blind study. JAMA 1983; 256:3110–3116.
6. Van Joost TH, Bos JD, Heule F, et al. Low-dose cyclosporine A in severe psoriasis: a double blind study. Br J Dermat 1988; 118:183–190.
7. Cooper KD, Voorhees JJ, Fisher GJ, et al. Effects of cyclosporine on immunologic mechanisms in psoriasis. J Am Acad Dermat 1990; 23:130–128.
8. Fairley J. Intracellular targets of cyclosporine. J Am Acad Dermat 1990; 23:1329–1334.
9. Valdimarsson H. Immunity during cyclosporine therapy. J Am Acad Dermat 1990; 23:1294–1300.

10. Baadsgaard O, Hansen E, Chan L, et al. Conditioned media from lesional psoriatic T-cell clones induces keratinocyte proliferation and expression of the surface activation molecule. Clin Res 1989; 37:688A.
11. Baadsgaard O, Tong P, Elder JT, et al. UM4D4+ (CDw 6o) T-cells are compartmentalized into psoriatic skin and release lymphokines that induce a keratinocyte-phenotype expressed in psoriatic lesions. J Invest Dermat 1990; 95:275–282.
12. Kronke M, Leonard WJ, Depper JM, et al. Cyclosporin A inhibits T-cell growth factor gene expression at the level of M-RNA transcription. Proc Natl Acad Sci USA 1984; 81:5214–5218.
13. Bunjes D, Hardt C, Wagner H, et al. Cyclosporine mediates immunosuppression of primary cytotoxic T-cell responses by impairing the release of interleuken-1 and interleukin-2. Eur J Immunol 1981; 11:657–661.
14. Cooper KD, Baadsgaard O, Ellis CN, et al. Mechanisms of cyclosporine A inhibition of antigen presenting activity in uninvolved and lesional psoriatic epidermis. J Invest Dermat 1990; 94:649–656.
15. Emmel EA, Verweij CL, Durand CB, et al. Cyclosporine A specifically inhibits function of nuclear proteins involved in T-cell activation. Science 1989; 246:1617–1620.
16. Saydjari R, Townsend CM, Barranco FL, et al. Effects of cyclosporine A and α-difluromethylornithine on the growth of hamster pancreatic cancer in vitro. J Natl Cancer Inst 1986; 77:1087–1092.
17. Urabe A, Kanatakis J, Viac J, et al. Cyclosporine A inhibits directly in vivo keratinocyte proliferation of living human skin. J Invest Dermat 1989; 92:755–757.
18. Handschumacher RE, Harding MW, Rice J, et al. Cyclophilin: a specific cytosolic binding protein for cyclosporine A. Science 1984; 226:544–547.
19. Watkins PB. The role of cytochromes P-450 in cyclosporine metabolism. J Am Acad Dermat 1990; 23:1301–1311.
20. Watkins PB, Wrighton SA, Mauler P, et al. Identification of an inducible form of cytochrome P-450 in human liver. Proc Natl Acad Sci USA 1985; 82:6310–6314.
21. Watkins PB, Wrighton SA, Schuetz EG, et al. Identification of glucocorticoid-inducible cytochromes P-450 in the intestinal mucosa of rat and man. J Clin Invest 1987; 80:1029–1036.
22. Kolars JC, Duel EA, Schmiedlin-ren P, et al. Cyclosporine metabolism by cytochrome P-450 IIIA in rat enterocytes: another determinant of oral bioavailability? Gastroenterology 1990; 98(5):A182.
23. Wilkel C, McDonald CJ. Cyclosporine for resistant bullous erythema multiforme. Arch Dermat 1990; 126:397.
24. Bennett WM. Renal effects of cyclosporine. J Am Acad Dermat 1990; 23:280–287.
25. Myers BD, Newton L, Boshkos C, et al. Chronic injury of human renal microvessels with low dose cyclosporine therapy. Transplantation 1988; 46:694–703.
26. Jackson NM, Hsu C, Visscher GE, et al. Alterations in structure and function in a rat model of cyclosporine nephrotoxicity. J Pharm Exp Ther 1989; 242:739–756.
27. Keusun G, Gmur J, Baamgartner D, et al. De novo hemolytic uremic syndrome in two renal allograft recipients treated with cyclosporine: successful therapy with plasma pheresis. Transplant Proc 1986; 18:9097–9098.

28. Gilbert SC, Emme HM, Menter A, et al. Cyclosporine therapy for psoriasis. Serum creatinine measurements are an unreliable predictor of decreased renal function. J Am Acad Dermat 1989; 21:470–474.
29. Messana JM, Rochar LL, Ellis CM, et al. Effects of cyclosporine on renal function in psoriasis patients. J Am Acad Dermat 1990; 23:1288–1293.
30. Feutren G. Risk factors of cyclosporine-induced nephropathy in patients with autoimmune disease. N Engl J Med 1992; 326:1654–1660.
31. Vathsalos A, Weinberg RB, Schoenberg L, et al. Lipid abnormalities in renal transplant recipients treated with cyclosporine. Transplant Proc 1989; 21:3670–3673.

11
Retinoids

Charles J. McDonald
Brown University, Providence, Rhode Island

I. GENERAL

For over half a century vitamin A and its family of derivatives, the retinoids, have been shown to exert profound effects on many biological functions. Vitamin A is an essential nutritional factor for a variety of vital physiological functions such as vision, growth, bone development, and reproduction. In recent years investigations in physiology, embryology, nutrition, and oncology have shown that vitamin A and the retinoids are intimately involved in the proliferation and differentiation of epithelial structures, particularly in the skin, and also play a critical role in normal immune function. The use of retinoids to treat dermatological diseases such as psoriasis and other disorders of keratinization and acne vulgaris is well known. Their effects on malignant disease have just recently come under intense investigation. Successful treatment of human malignancies, especially when used in combination with other agents, have been described in squamous cell cancer of the skin (1), cutaneous T-cell lymphoma (2), acute promyelocytic leukemia (3), cervical cancer (4), juvenile chronic myelogenous leukemia, and squamous cell carcinoma of the head and neck (5). Successes in these areas have stimulated the development of clinical trials to better define a spectrum of responsive tumors. Stimulated by the knowledge that retinoids were capable of reversing the progression of premalignant actinic keratoses (5), additional interest is being shown in the use of the retinoids in the chemoprevention of head and neck cancers.

II. CHEMISTRY

Both the natural forms and the synthetic analogs of vitamin A are designated retinoids (Figure 1). Carotenoids from vegetables and retinol esters from animal tissues in the diet are the main human sources of vitamin A (retinol). After oral ingestion enterocytes of the intestinal mucosa are responsible for the conversion of carotenoids and retinyl esters to retinol. Retinol is esterified with long-chain fatty acids to form retinyl esters. Retinol esters are incorporated into chylomicrons, which are exocytosed by the enterocytes and make their way to the liver where they are cleared and stored. Chemically unbound vitamin A and the retinoids consist of a three-part structure: a cyclic group, a polyene side chain, and a terminal polar group (Figure 1). Successive modification of these building units of the molecule allows one to obtain a variety of analogs of retinol (6). Within specific enterocytes retinol may be oxidized to all-*trans* retinoic acid by the enzyme nicotinamide-adenine-dinucleotide phosphate (NAD[P])-linked aldehyde dehydrogenase. All-*trans* retinoic acid may then undergo nonenzymatic photoisomerization, or enzymatic isomerization to 13-*cis*-retinoic acid. Both retinoic acid and its isometric form 13-*cis*-retinoic acid may be hydroxylated to 4-hydroxy metabolites that are subsequently oxidated to 4-oxo metabolites. The hydroxylation reaction is mediated by cytochrome P-450-dependent enzymes. The oxidized metabolites undergo conjugation with glucuronic acid and are secreted into the biliary tree and/or enterohepatic circulation. Inhibitors of cytochrome P-450-

Retinol

All- *trans*
Retinoic Acid

13 *cis*-
Retinoic Acid

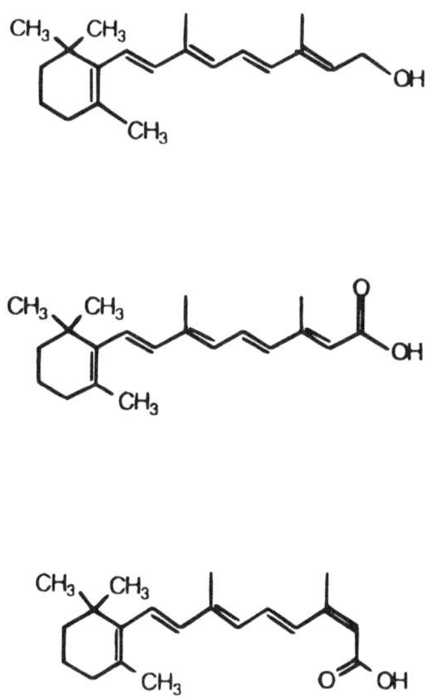

Figure 1 Chemical structure of common retinoids.

dependent enzymes will suppress hepatic metabolism of retinoids, thus delaying plasma clearance of these agents. Ketoconazole will inhibit cytochrome P-450-dependent enzymes. Lastly, retinol, but not its analogs, will accumulate in liver tissues, leading eventually to severe chronic liver disease. Retinol and retinoic acid circulate in the blood tightly bound to proteins, retinol-binding protein for retinol and albumin for retinoic acid.

III. MECHANISM OF ACTION

The retinoids, natural and synthetic, have a profound influence on epithelial differentiation and proliferation. However, other diverse effects occur in many normal and transformed epithelial cells. Thus, the true mechanism of action of this class of agents remains essentially unknown. The variety of analogs studied to date have been found to have individually different tissue reactivity, and thus observations on individual agent activity may not be universal to the class. Some interesting phenomena on the possible mechanism of action of the retinoids is cited below.

Cytoplasmic retinoid binding proteins exist within the cytoplasm of the cell and appear to be individually specific for retinol and retinoic acid (7). The exact role of these proteins is unknown, but they are believed to mediate transfer of retinol and retinoic acid from the cytoplasm to the nucleus, or alternatively may sequester retinoic acids in the cytoplasm. Some experiments have shown that overexpression of the retinoic acid binding protein within a cell can result in a diminished response of that cell to retinoic acid (8). Again, these responses are quite variable, depending on the tissue type and specific analog. It has been demonstrated that systemic administration of 13-*cis*-retinoic acid in patients with acne vulgaris does not cause increased epidermal retinoic acid binding protein levels, whereas systemic all-*trans* retinoic acid and acitretin will cause increased levels (9).

In contrast to retinoic acid cytoplasmic receptors, it appears that retinoic acid nuclear receptors are intimately involved in the differentiation-inducing effects of retinoic acid (10). There is evidence to suggest that some tissue effects of retinol are mediated by tissue oxidation of retinol to retinoic acid and subsequent binding of retinoic acid to nuclear retinoic acid receptors. Three nuclear retinoic acid receptors, all members of the steroid-thyroid superfamily of receptors, have been identified. They are labeled α, β, and γ receptors, each with molecular masses around 50,000 kD. The α receptor gene maps to the q21 band of chromosome 17. The β gene maps to the p24 band of chromosome 3, and the γ gene maps to chromosome 12. Multiple isoforms for retinoic acid receptors α, β, and γ have been demonstrated. It is suggested that each isoform has a distinctive functional role.

Retinoic acid nuclear receptors control gene transcription by direct interactions with specific DNA sequences. The resulting induced mRNA species direct synthesis of proteins that mediate the growth inhibition and differentiation effects of retinoic acid (11).

IV. PHARMACOLOGY

Most studies of the pharmacology of retinoids have been done with the two agents most commonly used for dermatological diseases: isotretinoin (13-*cis*-retinoic acid) and etretinate. Interestingly, it appears that the pharmacology of all-*trans* retinoic acid (tretinoin) differs significantly from 13-*cis*-retinoic acid. All analogs may be administered by the oral route.

A. Isotretinoin

After oral administration, peak plasma concentration occurs in 1.5–3 h. After a single oral dose of 80 mg, plasma concentrations may vary from 180–459 ng/ml, showing considerable individual variation in absorption. It is believed that no more than 25% of any given dosage is available for use in the human system. The terminal elimination half-life is between 10 and 20 h. It appears that the pharmacokinetics do not change after repeated administration. Oral absorption appears to be affected by drug formulation and by the relationship of dosing to food intake.

B. Etretinate

After a single oral dose it appears that between 30 and 70% of the drug becomes available. Peak plasma concentrations of 400–1600 mg/ml occur within 2–3 h. The threshold of detection in plasma is reached 24–36 h after administration. Mean half-life of administration ranges from 7–9 h. Although the final elimination half-life remains unknown, 100 d has been suggested. This implies that etretinate, unlike isotretinoin, may be stored in some deep-tissue compartment, returning slowly to the central compartment for excretion.

V. CLINICAL INDICATIONS

Collectively the retinoids have been used in the treatment of the following disorders of the skin: acne vulgaris, both topical and systemic; psoriasis, all forms; and disorders of keratinization, such as lamellar ichthyoses, congenital ichthyosiform erythroderma, Darier's disease, pityriasis rubra pilaris, porokeratosis, and a variety of keratodermas. Increasingly the retinoids are finding use in the treatment of a wide variety of cancers, including acute promyelocytic leukemia, juvenile chronic myelogenous leukemia, cutaneous T-cell lymphoma, squamous cell cancer of the head and neck, squamous cell cancer of the skin, and basal cell cancer of the skin (12). Although currently available agents have shown minimal to good effects in these tumors, the success rate and the potential for increasing the success rate in a number of tumors by using, for example, the receptor-specific targeted metabolites has spurred intensive searches for more new and effective retinoids. The potential for retinoid-cytokine synergism in human cancer is also under investigation (13).

VI. ADVERSE REACTIONS

Adverse reactions to the systemic administration of retinoids are quite common, but rarely are severe enough to stop use of the drugs. The most reactions are seen in the skin and mucous membranes, liver, musculoskeletal system, central nervous system, and lipid metabolism. A major manifestation, teratogenicity, limits the use of the retinoids in women of childbearing age.

Dryness of the skin and mucous membranes appear in nearly every patient treated with systemic retinoids, and is the most common complaint of a treated population. Dry skin, which can be problematic in winter, often dictates the dosage of the drug that is given. Dry lips often herald the onset of this problem, followed by dryness and fragility of the nasal mucosa, which may be manifest by frequent nasal bleeding. Dry eyes are the next most frequent complaint and may be particularly distressing to patients who wear contact lenses. Dryness and peeling of the palms and soles often occurs, but is less problematic to most patients. Often dryness of the skin is associated with an eczematous dermatitis, pruritus and a skin rash being the principle manifestations. Other complaints noted have been skin fragility, nail thinning, and reversible diffuse or partial alopecia. Patients should especially be warned of alopecia, since it appears that patients prone to the development of androgenic alopecia may not experience complete regrowth of hair in the classically balding areas when retinoid use is ended.

Frequent applications of emollients to the wet skin and mucous membranes, in other than patients treated for acne vulgaris, will generally suffice to reduce the number of complaints of skin dryness and pruritus. A small reduction in drug dosage is often warranted in the treatment of dry skin and pruritus. Artificial tears may aid in controlling the symptom of dry eyes.

Serum changes in lipid concentration are quite common after systemic administration of the retinoids. Every patient is suspect for developing hyperlipidemia. Serum cholesterol and triglycerides may reach astonishing levels. The cause of this phenomenon is unclear. Proper dietary consultation is often all that is needed to direct patient compliance with a diet devoid of those foodstuffs that may be responsible for the hyperlipidemia. Having had little or no success using lipid-lowering agents, I am loath to prescribe them in patients receiving retinoid therapy.

Musculoskeletal pain and cramps may occur without evidence of muscle or bone involvement, and often occur-after a prolonged period of drug intake. Occasionally, pain may be associated with diffuse hyperostoses, especially of the lumbar and thoracic spine, and calcifications of tendons and ligaments. The Achilles tendon often shows the most dramatic involvement with calcification. X-ray examination of this structure is used frequently in the evaluation of patients who complain of bone pain. The appearance of calcifications and bony spurs on x-rays are indications for ending retinoid treatment. Severe, unrelenting bone pain is another cause for ending long-term treatment with retinoids.

Liver function abnormalities are frequently transitory. Repeat laboratory testing after a discussion with the patient of possible causes generally cures this problem. Continuous abnormalities indicate toxicity and drug treatment should be discontinued. Increased intracranial pressure may be associated with complaints of headaches and visual difficulties. Funduscopic examination of the eye is indicated. If papilledema is noted or the eye examination cannot be completed, the drug should be discontinued.

Finally, *teratogenicity precludes the use of these agents in women of childbearing age who are not willing to practice an acceptable form of contraception* for a minimum of 1 mo after treatment with isotretinoin and 2 y after treatment with etretinate and acitretin.

REFERENCES

1. Lippman S, Parkinson D, Itril L, et al. 13-Cis-retinoid and acid and interferon alpha-2a. Effective combination therapy for advanced squamous cell carcinoma of the skin. J Natl Cancer Inst 1992; 84:235–241.
2. Claudy A, Delomier Y, Hermier C. Treatment of cutaneous T-cell lymphoma with a new aromatic tretinoid (R. 10-9359). Arch Dermat Res 1982; 273(1–2):37–42.
3. Huang M, Ye Y, et al. Use of all-trans retinoic acid in the treatment of acute promyelocytic leukemia. Blood 1988; 72:567–572.
4. Lippman S, Kavanaugh J, Parades-Espinoza M, et al. 13-Cis-retinoic acid plus interferon alpha-2A: highly active system for squamous cell carcinoma of cervix. J Natl Cancer Inst 1992; 84:241–245.
5. Meyskens F, Gilmartin E, Alberts O, et al. Activity of isotretinoin against squamous cell cancers and preneoplastic lesions. Cancer Treat Rep 1982; 66:1315–1319.
6. Bollag W, Geiger J. Historical development of retinoids in psoriasis. In: Roenigk HH Jr, Maibach HI, eds. Psoriasis. New York: Marcel Dekker, 1985:515–521.

7. Ceytil F, Ong D. Cellular retinoid binding proteins. In: Sporn M, Roberts A, Goodman D, eds. The retinoids. Orlando, Fla: Academic Press, 1984:90–125.
8. Boylan J, Gudas L. Over expression of the cellular retinoic acid binding protein 1(RABP-L) results in a reduction in differentiation-specific gene expression in Fg teratocarcinoma cells. J Cell Biol 1991; 112:965–979.
9. Hirschel-Scholz S, Siegenthaler G, Saurat J-H. Isotretinoin differs from other synthetic retinoids in its modulation of human cellular retinoic binding protein (RABP). Br J Dermat 1989; 120:639–644.
10. Collins S, Robertson K, Mueller L. Retinoic acid-induced granulocyte differentiation of H-L-60 myeloid leukemia cells is mediated directly through the retinoic acid receptor (RAR) alpha. Mol Cell Biol 1990; 10:2154–2163.
11. Petkovich M, Brand N, Krust A, et al. A human retinoic acid receptor which belongs to the family of nuclear receptors. Nature 1987; 330:444–450.
12. Smith MA, Parkinson DR, Cheson BD, Friedman MA. Retinoids in cancer therapy. J Clin Oncol 1992; 10:839–864.
13. DiGiovanna JJ. Retinoids for the future: oncology. J Am Acad Dermat 1992; 27:534–537.

12
Miscellaneous Agents—Vitamin D (Calcipotriol)

Sharon Zellis
Philadelphia College of Osteopathic Medicine, Philadelphia, Pennsylvania

Stephanie Pincus
State University of New York at Buffalo, Buffalo, New York

I. INTRODUCTION

Calcitriol and its analogs have recently proven successful in the treatment of skin disorders of proliferation and differentiation. The identification of tissue receptors on keratinocytes (1) fibroblasts (1), and immunologic cells (2) suggests that this active form of vitamin D_3 may exert a paracrine effect on the cutaneous environment, by regulating the differentiation and proliferation of epidermal cells and/or modulating the local immune response. A major clinical application of calcitriol has been in the treatment of psoriasis vulgaris (3). Consequently, a number of chemical analogs to calcitriol were developed, and appear to offer valuable therapeutic potential for safe clinical use in dermatology (4).

II. BACKGROUND

A. Effect on Calcium Hemostasis

The hormonal effects of 1,25-dihydroxyvitamin D_3 on calcium homeostasis have been well established. Vitamin D_3 is formed in the skin, mainly in the malpighian layer of the epidermis after 7-dehydrocholesterol is exposed to sunlight (5). Vitamin D_3 (cholecalciferol) is then transported to the liver where it is initially hydrolyzed to 25-hydroxyvitamin D_3, and subsequently transported to the kidney where it is further hydrolyzed to the active metabolite 1,25-dihydroxyvitamin D_3 (6). Calcitriol (1,25-dihydroxyvitamin D_3) is known to act on target cell receptors located on the intestines, bone, distal kidney, and parathyroid gland (see Table 1) in a regulatory feedback loop that functions to maintain serum calcium and phosphorous concentrations within physiologic parameters.

B. 1,25-$(OH)_2D_3$ Receptor

The 1,25-$(OH)_2$ receptor is classified among the class of steroid receptors that include estrogen, glucocorticoid and thyroid receptors. Target receptors have been identified on various tissues (see Table 2), and a similar structure is common to all sites (7,8). Cytosolic and nuclear receptors specific for 1,25-$(OH)_2D_3$ appear to mediate gene transcription by attaching to a vitamin D-specific DNA sequence (8,9). Evidence suggests that the 1,25-$(OH)_2D_3$ receptor also functions to raise intracellular levels of calcium and cyclic GMP through nontranscription mediated activities (9). Many believe that the regulatory properties of calcitriol arise from its ability to alter cytosolic calcium levels and effect gene transcription (8,10).

Table 1 Classical Physiologic Actions of 1,25-$(OH)_2D_3$

Intestine	Stimulates absorption of calcium and phosphorus from diet
Bone	Mobilizes calcium and phosphorous from the bone
Thyroid	Stimulates the synthesis of thyroid stimulating hormone
Parathyroid	Inhibits parathormone synthesis
Kidney	Stimulates renal reabsorption of calcium

Source: Ref. 7.

Table 2 Distribution of 1,25-$(OH)_2D_3$ Receptors

Osteoblasts
Gonads
Stomach
Epidermis
Hair follicle
Pancreas
Breast
Kidney
Parathyroid Hormone
Thymus
Monocytes
Brain

Source: Ref. 7.

The skin is now recognized as an alternate source for the production of 1,25-$(OH)_2D_3$ (11) and appears to function as a target organ for this hormone (1,12). An expanded role beyond that of calcium hemostasis is supported by the discovery of specific target cell receptors for calcitriol on epidermal keratinocytes, dermal fibroblasts, Langerhans cells, macrophages, and activated T lymphocytes (1,2).

III. REGULATORY EFFECTS OF 1,25-$(OH)_2D_3$

A. Effect on Cell Proliferation and Differentiation

In normal skin 1,25-$(OH)_2D_3$ inhibits keratinocyte proliferation and stimulates cell differentiation. Hosomi et al. studied mouse epidermal cells in vitro and found that physiologic concentrations of 1,25-$(OH)_2D_3$ resulted in increasing numbers of differentiated cell types, while decreasing the number of proliferating basal cells. Moreover, a dose dependent decline in the rate of DNA synthesis in keratinocytes was observed. Additionally, this study identified a stimulatory effect of 1,25-$(OH)_2D_3$ on the formation of a cornified envelope from proliferating basal cells, and on the calcium-dependent transglutamase activity which functions to cross-link proteins in the envelope (13). These findings were later confirmed by Smith et al. using cultured human keratinocytes in serum free extracts (14).

B. Effect on the Immunoregulatory System

The skin's immune system is similarly influenced by calcitriol. Intracellular receptors for 1,25-$(OH)_2D_3$ can be found on peripheral blood monocytes, macrophages (2), and activated lymphocytes (15). In vitro studies show the ability of calcitriol to induce the differentiation of myeloid stem cells, promote the maturation of monocytes to macrophages, and enhance the expression of MHC class II antigens (15).

The regulatory effect of 1,25-dihydroxyvitamin D_3 on the interaction between macrophages and lymphocytes is at least in part mediated by calcitriol's influence on cytokine production. Calcitriol's selective effect of stimulating the synthesis and release of IL-1 and IL-3 (16), while inhibiting the production of IL-2 (2,17,18), IL-6 (19–21), gamma interferon (9,15,22), EGF-β (23), and GCSF (15) is well documented.

Furthermore, a suppressive effect of 1,25-$(OH)_2D_3$ on the thymocyte proliferative response to IL-1 has also been recognized (23–25). It is believed that the predominant influence of calcitriol on the immune system, whether stimulatory or inhibitory, is dependent on the intensity of antigen stimulation as well as on local concentrations of this hormone (2).

IV. CLINICAL APPLICATION

A. Psoriasis Vulgaris

Psoriasis is a chronic papulosquamous disorder that is believed to have an increased epidermal proliferation and a decreased differentiation of epidermal cells. In psoriasis there is an increased expression of cytokeratin 6 and 16, which are markers of hyperproliferation, and a decrease in the levels of keratins 1 and 2, which are markers of differentiation (26). The epidermal cell turnover time is decreased and is associated with defective maturation and keratinization (27). Clinically, lesions appear as well demarcated red scaly plaques. Histologic changes include hyperkeratosis, parakeratosis and focal hypogranulosis. Additional findings include elongation of the rete ridges, tortuous capillaries in the dermal papillae, Munro microabscesses, and a perivascular lymphohistiocytic infiltrate (28). An interest in calcitriol for the treatment of hyperproliferative diseases of the skin followed the unexpected improvement in a patient's psoriasis condition after the administration of 1 alpha-cholecalciferol (a synthetic precursor of 1,25-$(OH)_2D_3$) for osteoporosis (29). Subsequently, a series of trials investigated the value of calcitriol and its analogs administered orally and topically in the treatment of psoriasis vulgaris (30–34).

Scattered reports suggest a partial resistance of keratinocytes and dermal fibroblasts to the antiproliferative effects of calcitriol in patients with psoriasis (3,14,35–37). This is in contrast to a study by Hashimoto et al. (38) who examined the effects of 1,25 dihydroxyvitamin D_3 on the growth and DNA synthesis of cultured human keratinocytes from samples of psoriatic skin and found a similar dose-dependent antiproliferative response in both normal and psoriatic skin samples. Thus, the question of whether there are inherent abnormalities in the cellular response of psoriatic skin to 1,25-$(OH)_2D_3$ is still unresolved, but may simply vary among individual patients.

1. Efficacy Trials

Several well-designed clinical trials indicate a positive clinical response of chronic plaque psoriasis to calcitriol (12,20,31,32). Morimito et al. (24) enrolled 40 patients in an open-design study using both topical and oral calcitriol. These authors found topical therapy to be more effective than oral dosing. A double-blind placebo-controlled trial using topical and oral doses was performed by Holick et al. (39). Among 100 patients treated topically at dosages of 0.5 μg/g of base, 60% showed complete clearing and an additional 30% demonstrated significant improvement. In contrast, only 60% of the 45 patients treated with oral calcitriol showed significant clearing, and 25% complete resolution. Three stages of improvement were noted. Firstly, a decrease in the amount of scale, secondly a decrease in erythema, and lastly central clearing. They report hypercalcemia and hypercalcuria as an untoward effect in 25% of patients who received oral treatment (39,40). Smith et al. (37) recommend a single dose at bedtime to reduce the incidence of hypercalcemia.

V. CALCIPOTRIOL—A CALCITRIOL ANALOG

A. Pharmacokinetics

A variety of vitamin D_3 analogs have been synthesized, each with a similar affinity for the vitamin D receptor and similar activity at the cellular level, but with less effect on calcium metabolism than calcitriol (7,30). The aim has been to find analogs that are antiproliferative but do not effect calcium uptake or excretion. Among these agents, calcipotriol (MC903) has undergone the most scrutiny. It is a 1,24-dihydroxyvitamin D analog that contains a double bond and a cyclopropane ring as a side chain (3) (see Figure 1). Oral calcipotriol undergoes hepatic metabolism and deactivation more rapidly than calcitriol and is considered to be 100 times less potent in inducing hypercalcemia (41). The half-life of oral calcipotriol is estimated at 12–60 min, with excretion primarily through the fecal route. Moreover, the topical form of calcipotriol demonstrates less than 1% systemic absorption, with merely trace amounts detectable in the urine and feces (42).

B. Adverse Effects

Dosing studies show that calcipotriol at a concentration of 50 μg/g in a petrolatum base, applied topically twice daily at a maximum dose of 100 g/wk provided its

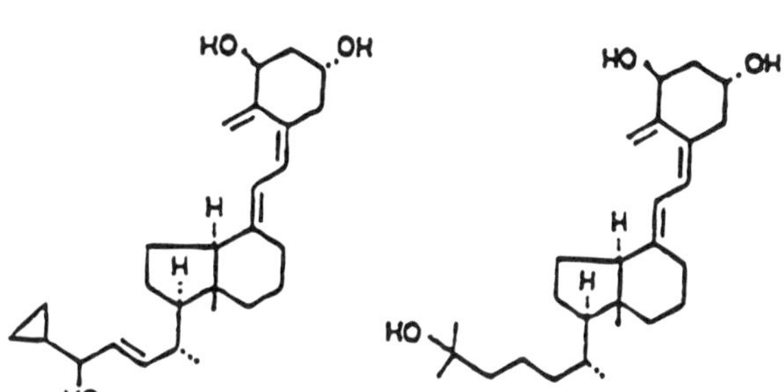

Calcitriol ($1,25(OH)_2D_3$) Calcipotriol

Figure 1 Calcipotriol is a 1,25-dihydroxyvitamin D analog that differs from calcitriol by the presence of a double bond and a cyclopropane ring. (From Kragballe, 1992.)

greatest benefit after 6–8 weeks of therapy. No changes in calcium levels occurred in patients who adhered to this recommended protocol (43). The most common side effect reported is that of an irritant dermatitis particularly involving the face and skin folds. Other adverse effects include transient stinging, burning, or itching at the site of application (32). Cases of allergic contact dermatitis to calcipotriol have also been reported (44,45). Klaber et al (46) assessed the long term effects of calcipotriol in a one year investigation of 118 patients who received continuous topical therapy. No significant alteration in serum calcium or renal or hepatic function was noted in this study.

C. Effect on Cytochemical Markers

Several studies applied immunohistochemical methods to analyze the effects of topical calcipotriol on cytochemical markers of epidermal proliferation and differentiation in psoriasis (47–49). Despite a lack of complete normalization in the keratin pattern, most authors found an improvement in the hyperproliferative keratin 16 expression. A study by Holland et al. demonstrated an increase in keratins 1 and 2 (markers of differentiation) and a decline in keratins 6 and 16 correlated with clinical improvement (50). Additional investigation by Berth-Jones noted a decline in the basal keratin marker k5 and an increase in the suprabasilar keratin marker k10 following 4 wks of therapy with 50 μg/g of calcipotriol ointment (47). De Jong et al. (51) analyzed parameters for epidermal growth and inflammation in patients receiving long term topical MC903 treatment. They report a significant decline in numbers of PMNs after 1 wk, followed by a decrease in the number of cycling cells as measured by Ki-67 positive nuclei beginning at 2 wk, and a decline in the number of T cells by 4 wk. They conclude that patients with the lowest clinical psoriasis area and severity index (PASI) scores after 12 wk of treatment demonstrated the most marked reduction in numbers of proliferating cells, epidermal PMNs and T lymphocytes.

D. Comparative Studies

Current therapy for psoriasis includes corticosteroids, tar, anthralin, methotrexate, oral retinoids, UV light, and PUVA. Each are limited in their effectiveness and may result in untoward side effects. Clinical trials have been performed to compare the effectiveness and safety profile of MC903 to many of the existing treatment modalities for psoriasis. In one such study, 50 μg/g of calcipotriol ointment was compared with betamethasone 17 valerate ointment 0.1% in a double blind randomized left/right comparison trial (52). Clinical assessments were based on the PASI, erythema, thickness, and scale. Results of this study show calcipotriol to be slightly more effective than betamethasone 17 valerate after 2, 4, and 6 weeks of treating mild to moderate psoriasis. Similar results were obtained in a double-blind parallel group study involving 409 patients randomized to receive either calcipotriol or betamethasone valerate. However, in this trial, the authors observed more frequent cutaneous side effects consisting of burning or itching at the site of application among patients who received calcipotriol. Additionally, one patient was withdrawn from the study after developing hypercalcemia following use of a quantity of calcipotriol in excess of the recommended dose. This abnormality rapidly corrected once treatment was withdrawn (53). In parallel group studies, twice daily application of calcipotriene ointment was superior to fluocinonide ointment.

Studies comparing calcipotriene with other agents are now available. Recent studies on 277 patients using 0.005% calcipotriene ointment confirmed the utility and safety of this treatment with 70% of treated patients showing greater than 75% improvement as compared to placebo (54). Recent studies have failed to demonstrate enhanced benefits of daily calcipotriene combined with moderate to high potency steroids (55). However, when direct comparisons were made between twice daily fluocinonide ointment and calcipotriene, calcipotriene was more effective for plaque psoriasis. Berth-Jones et al. compared short contact dithranol cream once daily at increasing doses (0.1–2%), to calcipotriol ointment (50 μg/g) in an 8-week trial. The authors found that efficacy and patient tolerability favored the use of calcipotriol (56). Calcipotriene appears to be better than tar and increases the effectiveness of PUVA when applied prior to treatment (58,59). Combination with UVB should be done cautiously since photosensitivity may be observed (60).

E. Other Therapeutic Applications

Topical calcipotriol has been successfully applied to individual cases of dermatologic conditions other than chronic plaque psoriasis. Grey et al. report on the use of calcipotriol in an HIV-positive patient with refractory erythrodermic psoriasis where therapeutic options were limited. Topical calcipotriol was added to the preexisting regimen of etretinate with subsequent clearing of the patient's condition (61). Berth-Jones et al. additionally report on the successful use of topical calcipotriol in three cases of generalized pustular psoriasis where pustular formation cleared within 48 hours of treatment (62). Finally, there are reports where oral 1,25-$(OH)_2D_3$ proved beneficial in treating palmoplantar keratoderma (63), and linear scleroderma (64). Further controlled trials will be required prior to advocating the use of calcipotriol in these conditions.

VI. SUMMARY

In conclusion, a number of analogs to calcitriol have been developed that selectively regulate cell growth and responsiveness and demonstrate low calcitropic potential. Furthermore, these analogs are well tolerated and have low side effect profiles. Comparative studies illustrate that calcipotriol is equal or more efficacious in treating mild to moderate psoriasis vulgaris than many existing therapeutic regimens. As results of clinical trials designed to determine the effects of calcipotriol in combination with standard antipsoriatic modalities become available, the appropriate role of calcipotriene ointment will be further defined.

REFERENCES

1. Feldman D, Chen T, Hirst M, Colston K, Karasek M, Cone C. Demonstration of 1,25-dihydroxyvitamin D_3 receptors in human skin biopsies. J of Clin Endocron and Metab 1980; 51:1463–1465.
2. Bhalla A, Amento E, Krane S. Differential effects of 1,25-dihydroxyvitamin D_3 on human lymphocytes and monocyte/macrophages: inhibition of interleukin-2 and augmentation of interleukin-1 production. Cell Immun 1986; 98:311–322.
3. Kragballe K. Treatment of psoriasis with calcipotriol and other vitamin D analogues. J Am Acad Dermatol 1992; 27:100–108.
4. Kragballe K, Iversen L. Calcipotriol a new topical antipsoriatic. Dermatologic Clin 1993; 11:137–140.
5. Holick MF, MacLaughlin JA, Clark MB, et al. Photosynthesis of previtamin D_3 in human skin and the physiologic consequence. Science 1980; 210:203–205.
6. Bell NH. Vitamin D-Endocrine System. The J of Clin Invest 1985; 76:1–6.
7. DeLuca HF, Krisinger J, Darwish H. The vitamin D system. Kidney International 1990; 38:S-2–S-8.
8. Ozono K, Sone T, Pike W. The genomic mechanism of action of 1,25 dihydroxyvitamin D^3. J of Bone and Mineral Research 1991; 6:1021–1027.
9. Baran DT, Mine ML. 1,25 Dihydroxyvitamin D increases hepatocyte cytosolic calcium levels. J Clin Invest 1986; 77:1622–1626.
10. Smith EL, Holick MF. The Skin: the site of vitamin D_3 synthesis and a target tissue for its metabolite, 1,25-dihydroxyvitamin D_3. Steroids 1987; 49:103–131.
11. Bikle D, Neumanic M, Gee I, Elias P. 1,25-Dihydroxyvitamin D_3 production by human keratinocytes. J of Clin Invest 1986; 78:557–556.
12. Holick MF, Smith E, Pincus SH. Skin as the site of vitamin D synthesis and target tissue for 1,25-dihydroxyvitamin D_3. Arch Dermatol 1987; 123:1677a–1683a.
13. Hosomi J, Hosoi J, Abe E, Suda T, Toshio D. Regulation of terminal differentiation of cultured mouse epidermal cells by 1,dihydroxyvitamin D_3. Endocrinology 1989; 125:1647–1652.
14. Smith EL, Walworth SB, Holick MF. Effect of 1,25-Dihydroxyvitamin D_3 on the morphologic and biochemical differentiation of cultured human epidermal keratinocytes grown in serum-free conditions. J of Investigative Dermatology 1986; 6:709–714.
15. Manolagas SC, Hustmyer FG, Yu XP. Immunomodulating properties of 1,25-dihydroxyvitamin D_3. Kidney International 1990; 29:S9–S16.

16. Hodler B, Evequoz V, Trechsel U, Fleisch H, Stadler B. Influence of vitamin D_3 metabolites on the production of interleukin 1,2, and 3. Immunobiology 1985; 170:256–269.
17. Rigby WF, Denome S, Fanger MW. Regulation of lymphokine production and human t lymphocyte activation by 1,25-dihydroxyvitamin D_3 (calcitriol). J Clin Investigation 1984; 74:1451–1455.
18. Tsoukas CD, Provedini DM. 1,25-Dihydroxyvitamin D_3: A novel immunoregulatory hormone. Science 1984; 224:1438–1440.
19. Hettmannsperger U, Detmar M, Owsianowski M, Tenorio S, Kammier H, Orfanos C. Cytokine stimulated human dermal microvascular endothelial cells produce interleukin 6-inhibition by hydrocortisone, dexamethasone, and calcitriol. J of Invest Derm 1992; 99:531–536.
20. Morimoto S, Onishi T, Imanaka D, et al. Topical administration of 1,25-dihydroxyvitamin D_3 for psoriasis: report of five cases. Calcif Tissue Int 1986; 38:119–122.
21. Oxholm A, Oxholm P, Staberg B, Bendtzen K. Expression of interleukin 6 like molecules and tumor necrosis factor after topical treatment of psoriasis with a new vitamin D analogue (MC 903). Acta Derm 1989; 69:385–90.
22. Rigby WF, Denome S, Fanger MW. Regulation of lymphokine production and human T lymphocyte activation by 1,25-dihydroxyvitamin D_3. J of Clin Investigation 1987; 79:1659–1664.
23. Kragballe K. Vitamin D analogues in the treatment of psoriasis. J of Cellular Biochemistry 1992; 49:46–52.
24. Morimoto S, Yoshikawa K. Psoriasis and vitamin D_3. Arch Dermatol 1989; 125:231–234.
25. Muller K, Svenson M, Bendtzen K. 1,25-dihydroxyvitamin D_3 and a novel vitamin D analogue MC903 are potent inhibitors of human interleukin 1 in vitro. Immunology Letters 1988; 17:361–366.
26. Holland D, Wood E, Goodfield M, Cunliffe W. Changes in epidermal keratin levels during treatment of psoriasis with the topical vitamin D_3 analogue MC903. Br J of Dermatol 1990; 122:284.
27. Araujo OE, Flowers FP, Brown KD. Vitamin D therapy in psoriasis. The Annals of Pharmacotherapy 1991; 25:835–839.
28. Lever WF, Schaumburg-Lever G. Noninfectious erythematous/papular, and squamous diseases. In: Lever WF, ed. Histopathology of the Skin, J.B. Lippincott Co, Philadelphia: 1990; 156–161.
29. Morimoto S, Kumahare Y. A patient with psoriasis cured by 1-hydroxyvitamin D_3. Med J Osaka Univ 1985; 35:51–54.
30. Dubertret L, Wallach D, Souteyrand P, et al. Efficacy and safety of calcipotriol (MC903) ointment in psoriasis vulgaris. J of the Am Acad of Derm 1992; 27:983–988.
31. Henderson CA, Papworth-Smith J, Cunliffe WJ, Highest AS, Shamy HK, Czarnetzki BM. A double blind, placebo-controlled trial of topical 1,25-dihydrocholecalciferol in psoriasis. Br J of Dermat 1989; 121:493–496.
32. Lugo-Somolinos A, Sanchez JL, Haddock L. Efficacy of 1,alpha 25-dihydroxyvitamin D in the treatment of psoriasis vulgaris: an open study. Bol Assoc Med P. Rico 1990; 82:450–453.

33. Morimoto S, Yoshikawa K, Kozuka T, et al. An open study of vitamin D_3 treatment in psoriasis vulgaris. Br J of Dermatol 1986; 115:421–429.
34. Morimoto S, Onishi T, Imanaka S, Yukawa H, et al. Topical administration of 1,25-dihydroxyvitamin D_3 for psoriasis: report of five cases. Calcif Tissue Int 1986; 38:119–122.
35. Abe J, Kondo J, Nishii S, Kuroki T. Resistance to 1,25-Dihydroxyvitamin D_3 of cultured psoriatic epidermal keratinocytes isolated from involved and uninvolved skin. J of Clin Endocrin and Metab 1988; 68:851–854.
36. MacLaughlin JA, Gange W, Taylor D, Smith E, Holick MF. Cultured psoriatic fibroblasts from involved and uninvolved sites have a partial but not absolute resistance to the proliferation-inhibition activity of 1,25-dihydroxyvitamin D_3. Proc Natl Acad Sci 1985; 82:5409–5412.
37. Smith EL, Pincus SH, Donovan L, Holick MF. A novel approach for the evaluation and treatment of psoriasis. J Acad of Dermatol 1988; 19:516–527.
38. Hashimoto, Matsumoto K, Higashiyama M, Nishida Y, Yoshikawa K. Growth-inhibitory effects of 1,25-dihydroxyvitamin D_3 on normal and psoriatic keratinocytes. Br J of Dermatol 1990; 123:93–98.
39. Holick M, Pochi P, Bhawan J. Topically applied and orally administered 1,25-dihyddroxyvitamin D_3 is a novel, safe and effective therapy for the treatment of psoriasis: a three year experience with histologic analysis. J of Clin Investigation 1989; 92:446.
40. Holick MF. 1,25-dihydroxyvitamin D_3 and the skin: a unique application for the treatment of psoriasis. Proceedings of the Society for Experimental Biology and Medicine 1989; 191:246–57.
41. Binderup L, Bramm E. Effects of a novel vitamin analogue MC903 on cell proliferation and differentiation in vitro and on calcium metabolism in vivo. Biochemical Pharmacology 1988; 37:889–895.
42. Murdoch D, Clissold SP. Calcipotriol. Drugs 1992; 43:415–429.
43. Kragballe K. Treatment of psoriasis by the topical application of the novel cholecalciferol analogue calcipotriol (MC903). Arch Dermatol. 1989; 125:1647–1652.
44. Bruynzeel DP, Hol CW, Nieboer C. Allergic contact dermatitis to calcipotriol. Br J of Dermatol 1992; 127:66.
45. Yip J, Goodfield M. Contact dermatitis from MC903, a topical vitamin D3 analogue. Contact Dermatitis 1991; 25:135–140.
46. Klaber MR, Hutchinson PE, Holden C, Price M, Ramsay CA. Long term treatment of psoriasis with calcipotriol. Br J of Derm 1992; 127(suppl. 40):17.
47. Berth-Jones J, Fletcher A, Hutchinson P. Epidermal cytokeratin and immunocyte response during treatment of psoriasis with calcipotriol and betamethasone valerate. Br J of Derm 1992; 126:356–361.
48. De Mare S, De Jong E, Van De Kerkhof. DNA content and Ks8.12 binding of the psoriatic lesion during treatment with the vitamin D_3 analogue MC903 and betamethasone. Br J of Dermatol 1990; 123:291–295.
49. Mallet B, Coulden I, Purkis P, Leigh I, Holden C. Immunohistochemical analysis of the changes in the immune infiltrate and keratin expression in psoriasis treated with calcipotriol compared with betamethasone ointment. Br J of Dermatol 1990; 122:837.

50. Holland D, Roberts S, Russel A, Wood E, Cunliffe W. Changes in epidermal keratin levels during treatment of psoriasis with the topical vitamin D_3 analogue MC903. Br J of Derm 1990; 122:284.
51. De Jong E, Van Kerkhof. Simultaneous assessment of inflammation and epidermal proliferation in psoriatic plaques during long-term treatment with the vitamin D_3 analogue MC903: modulations and interrelations. Br J of Derm 1991; 124:221–229.
52. Kragballe K, Gjertsen BT, DeHoop D, et al. Double-blind, right/left comparison of calcipotriol and betamethasone valerate in treatment of psoriasis vulgaris. The Lancet 1991; 337:193–196.
53. Cunliffe W, Berth-Jones J, Claudy A, et al. Comparative study of calcipotriol (MC903) ointment and betamethasone 17-valerate ointment in patients with psoriasis vulgaris. J Am Acad of Dermatol 1992; 26:736–43.
54. Highton A, Quell J. Calcipotriene ointment 0.005% for psoriasis: A safety and efficacy study. J Am Acad Dermatology 1995; 32:67–72.
55. Pincus SH. Combination therapy of psoriasis with calcipotriene and topical steroids. The Intnl J of Derm (submitted).
56. Berth-Jones J, Chui AC, Dodd WA, et al. A Multi-center parallel group comparison of calcipotriol ointment and short contact anthralin in chronic plaque psoriasis. Br J of Dermatol 1992; 127:266–71.
57. Bruce S, Epinette W, Funicella T, Ison A, Jones EL, et al. Comparative study of calcipotriene ointment (MC 903) ointment and fluocinonide ointment in the treatment of psoriasis. J Am Acad Derm 1994; 31:755–59.
58. Than SN, Lun KC, Cheong WK. A comparative study of calcipotriol ointment and tar in chronic plaque psoriasis. Br J Derm 1994; 131:673–77.
59. Speight E, Farr PM. Calcipotriol improves the response of psoriasis to PUVA. Br J Derm 1994; 130:79–92.
60. McKenna KE, Stein RS. Photosensitivity associated with combined UVB and calcipotriene therapy. Arch Dermatology 1995; 131:1305–1307.
61. Gray J, Bottomley W, Layton A, Cotterill J, Monteiro E. The use of calcipotriol in HIV-related psoriasis. Clinical and Experimental Dermatol 1992; 17:342–343.
62. Berth-Jones J, Bourke J, Baily K, Graham-Brown R, Hutchinson P. Generalized pustular psoriasis: response to topical calcipotriol. British Medical Journal 1992; 305:869.
63. Katayama H, Yamane Y. Improvement of palmoplantar keratoderma of nonhereditary type (eczema tyloticum) after oral administration of 1,25-dihydroxyvitamin D_3. Arch of Dermatol 1989; 125:1713.
64. Humbert PG, Dupond JL, Rochefort A, Vasselet R, Laurent R, Agache P. Localized scleroderma-response to 1,25-dihydroxyvitamin D_3. Endocrinology 1983; 3: 1950–1957.

13

Bullous Diseases: Pathogenesis and Treatment

Narciss Mobini and A. Razzaque Ahmed
Harvard School of Dental Medicine, Boston, Massachusetts

I. PEMPHIGUS

A. Introduction

Pemphigus vulgaris (PV) is an autoimmune blistering disease that affects the skin and mucous membranes (1). Patients have circulating antibody, mostly of the IgG type, to an intercellular cement substance (ICS). The in vivo deposition of this antibody is a hallmark of the disease (2). The antibody appears to be pathogenic, since newborn infants of mothers with pemphigus may have transient blisters (3), and newborn mice injected with the antibody from patients develop blisters (4).

B. Immunogenetics

The disease has a higher incidence in the Jewish population. There appears to be a genetic predisposition for developing PV. The major histocompatibility complex (MHC) alleles, especially the class II region, confer this susceptibility. Human histocompatibility leukocyte antigen (HLA) class II has a crucial role in antigen presentation to appropriate T lymphocytes of the immune system. These T cells, in turn, will help B cells produce the relevant autoantibody.

Studies on Ashkenazi Jewish PV patients have demonstrated significant association with the haplotype [HLA-A26, B38, SC21, DR4, DQ8] and [HLA-A26, B35, SC31, DR4, DQ1]. Most of the non-Jewish patients carry the haplotype [HLA-B55, SB45, DR6, DQ5] (5,6).

The PV antigen (PVA) has been identified to be a 130-kDa glycoprotein. It belongs to the cadherin superfamily of adhesion molecules, probably a desmoglein. These are transmembrane proteins that mediate calcium-dependent homophilic cell adhesion. The location of the PVA is in the desmosomal area in the cell membrane of the keratinocytes.

C. Pathology

Intercellular edema and disappearance of the intercellular bridges in the lowermost portions of the epidermis results in the loss of cohesion between the epidermal cells. This is called acantholysis, which eventually leads to blister formation. By indirect immunofluorescence (IIF) autoantibodies can be demonstrated in 80–90% of PV sera. Direct immunofluorescence (DIF) is of critical importance and benefit in making the diagnosis of PV. It shows intercellular deposition of IgG, with or without complement components, throughout the lower epidermis and the epithelium of the mucous membrane. Direct immunofluorescence is positive in the majority of the patients.

D. Pathogenesis

The initial events that trigger the production of the autoantibody are unknown. In genetically predisposed individuals the autoantigen (PVA) is presented to the relevant T cells bearing the specific receptor (TCR) for the antigen. There is production of an autoantibody by specific B cells against the autoantigen. Binding of autoantibody to autoantigen results in the release and activation of plasminogen activator which cleaves plasmin from plasminogen. Plasmin is believed to be responsible for the acantholysis by dissolving the ICS (Figure 1).

There are two major types of pemphigus: pemphigus vulgaris (PV) and pemphigus foliaceous (PF). The latter is the superficial variety of pemphigus with blister formation in the upper epidermis. The autoantigen in PF has been identified to be a 160-kD a protein referred to as desmoglein-1 (8).

Pemphigus vulgaris accounts for 80% of the patients, is often more difficult to treat, and does not have as good a prognosis as PF (9).

E. Indications for the Use of Immunomodulatory and Cytotoxic Agents

Based on the studies in the literature (10), the following indications for the use of chemotherapeutic agents in patients with PV should be considered.

Patients with severe, rapidly progressive disease.

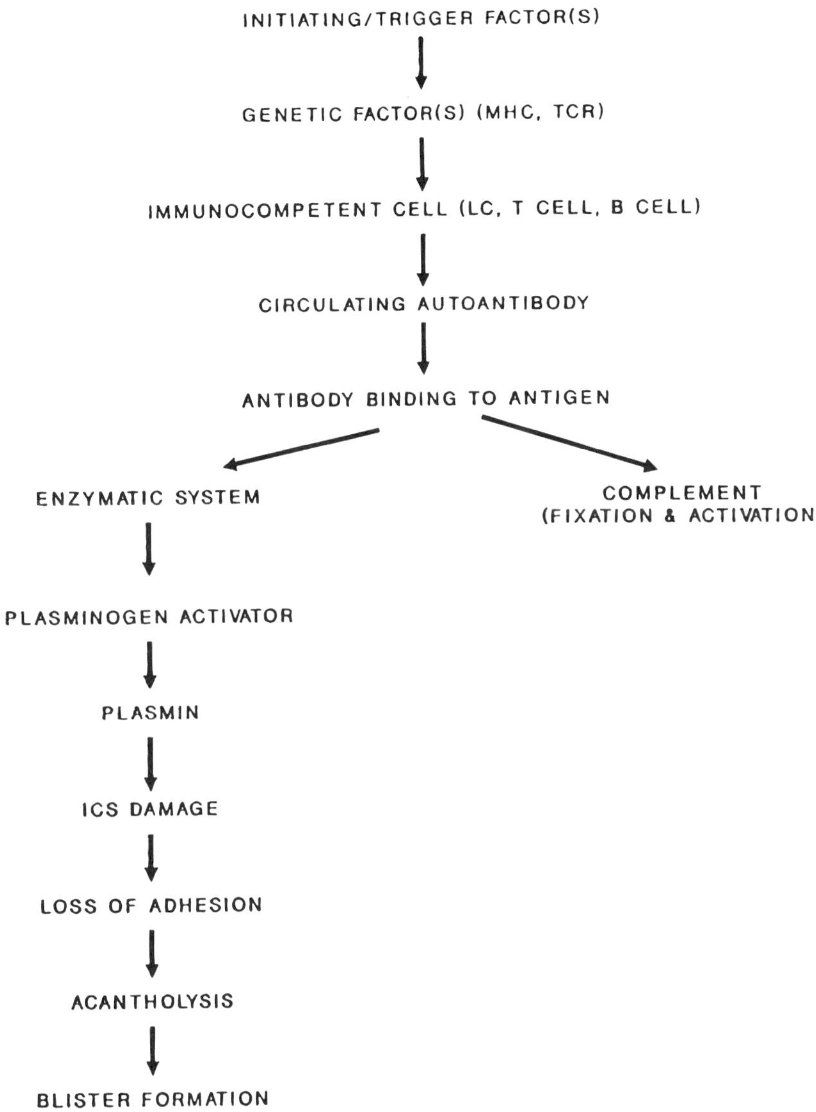

Figure 1 Schematic presentation of pathogenic events leading to blister formation in pemphigus.

Patients with severe disease and high titers of PV autoantibody. It should be mentioned that one treats the patient, not the antibody titer. This titer can serve as only a guide, especially in extensive forms of disease. The correlation between autoantibody titers and disease severity is not universal.

Multiple mucous membrane involvement. If more than two mucous membranes in addition to the skin are involved, the early use of such agents is advised.

Patients not responsive to a daily dose of 100 mg or higher of prednisone or equivalent. In the assessment of clinical effectiveness of any dose, the patient should be kept on the dose for a minimum of 5–7 d. Doubling the dose of corticosteroid is not recommended.

Patients in whom systemic corticosteroid therapy is not recommended (those who already have diabetes mellitus, hypertension, peptic ulcer, etc.). Use of high-dose systemic corticosteroid therapy will add to the existing problems.

Patients developing significant side effects from systemic corticosteroid therapy, for example, osteoporosis, myopathy, opportunistic infections, diabetes mellitus, and other effects.

Children in whom growth retardation has occurred due to systemic corticosteroids.

Patients with other associated autoimmune diseases.

Recent studies clearly demonstrate improved prognosis, decreased mortality, increase in prolonged remission rates, and the relative safety of immunosuppressive agents in the overall management of PV (10–12).

In this regard, some general guidelines in using various agents should be considered.

Before starting a patient on any of these agents, it is critical to have complete familiarity with the drug.

The patient must be informed of all the possible side effects in detail. It is advisable to have a conference with the patient and the family to define the goals at the very outset. It may not be possible to "cure" the patient. The patient may do quite well and maintain a near normal daily life, with the occasional blisters on a lower dosage, rather than use higher doses with lethal side effects and achieve complete clearance.

It is important to remain available and accessible to the patient. In case of serious side effects (e.g., septicemia), time is a critical factor.

A very careful and close follow-up is mandatory.

Adjunct therapy with topical or sublesional injection therapy with corticosteroids should be considered whenever appropriate and possible.

It is not necessary to cause myelosuppression in order to provide the desired immunosuppressive effect with any of these drugs (13).

Define the desired effect or goal. Once it is achieved the drug(s) should be slowly, cautiously, but definitely, withdrawn. Once a patient is in a sustained clinical remission, an attempt to withdraw all drugs is warranted. However, in some patients a single agent or combination in very low doses may be necessary to maintain the remission. In such patients side effects from long-term use of any of these drugs should be carefully monitored.

As far as possible, the use of cyclophosphamide and azathioprine should be definitely avoided in women in childbearing ages.

With most of these agents, patients with active infections should not be treated until the infection is cleared. Also, those patients who have the potential to reactivate a quiescent infection (tuberculosis) should be screened and offered effective prophylaxis if an immunosuppressive/cytotoxic agent is to be used (14).

Since the biochemical and pharmacological aspects of individual agents have been discussed in previous chapters, these will not be presented in detail here. Only some relevant features will be highlighted in particular diseases when needed.

F. Methods and Rationales of Treatment

Systemic corticosteroids have been extensively used in the majority of blistering diseases. They remain the mainstay of therapy for PV.

1. Azathioprine

Although cyclophosphamide is theoretically more effective, azathioprine is preferred because it has less short- and long-term toxicity (15). It is an antimetabolite that inhibits RNA and DNA synthesis. Azathioprine influences both humoral and cell-mediated immunity. It is started in a dose of 50 mg daily and may be increased up to 150 mg daily depending upon clinical response. Not uncommonly it may be necessary to use 200 mg daily. Side effects are frequent at a 300 mg daily dose. To monitor its most serious complication of bone-marrow suppression, a CBC should be ordered weekly for the first month, then every 2 wk for 2 mo, and then once a month for the subsequent 6 mo. Thereafter the frequency of the CBC is determined by the patients clinical response and overall general health. An SMA-12 should be performed monthly or more frequently if warranted (16). Drug-induced hepatitis is a frequent side effect.

The clinical effects of azathioprine manifest in 3–8 wk. This is best measured by cessation of all new blister formation and rapid healing of previous lesions. As the patient responds and a clinical remission is evident, systemic corticosteroids are tapered first and then azathioprine is gradually decreased and finally stopped. Recurrences occur when the tapering is rapid. Generally, reduction of the daily dose of prednisone by 10 mg every 5–10 d is effective, until a daily dose of 25 mg is reached. Thereafter, switching to alternate-day therapy for 6 wk before complete cessation is advised. This total process from initiation to cessation of therapy may take 15–36 mo. An attempt should be made to get every patient off both systemic corticosteroid and azathioprine.

Oral lesions are usually very difficult to eradicate completely. Topical therapy and sublesional corticosteroid injection therapy will expedite their healing.

If a minor recurrence of three to five blisters occurs, instead of reinstituting systemic therapy, it may be advisable to use sublesional triamcinolone injection and topical therapy for 4–6 wk. If new lesions continue to erupt then low-dose systemic therapy should be considered.

Not all patients with PV will respond to azathioprine. If a patient has shown no clinical response and continues to have new lesions after 12–16 wk of azathioprine at optimal doses, it should be considered a failure. The drug should be discontinued.

2. Cyclophosphamide

This is an alkylating agent that exerts its antineoplastic activity by inhibiting nuclear DNA replication in a nonphase-specific but cell cycle-specific manner (17). Chloracetaldehyde released during its side-chain oxidation is probably responsible for its immunosuppressive activity (17). Human B lymphocytes appear to be most sensitive to the pharmacological action of cyclophosphamide, followed in sensitivity by the suppressor T lymphocytes, while helper T lymphocytes appear to be relatively resistant (18). Compared to azathioprine, the mode of onset of cyclophosphamide is faster. Weekly CBC and urine analysis are necessary during the first month; then once in 2 wk for the subsequent 2 mo, and thereafter on a monthly basis until the drug is discontinued.

The onset of cystitis may be minimized by encouraging large daily fluid intake, frequent voiding, and taking the drug early in the morning so that most of it is excreted before bedtime. This reduces the presence of the drug or its metabolites in the bladder overnight. Damage to the bladder may be due to the direct effect of the toxic metabolites in the urine (19).

Studies have shown that cyclophosphamide is useful in patients who are nonresponsive to azathioprine (11,12). Patients respond to doses of 50–150 mg daily, but frequently require doses of 75 mg daily. Cyclophosphamide is usually effective within 4–6 wk of therapy at optimal doses. Once there is clinical remission keep the patient on the same dose for an additional 4–6 wk, then gradually decrease the dose. If the patient is on systemic corticosteroids simultaneously, the corticosteroids should be reduced and gradually withdrawn first. Cyclophosphamide should be reduced slowly and cautiously at a rate of 25 mg every month until reducing to a dose of 25 mg daily, then briefly be switched to alternate-day therapy, followed by thrice weekly therapy before stopping. Usually the total duration of cyclophosphamide therapy is 10–12 mo. If there are minor recurrences, treatment with topical and sublesional corticosteroid injection therapy is suggested.

3. Gold

Since biochemistry and clinical pharmacology of gold salts has not been previously discussed we will briefly present these aspects.

Gold is available as two water-soluble compounds: aurothiomalate (Myochrysine) and aurothioglucose (Solganol) that are used parenterally. Recently a lipid-soluble, orally absorbed compound auranofin (Riduara) has been available. Since the availability of oral gold, most patients with autoimmune blistering skin disease are treated with oral gold, rather than parenteral gold, if and when chrysotherapy is indicated.

The parenteral preparations are 100% absorbed, bind to plasma proteins, and are excreted very slowly by the kidney. At least 30% of the administered dose is retained in the body in various tissues, but it is particularly high in the reticuloendothelial system, kidneys, and adrenal glands (20). Oral gold has a 25% absorption rate. It has a predictable plasma concentration. The half-life of oral gold is 21 d. It binds to plasma proteins and to the membranes of red blood cells. Oral gold is principally excreted in the feces. It is not retained in the body and is nondetectable in keratinous tissues after cessation of therapy (20).

The clinical response observed in patients with autoimmune diseases treated by gold is due to the potent antiinflammatory and immunosuppressive effects of the agent. Gold reduces the release of inflammatory mediators (21). It also inhibits chemotactic and phagocytic responses of macrophages and polymorphonuclear leukocytes (22). Oral gold has been shown to inhibit antibody-dependent cell-mediated cytotoxicity, and complement lysis in vitro and suppress antibody production and the immune response (23).

The major limiting factor in the use of parenteral gold therapy is the high incidence of adverse reactions that are experienced by approximately one-third of the patients (20). While 80% of the complications are of no grave significance, 10–15% are usually reasonably severe and frequently require discontinuation of therapy. While they can occur at any time, they are most likely to occur during the initial phase of therapy. The frequency of side effects is much less with the oral preparation compared to the parenteral form.

Mucocutaneous side effects ranging from stomatitis to toxic epidermal necrolysis represent about 50% of complications with parenteral and approximately 30% with oral gold therapy. They are best managed by early recognition, cessation of therapy, and supportive care. Diarrhea is the most common side effect, noted in 35–40% of patients being treated with oral gold. Proteinuria usually secondary to a nephropathy has been reported with a frequency of 2–10%.

Hematological (thrombocytopenia, eosinophilia), ocular (keratitis, corneal ulceration), pulmonary (chronic fibrosis), or vasomotor side effects also can be quite distressing, and the dermatologist should be aware of them and maintain close follow-up on patients receiving chrysotherapy.

In the past, patients receiving parenteral gold were first given a test dose. If no idiosyncratic reactions were observed, 50 mg was administered weekly. However, since the oral preparation is now available, the use of parenteral gold is discouraged. When using oral gold, it is advisable to start with 3 mg a day for the first 3–5 d. If no undesirable effects are observed, increase the dose to 6 mg daily. In the majority of patients a good clinical response is seen at a daily dose of 6 mg, preferably in two divided doses (24).

The best method of preventing adverse or toxic effects is close follow-up of the patient. CBC with platelet counts and urine analysis should be done weekly for 6 wk, then once in 2 wk for the next 6 wk of therapy, and monthly thereafter throughout the course of therapy. In cases where a mild reaction is observed, a slight reduction in the dose of the drug frequently results in a better tolerance for the drug and also alleviates the reaction (20).

In patients who have not responded to azathioprine or to a subsequent trial of cyclophosphamide, gold may be a good alternative. Several studies indicate that chrysotherapy is effective as adjuvant therapy of PV, however there may be recurrences upon discontinuation of therapy (25,26). Treatment is usually 6 mg daily and may be needed for 9–18 months. If after 4 mo of consecutive use of optimal doses a clinical improvement is not clear, then the chrysotherapy should be discontinued.

4. Cyclosporin A

The dermatological applications of cyclosporin A have been reviewed recently (27,28). It is a cyclic polypeptide composed of 11 amino acids. Cyclosporin targets primarily the T helper lymphocytes. It inhibits them in their G0 and G1 phases (29). It decreases the production of IL-1, IL-2, and other cytokines. It may also abrogate the interaction of T-cell receptor (TCR) with the antigen. It also suppresses humoral immunity in a reversible manner. Suppressor cells appear to be unaffected by cyclosporin and perhaps even favored (29).

In treating autoimmune blistering skin disease, only the oral preparation (Sandimmune) is recommended. It is available in an olive oil base at 100 mg/ml. Reported studies in autoimmune blistering disease have used 6–8 mg/kg/d. However, doses in the range of 4–6 mg/kg/d are frequently adequate. In patients who do not respond to azathioprine, cyclophosphamide, or gold, especially when the disease is widespread and involves multiple mucous membranes, the use of oral cyclosporin A is particularly recommended. The clinical effects are usually evident in about 3–4 wk of maximum therapy.

Monitoring serum levels is the best way to determine the exact dose that a patient requires. A serum level of 100–125 ng/ml is usually an adequate level to obtain the desired clinical results. Once the desired clinical response is achieved, the dose should be gradually reduced, not abruptly stopped. Once started the therapy should be continued for at least 3 mo. The total duration of therapy is usually 6 mo. During the initial therapy serum levels, CBC, BUN, creatinine, and urine analysis must be performed weekly for 6 wk, then once in 2 wk for the subsequent 6 wk. Thereafter the frequency will depend on the response of the patient and the dosage used.

It is clear that cyclosporin A has no role as a single drug in controlling the acute stage of PV, but it is useful as an adjunct to systemic corticosteroids. There are reports of treating PV patients with cyclosporin (30).

5. Methotrexate

This agent competitively inhibits the enzyme dihydrofolate reductase, thus this blocker of purine synthesis is effective in inhibiting both DNA and RNA synthesis. In 1969, Lever and Goldberg described the use of methotrexate for control of PV (31). Subsequently the use of this agent has lessened, while the use of the other immunosuppressives has increased. Recently Bystryn summarized the treatment of pemphigus and believed that methotrexate was the least favored of the immunosuppressive agents (10).

6. Plasmapheresis

In some recalcitrant patients, immunosuppressive agents are used in combinations with other modalities like plasma exchange (32). Plasma exchange causes two types of rebound phenomenon. The first rebound occurs in the first 24–48 h of initiation of therapy. This is caused by a passive diffusion of immunoglobulins from the extracellular environment into the circulation. The second rebound is caused by an active physiological feedback mechanism that controls the serum levels of specific antibodies. Depletion of the specific PV antibodies induced by plasma exchange stimulates autoantibody synthesis. This rebound can be prevented by simultaneous use of corticosteroids and/or immunosuppressive agents (e.g., cyclophosphamide or azathioprine) that block autoantigen synthesis. It has been suggested that plasmapheresis be used in three sessions every week with exchange of 1.8–2 l of plasma each time.

7. Tranexamic Acid

Since experimental evidence suggests that plasminogen activator is involved in the pathogenesis of PV, recently tranexamic acid, which competitively inhibits conversion of plasminogen to plasmin, was used in treating two patients. It was found to be ineffective in preventing relapses during corticosteroid withdrawal (33).

Extracorporeal leukopheresis, intravenous immunoglobulin, and extracorporeal photopheresis are other forms of therapies; their effectiveness has not been confirmed.

8. Dapsone

Administered orally, dapsone is rapidly and almost completely absorbed, reaching peak concentration in 4–8 h. About 85% of it is excreted as metabolites in the urine. It has a rapid onset of action, and in the majority of patients clinical results can be observed with in 72 h of administration. It is reasonably safe in dosages of 50–200 mg daily. Side effects are more frequent when 300 mg or more daily doses are used.

Besides its antimicrobial potency, dapsone suppresses the generation of potentially damaging oxygen intermediates in neutrophils, particularly the hydroxyl radical, and inhibits the myeloperoxidase-H_2O_2-halide system, which is known to mediate cytotoxicity in mammalian cells (34). There is significant data to suggest that it interferes with cell-mediated immunity, diminishes specific immunoglobulin production, and is beneficial in treating immune complex mediated diseases (35).

The most significant side effect of dapsone is dose-related hemolysis. The majority of the patients treated with dapsone will demonstrate a 1–2 g reduction in hemoglobin levels, single-digit meth-hemoglobinemia, and 2–12% reticulocyte count. Such responses are greater in G6PD-deficient patients.

A reversible motor-loss peripheral neuropathy is a distressing but uncommon complication. Gastrointestinal distress, especially nausea is very common. Vertigo, blurred vision, and headaches are other side effects that frequently bother patients.

The mode of administration depends upon the condition treated. In treatment of autoimmune blistering diseases, therapy is initiated cautiously (36). The average patient responds to 100–150 mg daily doses. In patients with body weights exceeding 80 kg, it may be necessary to use 200–250 mg daily doses. The therapy has to be carefully monitored. Before initiation of dapsone the G6PD enzyme level must be checked in every patient irrespective of race. CBC with reticulocyte and platelet counts, SMA-12, and urine analysis should be monitored every week for the first 5–6 wk, then once a month for about 6 mo. The frequency of laboratory tests thereafter depends on the clinical response, the dose of the drug, and factors pertaining to the patients general medical condition. Careful monitoring of the patient is the best way to avoid side effects.

G. Treatment of Pemphigus Foliaceous

Pemphigus foliaceous and its variant pemphigus erythematosus (PE) respond quite well to lower doses of systemic corticosteroids and rarely require immunosuppressive therapy (37). Since the disease is less hazardous than PV, the clinician should use lower doses of systemic corticosteroids and accept the presence of a scattered few lesions in some areas. The dose of corticosteroids is rarely higher than 60–80 mg/d of prednisone. If this dose does not control the disease, it is worthwhile to try dapsone. Dapsone as a single agent, may be effective in treating PF and PE (38). Recurrences upon cessation of treatment may easily be controlled by resumption of the drug. If an immunosuppressive agent is needed, the first drug of choice should be oral gold (10,39).

II. BULLOUS PEMPHIGOID

A. Introduction

Bullous pemphigoid (BP) is an autoimmune subepidermal blistering disease that is usually observed in the elderly population. The presence of antiepidermal basement membrane zone (BMZ) autoantibodies is now a hallmark in the diagnosis of BP (40).

B. Etiology

The sera of 70–75% of the patients demonstrate the anti-BMZ antibody, the titer of which does not correlate with disease activity or severity (41). It is predominantly of the IgG4 subclass (42). In DIF, there is a deposition of immunoglobulins and/or complement components (mostly C3) at the BMZ in approximately 100% of patients.

C. Bullous Pemphigoid Antigen

Bullous pemphigoid antigen is a component in the BMZ of normal skin and is associated with hemidesmosomes. It is also found in the basement membrane of gallbladder, urethra, bladder, trachea, bronchi, and amnion. Bullous pemphigoid antigen is distributed in two pools, a large intracellular and a small extracellular pool (43–46). By direct immunoelectron microscopy, in vivo bound autoantibody deposits are seen only in the upper part of lamina lucida (44,45,47,48). In general, BP antigen was identified as a unique 230-kDa protein by immunoprecipitation (49–51). However, immunoblot analysis showed several different BP antigens, mainly the 230-kDa and 170- or 180-kDa proteins (52–56). There may be a difference in the 230-kDa BP antigen and the 170-kDa antigen (57).

D. Pathogenesis

Bullous pemphigoid is characterized by the presence of autoantibodies that bind to the BP antigen. IgG4 stimulates mast cells, and IgG1 and IgG3 activate complement. The complement system is activated by both classic and alternative pathways. C3a and C5a, act as chemoattractants for PMN leukocytes, eosinophils, and monocytes. Mast cells and eosinophils degranulate and release histamine, which may explain the early urticarial, pruritic lesions of BP. Proteolytic enzymes are then released from the PMN leukocytes, eosinophils, and mast cells. Separation at the lamina lucida occurs as a result of damage from these enzymes and/or from the direct cytotoxic effects of these cells. The ultimate result is the formation of a subepidermal blister.

E. Pathology

The disease is characterized by a subepidermal bulla, superficial dermal infiltrate mostly consisting of eosinophils, with varying numbers of lymphocytes and neutrophils.

The clinical presentation is heterogeneous and the course is considerably variable. In the majority of patients it has a self-limiting benign course. In some patients it can have a rapid turbulent course marked by relapses and remissions. Since these patients are usually elderly, some degree of difficulty is experienced in controlling the disease and in the overall management of the patient.

F. Indications for the Use of Immunomodulatory Agents

The indications for the use of immunosuppressive drugs in patients with BP are similar to those for patients with PV.

Widespread severe disease.

Patients not responding to 80 mg daily of prednisone.

Patients who have developed significant complications of systemic corticosteroid therapy.

Patients in whom high doses of systemic corticosteroids are not recommended (e.g., diabetes mellitus, uncontrolled hypertension, peptic ulcer, etc.).

Association with other autoimmune diseases.

G. Methods of Treatment

A careful decision should be made. The age, disease severity, clinical evolution, and course must be considered before initiating therapy. Many patients respond to 40–60 mg daily of prednisone alone (41,58). If successful management is not achieved, the first drug that should be added to the therapeutic armamentarium is dapsone. The therapy should be cautiously initiated as described earlier (37). A clinical response is observed in most patients with a 100–150 mg daily dose. The systemic corticosteroid should be tapered first, and once a dose of 30 mg of prednisone on alternate-day therapy is reached, a gradual and slow reduction of dapsone should be initiated. The slow withdrawal of dapsone is necessary to avoid recurrences. Recently in one study of 18 patients with BP, dapsone was used as the first or primary drug of choice for initial therapy (59). Whenever any adjuvant therapy is used to treat BP patients along with systemic corticosteroids, the adjuvant therapy should be continued until the dose of prednisone is reduced to 15 mg daily or equivalent.

If a combination of dapsone and prednisone are ineffective, then dapsone must be discontinued and azathioprine therapy instituted. Azathioprine in doses of 1–1.5 mg/kg/d reduces both the daily dose of prednisone needed to control the disease and the total duration of maintenance therapy with prednisone (60). The beneficial clinical effect of the azathioprine usually occurs in approximately 3–8 wk and should be maintained for an additional 8–10 wk. Systemic corticosteroids should be tapered and discontinued first. The total duration of therapy is usually 15–20 mo. In BP patients the same guarded and slow approach to dose reduction and tapering is suggested as in PV patients.

If the patient continues to have new lesions or previous lesions do not show signs of healing, in spite of 4 mo of maximum therapy with azathioprine, it should be considered a therapeutic failure. In such cases cyclophosphamide may be useful.

Nicotinamide (2500 mg/d) in combination with tetracycline (1500 mg/d) has been reported to be effective in BP (61,62). Such high doses of these two agents can have significant and distressing side effects in the elderly population. It is critical to emphasize that some of these patients had localized disease. In many patients the clinical course was of short duration and the disease was not widespread or recurrent in nature. The mechanism of action of these two agents is unknown. Nicotinamide inhibits polymorphonuclear and eosinophil chemotaxis and blocks IgE-mediated histamine release and mast cell degranulation (63). In addition, both tetracycline and nicotinamide inhibit lymphocyte blast transformation in vitro (64,65).

In patients nonresponsive to azathioprine and cyclophosphamide when the disease is clinically still active, a trial of cyclosporin A is suggested. Cyclosporin A has been reported to be effective in some patients (28,29). It should not be used as the first drug and should only be used in patients that are recalcitrant to other chemotherapeutic agents. Pulse therapy with methylprednisone (66), plasmapheresis (67), and intravenous gammaglobulin (68) have been used in limited treatment at special centers. The clinical benefit of the therapies has not been confirmed or established.

III. EPIDERMOLYSIS BULLOSA AQUISITA

A. Introduction

Epidermolysis bullosa aquisita (EBA) is an autoimmune subepidermal bullous disease of adult onset characterized by skin fragility. Trauma-induced blisters on the skin and mucosal surfaces, which resemble dystrophic epidermolysis bullosa, heal with scarring and milia formation (69). An increased frequency of HLA-DR2 has been reported in patients with EBA (70).

B. Immunopathological Findings

Direct immunofluorescence most frequently reveals the deposition of IgG and C3 in a linear pattern along the BMZ (71). The presence of three or more immunoreactants at the BMZ may be more indicative of EBA than of BP, which usually has only IgG and C3 (72). Indirect immunofluorescence reveals circulating anti-BMZ autoantibodies of the IgG class in nearly 50% of patients. Using the saline-split skin technique, these antibodies bind to the dermal (lower) portion of the split (73). This method differentiates EBA from BP where the anti-BMZ antibodies bind to the epidermal (upper) portion of the split. By immunoelectron microscopy, immunoglobulin deposition at the BMZ is specifically localized in the sublamina densa region. In BP this deposition can be demonstrated in the lamina lucida. Western immunoblot reveals that the autoantibodies are directed against the 290-kDa or 145-kDa protein, the EBA antigen (74).

C. Epidermolysis Bullosa Aquisita Antigen

The EBA antigen is present in normal stratified squamous epithelium. In normal skin, EBA antigen is thought to play a role in adherence of the BMZ to the papillary dermis (75). It is a 290-kDa glycoprotein composed of a 145-kDa globular, carbohydrate rich, collagenase-resistant domain identical to type VII collagen and a 145-kDa rod-like, collagenase-sensitive domain. The globular domain is in the lamina densa, and the collagen tail hangs perpendicularly into the sublamina densa, where it aggregates into anchoring fibrils.

D. Pathogenesis

The EBA IgG antibody binds to the EBA antigen type VII collagen and directly decreases the number of type VII collagen anchoring fibrils, activates complement, or both. Polymorphonuclear leukocytes are recruited which release proteolytic enzymes, causing BMZ damage (72). Several alterations in dermal connective tissue are found, including a decrease in mature collagen, an increase in the number of new collagen fibrils, and a decrease in elastin (76,77). These alterations may be secondary phenomena caused by BMZ inflammation.

E. Therapy

Spontaneous remissions are exceedingly rare and the clinical course is typically chronic and relentless. It is characterized by being relatively resistant to most therapies and by demonstrating only partial or temporary responses with eventual scarring and dystrophic changes (78). Cyclosporin A has been reported to be effective in some patients with this disease and warrants further trial and confirmation (79,80).

In resistant, recalcitrant cases, treatment with low-dose (10 mg on alternate-day) prednisone, 100 mg daily of dilantin, 75,000–100,000 units daily of vitamin A, or 10 mg daily of accutane may be an avenue of last resort. Most of these agents have some demonstrable activity against collagenase and may impede or deter scar formation.

Recently there has been a report of the successful use of high-dose intravenous immunoglobulin G (IgG) in the treatment of a resistant case of EBA to multiple therapies such as cyclosporin A, vitamin E, and prednisolone (81). Intravenous IgG was used in addition to prednisolone and cyclosporin. The dosage was 400 mg/kg/d for 4 d repeated every 2 wk. After four courses, there was a disappearance of circulating antibodies.

The mechanism of action of intravenous immunoglobulins may be due to the effects they have on the function of the immune system through antidiotypic activity or the modulation of T and B lymphocytes (82).

IV. BULLOUS ERYTHEMA MULTIFORME

Bullous erythema multiforme, or Stevens Johnson Syndrome (SJS), is a severe and at times fatal variety of erythema multiforme.

A. Etiology

There are number of etiological and precipitating factors that lead to this disease. They include drugs, infections (viral, bacterial, mycotic, protozoal), vaccines, allergic skin contacts, internal malignant diseases, x-ray irradiation of tumors, and other miscellaneous causes.

B. Pathogenesis

The immune system of the host may play an important role in the pathogenesis. It is hypothesized that foreign antigens are sequestered in the epidermis. These are a stimulus for the specific cytotoxic responses in the immune system that lead to epidermal cell damage. While circulating immune complexes have been documented in some cases of erythema multiforme, and DIF may show vascular deposits of IgM and C3, a true vasculitis does not appear to occur in the process of the disease.

Studies in recent years have provided evidence that supports the hypothesis that the major immunological mechanism of tissue damage in erythema multiforme is cell mediated. Such evidence includes the predominantly mononuclear inflammatory infiltrate present in the skin. T lymphocytes (T4 helper cells predominantly in the dermis and T8 cells in the epidermis), monocytes, and macrophages are the major inflammatory cells (83–85).

The keratinocytes in the lesions stain positively for cell surface HLA-DR antigens. The antigen(s) involved in the pathogenesis are not known. However, there are clues that pertinent foreign antigens may be present at the sites of tissue injury. In certain instances, cultures for herpes simplex virus and mycoplasma pneumonia have been positive in erythema multiforme skin lesions (86–89). There is also evidence demonstrating the presence of HSV DNA in the lesions (90).

C. Pathology

The pathological features consist of epidermal necrosis. The epidermis in early lesions contains groups of keratinocytes with eosinophilic necrosis. Such necrotic cells with the adjoining mononuclear cells is referred to as satellite cell necrosis. The dermal changes consist of a mononuclear infiltrate around superficial blood vessels. In severely affected areas, hydropic degeneration of the basal cells may result in subepidermal separation. In immunoelectron microscopy, the basal lamina, if present, is located at the floor of the bulla.

D. Therapy and Its Indications

By definition, erythema multiforme of the minor type is an acute, self-limited illness, resolving within 3–4 wk. However, in the SJS variety the tissue damage is more extensive and the illness may be more prolonged. Complications rarely seen in typical erythema multiforme may be significant in the bullous variety (91). Keratitis, dysphagia secondary to severe oral and pharyngeal erosions, and pneumonia in association with upper airway involvement have been reported.

Medical management of erythema multiforme attempts to bring about a suppresion of the host immune response and immune-mediated tissue damage and requires symptomatic and supportive therapies. Since it is believed that the host immune system is involved in the pathogenesis, it would seem reasonable that drugs that suppress this system might be of benefit in therapy. However, this issue is controversial and convincing data is not available. In severe cases of SJS, systemic corticosteroid therapy with 1.5–2 mg/kg/d (60–100 mg/d) of prednisone orally should be considered. Patients unable to tolerate oral intake should be treated with 1 mg/kg of triamcinolone acetonide in a single IM dose, repeated after 3–4 d. It should be emphasized that the therapy should be given early in the course of the disease. Such therapy may not be of benefit once the tissue damage has already occurred and may lead to complications or can retard healing (92). Other immune suppressive drugs such as azathioprine probably do not act rapidly enough to be useful in therapy. Wilkel and McDonald have reported on the use of cyclosporin in severe bullous erythema multiforme that had proven resistant to all other therapeutic interventions (93). In severe cases with widespread cutaneous damage, aggressive therapy in a specialized burn unit is appropriate. Intravenous fluids, respiratory care, narcotic analgesics, moist dressings, antibiotics, and even skin grafts may be indicated (94).

While the guidelines provided are effective in most patients, it is important to emphasize that these diseases are rare. Hence, each patient should be carefully and individually evaluated and therapy should be adjusted to meet the needs of the individual patient. Whenever possible, advice and suggestions from individuals with more experience should be obtained. Such advice may be more beneficial if obtained early. As the immune system and especially the pathogenesis of autoimmunity is better understood, agents with specific modes of actions will become available. Advances in molecular biology coupled with advances in molecular pharmacology may result in agents or drugs that might be highly selective in treating such diseases.

REFERENCES

1. Ahmed AR, Graham J, Jordon RE, Provost TT. Pemphigus current concepts. Ann Intern Med 1980; 92:396–405.
2. Korman N. Pemphigus. J Acad Dermat 1988; 18:1219–1238.
3. Wasserstrum N, Laros RK. Transplacental transmission of pemphigus. JAMA 1983; 249:1480–1482.
4. Anhalt GJ, Labib RS, Voorhees JJ, et al. Induction of pemphigus in neonatal mice by passive transfer of IgG from patients with the disease. N Engl J Med 1982; 306:1189–1196.
5. Ahmed AR, Yunis EJ, Khatri K, Wagner R, et al. Major histocompatability complex haplotype studies in Ashkenazi Jewish patients with pemphigus vulgaris. Proc Natl Acad Sci USA 1990; 87:7658–7662.
6. Ahmed AR, Wagner R, Khatri K, Notani G, et al. Major histocompatibility complex haplotypes and class II genes in non-Jewish patients with pemphigus vulgaris. Proc Natl Acad Sci USA 1991; 88:5056–5060.
7. Amagai M, Klaus-Kovtun V, Stanley JR. Autoantibodies against a novel epithelial cadherin in pemphigus vulgaris, a disease of cell adhesion. Cell 1991; 67:869–877.

8. Stanley JR, Klaus-Kovtun V, Sampaio SA. Antigenic specificity of fogo selvagem autoantibodies is similar to North American pemphigus and distinct from pemphigus vulgaris autoantibodies. J Invest Dermat 1986; 87:197–201.
9. Ahmed AR. Clinical features of pemphigus. Clin Dermat 1983; 1(2):13–21.
10. Bystryn JC. Adjuvant therapy of pemphigus. Arch Dermat 1985; 120:941–951.
11. Aberer W, Wolf-Schreiner EC, Stingl G, Wolff K. Azathioprine in treatment of pemphigus vulgaris. J Am Acad Dermat 1987; 16:527–533.
12. Ahmed AR, Hombal SH. Use of cyclophosphamide in azathioprine failures in pemphigus. J Am Acad Dermat 1987; 17:437–442.
13. McDonald CJ. Cytotoxic agents for use in dermatology I. J Am Acad Dermat 1985; 12:753–775.
14. Callen JP. Immunosuppressive and cytotoxic drugs: uses in the dermatologic patient. In: Callen JP, Dahl MV, Golitz LE, Schachner LA, Stegman SJ (eds.), Advances in dermatology. Vol. 5. Chicago: Year Book Medical Publishers, 1990:5.
15. McDonald CJ. Use of cytotoxic drugs in dermatologic disease II. J Am Acad Dermat 1985; 12:965–975.
16. Gendler E. Azathioprine for use in dermatology. J Dermat Surg Oncol 1984; 10:462–464.
17. Ahmed AR, Hombal SH. Cyclophosphamide. J Am Acad Dermat 1984; 11:1115–1126.
18. Stevenson HC, Fauci AS. Activation of human B lymphocyte XII differential effect of in vitro cyclophosphamide on human lymphocyte sub-population involved in B cell activation. Immunology 1980; 39:391–397.
19. Cox PJ. Cyclophosphamide cystitis and bladder carcinoma-a hypothesis. Eur J Cancer Clin Oncol 1979; 15:1071–1072.
20. Thomas I. Gold therapy and its indications in dermatology. J Am Acad Dermat 1987; 16:845–854.
21. Persellin RH, Ziff M. The effects of gold salts on lysosomal enzymes of peritoneal macrophages. Arthr Rheum 1966; 9:57–65.
22. Wolach B, DeBoard JE, Coates TD. Correlation of in vitro and in vivo effects of gold compounds on leukocyte functions: possible mechanism of action. J Lab Clin Med 1982; 100:37–44.
23. Walz DT, Dimartino MJ, Griswold DE. Mechanism of action of auranofin. J Rheum 1982; 9(suppl):32–36.
24. Weiss TE. Auranofin: dose-related risk to benefit. Am J Med 1983; 75:128–132.
25. Poulin Y, Perry HO, Muller SA. Pemphigus vulgaris: results of treatment with gold as a steroid-sparing agent in a series of 13 patients. J Am Acad Dermat 1984; 11:851–857.
26. Salomon D, Saurat JH. Oral gold therapy (auranofin) in pemphigus vulgaris. Dermatologica 1986; 172:310–314.
27. Biren CA, Barr RJ. Dermatologic applications of cyclosporin. Arch Dermat 1986; 122:1028–1032.
28. Page EH, Wexler DM, Guenther LC. Cyclosporin A. J Am Acad Dermat 1986; 14:785–789.
29. Wagner H. Cyclosporin A: mechanism of action. Transplant Proc 1983; 15:523–526.

30. Barthelemy H, Frappaz A, Cambarard F, Maudit G. Treatment of nine cases of pemphigus vulgaris with cyclosporin. J Am Acad Dermat 1988; 18:1262–1266.
31. Lever WF, Goldberg HS. Treatment of pemphigus vulgaris with methotrexate. Arch Dermat 1969; 100:70–78.
32. Guillaume JC, Roujeau JC, Morel P, et al. Controlled study of plasma exchange in pemphigus. Arch Dermat 1988; 124:1659–1663.
33. Marsden J. Lack of response of pemphigus to tranexamic acid. Br J Dermat 1987; 116:882–883.
34. Clarke RA, Klebanoff SJ, Einstein AB. Peroxidase-H_2O_2 halide system: cytotoxic effect on mammalian tumor cells. Blood 1975; 45:161–170.
35. Das PK, Uytdehaag F, Westerhof W. DDS inhibits in vitro synthesis of specfic IgA and IgG antibodies by sensitized human PBL. J Invest Dermat 1985; 84:434–439.
36. Rogers RS. Dapsone and sulfapyridine therapy of pemphigoid disease. Aust J Dermat 1986; 68:58–63.
37. Amerian ML, Ahmed AR. Pemphigus erythematosus. Int J Dermat 1985; 24:16–25.
38. Basset N, Guillot B, Michel B, et al. Dapsone as initial treatment in superficial pemphigus. Arch Dermat 1987; 123:783–785.
39. Lynch PJ, Gallego RE, Saied NK. Pemphigus: a review. Ariz Med 1976; 33:1030–1037.
40. Jordon RE, Beutner EM, Witebsky E, et al. Basement membrane zone antibodies in bullous pemphigoid. JAMA 1967; 200:91–96.
41. Hadi SM, Barnetson SR, Gankrodger DJ, et al. Clinical, histologic, and immunological studies in 50 patients with bullous pemphigoid. Dermatologica 1988; 176:6–17.
42. Bird P, Friedmann PS, Ling N, Bird AG, Thompson RD. Subclass distribution of IgG autoantibodies in bullous pemphigoid. J Invest Dermat 1986; 86:21–25.
43. Yamasaki Y, Nishikawa T. Ultrastructural localization of in vitro binding sites of circulating antibasement membrane zone antibodies in bullous pemphigoid. Acta Dermat Vener 1983; 63:501–506.
44. Mutasim DF, Takahashi Y, Labib RS, Anhalt GJ, Patel H, Diaz LA. A pool of bullous pemphigoid antigen is intracellular and associated with the basal cell cytoskeleton-hemidesmosome complex. J Invest Dermat 1985; 84:47–53.
45. Horigushi Y, Imamura S. Discrepancy between the localization of in vivo bound immunoglobulins in the skin and in vitro binding sites of circulating anti-BMZ antibodies in bullous pemphigoid: immunoelectron microscopic studies. J Invest Dermat 1986; 87:715–719.
46. Shimizu H, McDonald J, Kennedy A, Eady R. Demonstration of intra and extracellular localization of bullous pemphigoid antigen using cryofixation and freeze substitution for post-embedding immunoelectron microscopy. Arch Dermat Res 1989; 281:443–448.
47. Prost C, Labeille B, Chaussade V, Guillaume JC, Dubertret L. Immunoelectron microscopy in subepidermal autoimmune bullous diseases: a prospective study of IgG and C3 bound in vivo in 32 patients. J Invest Dermat 1987; 89:567–573.
48. Shimizu H, Hayakawa K, Nishikawa T. A comparative immunoelectron microscopic study of typical and atypical cases of pemphigoid. Br J Dermatol 1988; 119:717–722.

49. Stanley JR, Hawley-Nelson P, Yuspa SH, Shevach EM, Katz SI. Characterization of bullous pemphigoid antigen: a unique basement membrane protein of stratified squamous epithelia. Cell 1981; 24:897–903.
50. Stanley JR, Woodley DT, Katz SI. Identification and partial characterization of pemphigoid antigen extracted from normal human skin. J Invest Dermat 1984; 82:108–111.
51. Mueller S, Klaus-Kovtun V, Stanley JR. A 230-kd basic protein is the major bullous pemphigoid antigen. J Invest Dermat 1989; 92:33–38.
52. Labib RS, Anhalt GJ, Patel HP, Mutasim DF, Diaz LA. Molecular heterogeneity of the bullous pemphigoid antigens as detected by immunoblotting. J Immunol 1986; 136:1231–1235.
53. Robledo MA, Kim SC, Korman NJ, Stanley JR, Labib RS, Futamura S, Anhalt GJ. Studies of the relationship of the 230-KD and 180-KD bullous pemphigoid antigens. J Invest Dermat 1990; 94:793–797.
54. Cook AL, Hanahoe THP, Mallett RB, Pye RJ. Recognition of two distinct major antigens by bullous pemphigoid sera. Br J Dermat 1990; 122:435–444.
55. Meyer LJ, Taylor TB, Kadunce DP, Zone JJ. Two groups of bullous pemphigoid antigens are identified by affinity-purified antibodies. J Invest Dermat 1990; 94:611–616.
56. Meyer LJ, Taylor TB, Kadunce DP, Thuong-Nguyen V, Zone JJ. Bullous pemphigoid antigens: extraction and degradation of antigens during epidermal preparation. J Invest Dermat 1991; 96:991–993.
57. Hashimoto T, Ebihara T, Ishiko A, Shimizu H, Bhogal BS, Black MM, Stanley JR, Nishikawa T. Comparative study of bullous pemphigoid antigens among Japanese, British, and U.S. patients indicates similar antigen profiles with the 170-KD antigen present both in the basement membrane and on the keratinocyte cell membrane. J Invest Dermat 1993; 100:385–389.
58. Korman N. Bullous pemphigoid. J Am Acad Dermat 1987; 16:907–924.
59. Venning VA, Millard PR, Wojnarowska F. Dapsone as first line therapy for bullous pemphigoid. Br J Dermat 1989; 120:83–92.
60. Lever WF. Pemphigus and pemphigoid. J Am Acad Dermat 1979; 1:2–31.
61. Berk MA, Lorincz AL. The treatment of bullous pemphigoid with tetracycline and nicotinamide: a preliminary report. Arch Dermat 1986; 122:670–674.
62. Thornfeldt CR, Menkes AW. Bullous pemphigoid controlled by tetracycline. J Am Acad Dermat 1987; 16:305–310.
63. Berkier E, Masinski C. Antihistaminic action of nicotinamide. Agent Action 1974; 4:196.
64. Burger DR, Vandenbark AA, Daves D, et al. Nicotinamide: suppression of lymphocyte transformation with a component identified in human transfer factor. J Immunol 1976; 117:797–801.
65. Thong YH, Ferrante A. Inhibition of mitogen-induced human lymphocyte proliferative responses to tetracycline analogues. Clin Exp Immunol 1979; 35:443–446.
66. Siegel J, Eagelstein WH. High close methylprednisolone in treatment of bullous pemphigoid. Arch Dermat 1984; 120:1157–1165.

67. Roujeau JC, Morel P, Dalle E, Guillot B, Gorin I, Revuz L. Plasma exchange in bullous pemphigoid. Lancet 1984; 1:486–489.
68. Adoue D, Vilain C, Fontan B, LeTallec Y, Albarede JL, Oksman F. Utilisation de tres faibles doses d'immunoglobulines intraveneuses pour le traitment des pemphigoides bulleuses. Press Med 1987; 16:1625–1627.
69. Gammon RW, Briggaman RA, Woodley DT, Heald PW, Wheeler CE. Epidermolysis bullosa aquisita: a pemphigoid-like disease. J Am Acad Dermat 1984; 11:820–832.
70. Gammon RW, Heise ER, Burke WA, et al. Increased frequency of HLA-DR2 in patients with autoantibodies to EBA antigen. J Invest Dermat 1988; 91:228–232.
71. Yaoita H, Briggaman RA, Lawley TJ, et al. Epidermolysis bullosa aquisita: ultrastructural and immunological studies. J Invest Dermat 1981; 76:288–292.
72. Fine JD, Tyring S, Gammon WR. The presence of intralamina lucida blister formation in epidermolysis bullosa aquisita: possible role of leukocytes. J Invest Dermat 1989; 92:27–32.
73. Woodley DT. Immunofluorescence on salt-split skin for the diagnosis of epidermolysis bullosa aquisita. Arch Dermat 1990; 126:229–231.
74. Zhu XJ, Niimi Y, Bystryn JC. Epidermolysis bullosa aquisita: incidence in patients with basement membrane zone antibodies. Arch Dermat 1989; 126:171–174.
75. Woodley DT. Epidermolysis bullosa aquisita. Prog Dermat 1988; 22:1–13.
76. Kushniruk W. The immunopathology of epidermolysis bullosa aquisita. Can Med Assoc J 1973; 108:1143–1146.
77. Gibbs RB, Minus HR. Epidermolysis bullosa aquisita with electron microscopical studies. Arch Dermat 1975; 111:215–220.
78. Caughman SW. Epidermolysis bullosa aquisita. Arch Dermat 1986; 122:159–161.
79. Crow LL, Finkle JP, Gammon RW, Woodley DT. Clearing of epidermolysis bullosa aquisita with cyclosporine. J Am Acad Dermat 1988; 19:937–942.
80. Merle C, Blanc D, Zultak M, et al. Intractable epidermolysis bullosa acquisita: efficacy of cyclosporin A. Dermatologica 1990; 181:44–47.
81. Meier F, Sonnichsen K, Schaumburg-Lever G, Dopfer R, Rassner G. Epidermolysis bullosa aquisita: efficacy of high-dose intravenous immunoglobulins. J Am Acad Dermat 1993; 29:334–337.
82. Gordon DS. Intravenous immunoglobulin therapy: new directions and unanswered questions. Am J Med 1987; 83:52–56.
83. Tonnesen MG, Harrist TJ, Wintrub BU. Erythema multiforme microvascular damage and infiltration of lymphocytes and basophils. J Invest Dermat 1983; 80:282–286.
84. Margolis RJ, Tonnesen MG, Harrist TJ, et al. Lymphocyte subsets and Langerhans cells/indeterminate cells in erythema multiforme. J Invest Dermat 1983; 81:403–406.
85. Zaim MT, Giorno RC, Golitz LE, et al. An immunopathologic study of herpes-associated erythema multiforme. J Cutan Pathol 1987; 14:252–262.
86. Foerster DW, Scott LV. Isolation of herpes simplex virus from a patient with erythema mulfiforme exudativum (Stevens Johnson Syndrome). N Engl J Med 1958; 159:473–475.
87. McDonald A, Feiwel M. Isolation of herpes simplex virus from erythema multiforme. Br Med J 1972; 2:570–571.

88. Lyell A, Gordon AM, Dick MM, Sommerville DG. Mycoplasmas and erythema multiforme. Lancet 1967; 2:1116–1118.
89. Stutman HR. Stevens-Johnson Syndrome and mycoplasma pneumoniae: evidence for cutaneous infections. J Pediatr 1987; 111:845–847.
90. Brice SL, Krzemien D, Weston WL, Huff JC. Dectection of herpes simplex virus DNA in cutaneous lesions of erythema multiforme. J Invest Dermat 1989; 93:183–187.
91. Huff JC, Weston WL, Tonnesen MG. Erythema multiforme: a critical review of characteristics, diagnostic criteria and causes. J Am Acad Dermat 1983; 8:763–775.
92. Goldschmidt H, Grekin RC. Erythema and urticaria. In: Arnold HL, Odom RB, James WD (eds.), Andrew's diseases of the skin. Philadelphia: W.B. Saunders, 1990:137.
93. Wilkel C, McDonald CJ. Cyclosporin for resistant bullous erythema multiforme. Arch Dermat 1990; 126:397.
94. Marvin JA, Heimbach DM, Engrov LH, Harnas TJ. Improved treatment of the Stevens-Johnson Syndrome. Arch Surg 1984; 119:601–605.

14
Connective Tissue, Autoimmune Rheumatic Diseases

Charles J. McDonald
Brown University, Providence, Rhode Island

I. INTRODUCTION

There are an infinite number of diseases in which altered immunity and inflammation contribute to disease manifestations. Among these, the connective tissue or autoimmune rheumatic diseases are characterized by high levels of morbidity and mortality. In the following discussion, treatment of three of the most common and potentially most devastating diseases will be reviewed: systemic lupus erythematosus, progressive systemic sclerosis, and dermatomyositis. Although each of the three diseases presents with unique clinical manifestations, and it is probable that there are multiple factors involved in their initiation, promotion, and progression that are unique, all are in some measure caused by or are associated with abnormal T- and/or B-lymphocyte function.

II. SYSTEMIC LUPUS ERYTHEMATOSUS

Systemic lupus erythematosus (SLE) is a systemic autoimmune disorder characterized by chronic inflammation and immune-complex-mediated injury to a large and diverse number of organ systems within the human body. Within this segment or subset of lupus erythematous (LE) is a small number of patients with relatively severe internal manifestation of the disorder.

SLE occurs most commonly in females, tending to be more prevalent and severe in females of African American descent (1,2). The genetics of LE and the SLE subset are unclear at best. Some LE subsets have well-defined and strong HLA associations such as those groups that produce anti-RO and anti-LA antibodies (3–6). However, in many patients with active systemic disease, genetic linkages are weak or nonexistent (7).

A. Etiology and Pathogenesis

A vast array of immunological abnormalities occur in patients with SLE, some of which appear to be responsible for many of its clinical manifestations, and yet real pathogenetic mechanisms for the disease have not been identified. It appears that the disease occurs as a result of an immunomodulatory disturbance in a genetically predisposed host upon which a number of endogenous and exogenous factors interplay. A significant endogenous factor may be hormonal. Experimental studies in human and animal models have identified abnormalities in estrogen metabolism as an activating factor in this disease (8,9).

Among factors considered exogenous, excessive ultraviolet (UV) light exposure (UVA and UVB), drugs, stress, and infections have been associated with the precipitation or exacerbation of clinical disease in patients with SLE (10–12). The influence of UV light on the initiation and exacerbation of cutaneous disease has been most widely studied. It has been proposed that exposure to UV light enhances production and release of T-lymphocyte activated cytokines, inflammatory mediators, and adhesion molecules such as interleukin-1 and -6 (IL-1, IL-6), intercellular adhesion molecule-1 (ICAM-1), and prostaglandins (13–16). IL-1 exerts multiple effects on a wide variety of cell types. It activates antigen presenting cells causing the production of IL-2 through IL-6. IL-1 mediates cytotoxicity of lymphocytes through the production of tumor necrosis factor (TNF). It is involved in the maturation of B cells, and in synergy with other cytokines promotes B-cell proliferation and differentiation. IL-6 is a proinflammatory cytokine that up-regulates the production of acute phase proteins as well as stimulates T-cell proliferation. ICAM-1 is an important mediator of cell-to-cell adhesions. It is not difficult for one to postulate that the initiation and exacerbation of SLE begins with UV light exposure and injury to cutaneous epidermal cells causing release of IL-1 and IL-6. Lymphoid effector cells, both T and B cells, and macrophages are recruited to the affected epidermis by IL-1 and IL-6 and are bound to keratinocytes through the action of ICMA-1. Activated T cells and macrophages that have been recruited to the site through a mechanism of antibody-dependent, cell-mediated cytotoxicity produce further cellular damage and inflammation to initiate the first step in the disease process.

B. Pathology

The most conspicuous feature in patients with SLE is the regularity with which they produce autoantibodies against numerous cellular components. Within the cell these may be antinuclear antibodies (ANA), antibodies to double-stranded DNA (dsDNA) and single-stranded DNA (ssDNA), and antibodies directed toward the Smith antigen (Sm) and the Robert nuclear antigen (Ro) or soluble substance-A (SS-A). Other antibodies produced in LE include those directed toward the Lane soluble substance-B (SS-B) antigen, antiphospholipid antibodies, and antibodies to red blood cells, lymphocytes, and other cellular components in almost any organ or tissue in the body. Significantly, most of these autoantibodies are not specific to LE and are shared with one or more of the other autoimmune rheumatic diseases. However, there are some circulating antibodies, when found in high titers, that are very indicative of SLE (i.e., high titers of antibodies to double-stranded DNA, antibodies to Sm antigen, and antibodies to SS-A).

Tissue injury in SLE is believed to be initiated by complement-mediated immune complex deposition at a variety of organ sites. Deposition of immunoglobulins and complement can best be visualized using direct immunofluorescence at the dermal-epidermal junction (17). Finding immunoglobulin and complement at the dermal-epidermal junction in non-sun-exposed skin (buttocks) is often predictive of very serious SLE, especially LE nephritis (18). Likewise, the presence of antibodies to dsDNA within the renal glomerular basement membrane is indicative of the severity of SLE associated kidney disease. The predictive value of the lupus band test relative to the presence or absence of lupus nephritis has been debated. Based on the accumulated findings of the majority of studies, it appears that the specificity of the test increases with the number of immunoglobulins and the amount of complement detected at the basement membrane (19). It must be remembered that the lupus band test is one of a battery of tests necessary to make a firm diagnosis of SLE.

Immune complex deposition in SLE is mediated by complement. Therefore the level of complement in the serum often reflects disease activity. In very active disease complement levels can be depressed due to complement deposition in areas of increased disease subsequent to its consumption in the production of immune complexes. Reduced complement serum levels may also relate to decreased complement production, principally in the liver. Although decreased production occurs primarily in active disease, it does not appear that the level of immune complexing is decreased. Patients with reduced serum complement levels are at greatest risk of developing severe renal and central nervous system disease.

1. Skin

Patients with SLE may present with a variety of cutaneous lesions. Approximately 15% will present with typical discoid lupus lesions. Others show erythematous or edematous patches of varying size; surface scaling and epidermal atrophy are usually absent. Any area of the skin may be involved, including the malar region, although involvement of the malar region of the face does not occur as often as has been implied. Some patients present with urticaria, petechiae, vesicles, and telangiectasias. Often the latter lesions are signs that are indicative of disease with poor prognosis.

Early erythematous or edematous lesions may show nonspecific histopathological changes in the skin. Later stages are characterized by hydropic degeneration of the basal cell layer of the epidermis and proliferation of small blood vessels within the dermis. Edema and extravasation of red blood cells through blood vessels walls may be seen. Fibrinoid deposits in the dermis are quite common and are located principally between and within collagen bundles, but may also be seen in the subepidermal basement membrane and in the walls of dermal capillaries. Fat cells show signs of inflammation and focal mucoid degeneration.

2. Systemic Organs

Patients with SLE often show histological abnormalities in the kidney, heart, lung, spleen, and serous membranes. Renal changes are found in two-thirds of patients affected and consist of glomerular hypercellularity of the mesangium; diffuse, uniform thickening of the glomerular capillary wall; intracapillary or extracapillary cellular proliferation; mesangial and subendothelial deposition of fibrinoid; and glomerular sclerosis. These changes may be localized (focal) or may involve most of the renal glomeruli (diffuse). Small loci of inflammation and degeneration of muscle fibers can be seen in the myocardium and in skeletal muscle. In the spleen, fibrosis around follicular arteries can be seen. The submucosa of serous membranes, such as the pleura and epicardium, show fibrinoid deposits and a chronic inflammatory infiltrate. Small vegetations of the valve leaflets are associated with inflammation, deposition of fibrinoid, and fibrosis in subendothelial connective tissue.

C. Indications for Use of Cytotoxic Drugs

Treatment of SLE is directed toward reducing morbidity and mortality through appropriate treatment of the disease in major organ systems. The end result is relief of symptoms and prevention of organ damage as indicated by improvement in abnormal laboratory values.

Antiinflammatory agents such as aspirin, nonsteroidal antiinflammatory drugs, and antimalarials are drugs of choice in patients demonstrating disease of mild to moderate severity. Patients with mild disease characteristically show low-grade fevers, malaise, myalgias, arthralgias, and on occasion frank arthritis. Small doses of corticosteroids, 10–20 mg/d, may be required to supplement nonsteroidal and antimalarial drugs in these patients. Infrequently, high doses of corticosteroids may be required to control severe symptoms in patients with fulminant SLE, that is, patients with nephritis, central nervous system disease, vasculitis, pneumonitis, thrombocytopenia, and/or acute hemolytic anemia. Patients with severe disease are often refractory to even high dosages of corticosteroids. In such cases the use of cytotoxic drugs is almost mandatory, and the need for protracted use of moderate to high dosages of corticosteroids in patients with vasculitis, nephritis, pneumonitis, and CNS disease should prompt one to consider the alternate use of cytotoxic drugs.

Although the largest amount of data on the use of cytotoxic drugs in SLE have been accumulated in the treatment of renal disease (20–24), there is substantial positive data accumulating from controlled and open studies of cytotoxic drug use in CNS disease, vasculitis, thrombocytopenia, and pneumonitis (25–27). Boumpas et al. (27) have studied the effect of parenteral pulse cyclophosphamide therapy in patients with active SLE and severe central nervous system involvement. Using cyclophosphamide infusions, 0.75–1.0 g/m^2, once monthly for at least 2 mo, his group was able to conclude that " 'parenteral' pulse cyclophosphamide is an effective adjunctive therapy for the management of patients with SLE and especially to reduce central nervous system symptoms"(27). Simeon-Aznar et al. have reported on the positive response of patients with transverse myelitis in SLE after treatment with corticosteroids and cyclophosphamide (28). Klaiman and Miller have likewise reported a good clinical response in a single patient with SLE and transverse myelitis treated in a similar manner (29). Godeau, et al. (26) reported a positive response in a patient with bronchiolitis obliterans in SLE. The patient was treated initially with prednisone and experienced a transitory response. With the addition of cyclophosphamide at 2–4 mg/kg/d there was a dramatic and prolonged improvement of pulmonary disease (26).

As noted earlier, it is in the treatment of SLE nephritis in which the greatest amount of experimental data has been accumulated. Hence, much of the discussion of the use of cytotoxic and immunomodulatory agents in SLE will be limited to their use in lupus nephritis. In spite of extensive and mostly anecdotal literature describing the beneficial use of cytotoxic agents in lupus nephritis, controversy continues to exist. Is there a place for so-called aggressive therapy in the treatment of patients with SLE? Most authorities who care for patients with severe SLE will respond that there is. However, it is in the area of patient selection that disagreement is most profound. As years pass and more and more cases of SLE are uncovered, a substantial number of rheumatologists have concluded that most patients with SLE have benign, non-life threatening disease, and even among patients with renal disease a substantial number have disease that is not life threatening. Therefore, most treatment regimens for patients with SLE, even SLE with less than severe renal disease, should consist of agents that are qualitatively benign (30, 31).

Among patients with lupus renal disease it is possible to isolate a population whose disease is of such severity that it has the potential to cause substantial morbidity and mortality. It is within this group of patients that nearly everyone agrees cytotoxic or immunosuppressive therapy can be beneficial. Patients who show World Health Organization (WHO) class III or IV renal pathology, have significant glomerular disease, focal or diffuse, and who experience a fall in creatinine clearance to 70 ml/min/1.75 ml^2 should be considered for treatment with cytotoxic and immunosuppressive agents. Which agent is most beneficial has also been debated. Is it cyclophosphamide, methotrexate (MTX), azathioprine, or cyclosporine? To date, there is insufficient experience using MTX and cyclosporine to establish a reliable estimate of their efficacy.

Although azathioprine was the first of this class of agents to undergo controlled investigation in lupus nephritis, and it is considered the least toxic of the four, its activity does not appear to be sufficient to control but the most moderate forms of renal disease (32). Average daily dosages up to 90 mg/m^2 or 150 mg total are administered. Often prednisone at a total daily dosage approximating 60–80 mg is given along with azathioprine. Cyclophosphamide is by far the most widely used agent to achieve immunosuppression in SLE. It can be given by mouth or by intravenous infusion. Total oral dosages approximate 100–200 mg/d. In most centers that treat lupus nephritis with cytotoxic drugs, intravenous administration of cyclophosphamide has almost completely supplanted the use of oral drug.

Intravenous cyclophosphamide is usually given in pulse fashion. In a study conducted by Austin et al. (33), pulsed intravenous cyclophosphamide treatment was found to be superior to oral treatment. It appears that patients receiving intravenous pulse cyclophosphamide develop fewer cases of end stage renal disease than those receiving oral treatment. This is especially true for treatment during the early or initial phase of renal disease. Not only is cyclophosphamide more efficacious when administered in pulse fashion, it also appears that some of the known toxicities associated with this drug are obviated. On occasion, intravenous or oral corticosteroids may be added to a regimen using cyclophosphamide.

What is the expected outcome of treating patients with severe renal disease using cyclophosphamide. It is generally agreed that the early use of cyclophosphamide rather than corticosteroids leads to an improved prognosis (32). Renal function is statistically better preserved in patients receiving intravenous cyclophosphamide early in the course of the disease (33). There is a significant reduction in the probability of the disease progressing to renal failure, even in severe lupus nephritis (33). Although treatment outcome is better in early renal disease, significant benefits of cyclophosphamide use are seen in all patient groups with renal disease. The real benefit of treatment with cyclophosphamide becomes most apparent sometime after 5 y of treatment. Patients with normal serum creatinine levels at the beginning of treatment, or patients whose initial elevated serum creatinine returns to normal within 48 wk, are at low risk of developing progressive renal failure (34). Therefore, they may not require long-term treatment with cyclophosphamide. While certain patients appear to undergo complete remission with pulse cyclophosphamide, some require maintenance therapy indefinitely at 3 mo intervals (32). Not withstanding the significant effect of immunosuppressive treatment on the patient with lupus renal disease, McInnes et al. (35) have examined the economic impact of treating severe renal disease with cytotoxic agents. His group has concluded that over a 10 y period as much as $93 million in health care is saved by the use of combination therapy for severe lupus nephritis (35).

Indications for the use of cytotoxic and immunomodulatory agents in childhood SLE is of utmost interest to the dermatologist and rheumatologist, especially those who specialize in childhood diseases. Like in adult SLE, the use of immunosuppressive drugs to treat childhood disease is controversial. Lehman has addressed may of the issues surrounding treatment of childhood SLE and I shall quote liberally from him (36). Corticosteroid therapy, whether given on alternate days or daily, when given in sufficient dosages to control active disease will result in a large number of undesirable effects such as altered facial appearance, hirsutism, emotional lability, acne, short stature, striae, aseptic necrosis, and steroid cataracts. It appears that the properly monitored patient who is treated with cytotoxic drugs will experience considerably fewer adverse reactions during the course of treatment, thus immunosuppressive drugs are increasingly being used as an alternative to corticosteroids in severe childhood SLE. There are data to support the use of cyclophosphamide in childhood renal disease. Lehman (36) suggests that the use of criteria established for adults to select children for treatment with immunosuppressives may not be appropriate. He states that preservation of adequate renal function just to assure normal growth may require earlier treatment in children with aggressive diffuse proliferative glomerulonephritis. The efficacy of cyclophosphamide and other immunomodulatory drugs in controlling central nervous system, pulmonary, and other severe organ disease in children is not well established. It is considered permissible by some investigators to use immunomodulatory drugs in life-threatening disease affecting any and all vital organ systems in childhood.

D. Rationale for Treatment

Although often postulated, the how and why of immunosuppressive therapy in SLE remains unknown. To recapitulate, SLE like other rheumatic diseases occurs when self-recognition (tolerance) mechanisms break down and self-structures become the target (antigen) for protective substances (antibodies). Antigen and antibody complexing initiate a vast series of events within the host immune inflammatory system, which in turn stimulates the increased production of cytokines and the recruitment of macrophages, T lymphocytes, B lymphocytes, and other antigen-presenting and cytokine-producing cells to the affected site. Inflammation resulting from interactions of this type are locally destructive, and the end result is substantial damage to the affected organ. T lymphocytes (T cells) play a very important role in the initiation and perpetuation of the SLE immune response. Helper T cells stimulate B-cell proliferation and the production of immune globulins. T cells also potentiate the function of other activated T cells. A normal immune response as well as an autoimmune response does not occur in the absence of T-cell augmentation. It has been shown in animal systems during transient T-cell depletion that tolerance can be induced toward a specific antigen that is introduced during the period of helper T-cell depletion (37). Takeno et al. (38) in comparing the effects of two different treatment regimens on immune function—prednisone alone versus cyclophosphamide plus prednisolone—found that cyclophosphamide caused a selective reduction of serum IgM, and that combined cyclophosphamide and prednisolone interfered with cell-cycle progression of resting B cells to an activated point after immune stimulation.

Potentially an agent such as cyclophosphamide may exert a variety of effects on the immune inflammatory system. It can inhibit T-cell replication, probably not selectively, that is, T helper versus T suppressor, but sufficient to induce a state of tolerance in the host. Its effect on B-cell function has been known for a fairly long time and has recently been corroborated and extended by Takeno et al. (38). A cyclophosphamide-caused reduction in B-cell function would in effect reduce antigen-antibody complexing and any further inflammatory responses and would reduce tissue injury secondary to such responses.

Lastly, the cytotoxic agents have profound effects on cell replication, growth, and protein production. Any sustained action by either of the cytotoxics could ultimately cause suppression of macrophage, T- and B-cell replication, and protein, globulin, cytokine, and other factor production, in effect totally disrupting the normal tissue response to inflammation.

III. PROGRESSIVE SYSTEMIC SCLEROSIS

Progressive systemic sclerosis (PSS) is a variety of scleroderma in which extensive fibrotic changes in the skin and subcutaneous tissue are associated with the development of fibrosis in multiple internal organs. The lungs, gastrointestinal tract, kidneys, and heart are the organs most often involved in systemic scleroderma. Raynaud's phenomenon, or paroxysmal occlusion of digital blood vessels precipitated by cold or stress, is found in over 95% of patients with PSS. Progressive systemic sclerosis must be distinguished from localized scleroderma in which cutaneous lesions exist in the absence of Raynaud's phenomenon and internal organ involvement.

The typical patient with PSS presents with the complaint of Raynaud's phenomenon of varying duration and severity ranging from mild cyanosis of the fingers and toes to marked color changes of red, white, and blue. Often, painful or burning digits are described. Raynaud's syndrome, vascular signs and symptoms without accompanying disease, has been described in 20% or more of young females (39). Women are affected with PSS three times more often than men. However, disease severity appears to be greater in men. There are no apparent racial predilections, although overall black women suffer with the most severe disease, including renal involvement and malignant hypertension. Cutaneous disease ends with sclerosis, ulceration, increased pigmentation, edema, telangiectasia, and calcinosis. There appear to be three stages: edematous (inflammatory), sclerotic or fibrotic (fibrosis is occurring), and atrophic (sclerotic tissue predominates). In the edematosis stage the skin is swollen and tight. In the fibrotic stage the skin is smooth, waxy, and shiny. In the atrophic stage the skin is bound tightly to the underlying structures. Calcinosis and cutaneous ulcerations, particularly over joints, occur quite commonly. Facial and digital telangiectasias occur during any stage.

Gastrointestinal disease is characterized by symptoms such as dysphagia, heartburn, nausea, vomiting, sour eructations, and regurgitation of liquids. These symptoms are related to destruction of smooth muscle at the cardioesophageal junction, diminished peristalsis, and diffuse dilatation of the esophagus. Other complaints relate to an atonic stomach and delayed emptying time, mucosal and muscular defects in the small bowel leading to malabsorption, muscular defects in the small bowel wall leading to large wide-mouthed diverticula, and smooth muscle defects in the rectal sphincter accompanied by an inability to control the loss of feces through the rectum. Pulmonary symptoms include progressive exertional dyspnea and a productive cough. Extensive pulmonary fibrosis, not unlike that seen in primary idiopathic pulmonary fibrosis, is associated. Renal failure is the end result of sclerodermal renal disease. Patients show azotemia proteinuria, malignant hypertension, seizures, and rapid death. Cardiac symptoms of dyspnea, palpitation, and congestive heart failure are often thought to be related to primary pulmonary disease. Conduction defects directly attributable to sclerodermatous involvement of cardiac conduction fibers may lead to a variety of cardiac arrhythmias. Bone and joint disease are commonly experienced, leading to articular pain, swelling, and tenderness, as well as osteoporosis, destruction of bones in the distal phalanges, deposition of calcium in the soft tissue of the digits, soft tissue swelling, and narrowing of bony articulations.

Progressive systemic sclerosis may present in one of four clinical forms: a) CREST syndrome, that is, calcinosis, Raynaud's phenomenon, esophageal dysmotility, sclerodactyly, and telangiectasias predominate; b) Extremity ascending form in which sclerosis is confined to the arms and legs. The early appearance of Raynaud's phenomenon is followed by ascending sclerosis; c) Diffuse form. Extremity involvement with Raynaud's phenomenon and sclerosis is associated with truncal sclerosis; and d) Overlap syndrome. Progressive systemic sclerosis is associated with SLE or dermatomyositis. CREST syndrome has been characterized as having a better prognosis than other forms of PSS; however, patients with CREST may be plagued with severe pulmonary and/or renal disease and may experience death from either.

Epidemiological and survival studies show there is an average annual incidence of 2.7 cases per million population, and there is a 7 y cumulative survival rate of 35%. Poor prognosis is correlated with increasing age, maleness, black skin, and renal, cardiac, or pulmonary disease. Cutaneous disease does not appear to affect longevity (40,41).

A. Etiology and Pathogenesis

Progressive systemic sclerosis is a rheumatic disease in which large quantities of collagen, principally types I and III, are produced and deposited in unusual sites throughout the body. The etiology of PSS is unknown, but it is generally believed that alterations in the vascular system, changes in the reactivity of the immune system, and disturbance in the regulation of collagen synthesis combine to produce the vast array of defects seen in PSS.

Raynaud's phenomenon of varying degree is seen in nearly every patient presenting with PSS. Although there is considerable literature addressing the physiological mechanisms associated with Raynaud's phenomenon there are few that detail the morphological features of the vasculature in active disease (42–44). According to Burch et al. (42) patients with primary Raynaud's show lesions characteristic of segmental vasculitis and capillary degeneration with fibrinoid necrosis and fibrocytic replacement of capillaries. Patients with Raynaud's phenomenon and PSS show a diminution in the number of cutaneous capillaries and blood vessels and extensive deposition of collagen in the dermis. Additionally, fibrinoid degeneration of the type found in patients with primary Raynaud's, as well as thickened blood vessel walls, is quite common. He concluded that the very prominent vascular abnormalities seen in the capillaries of patients with Raynaud's phenomenon "indicate a prime relationship of vascular and capillary lesions to the pathogenesis of Raynaud's disease" (42). Capillary blood flow as well as capillary morphology is abnormal in patients with primary and secondary Raynaud's (45,46). Blood flow abnormalities are associated with vasospastic and morphological changes to the cutaneous vasculature. The degree of vasospasm appears to be highest in secondary disease. A positive correlation exists between the degree of vasospasm in Raynaud's and the level of phagocytosed immune complexes in circulatory polymorphonuclear leukocytes (47,48). Higher levels of phagocytized immune complexes are found in patients with secondary Raynaud's.

Cutaneous vascular changes in scleroderma have been further described by Fleischmajer and Perlish (49,50), who divided the observed abnormalities into three categories: a) activation of capillary components, b) perivascular cellular infiltrates, and c) perivascular fibrosis. Among early changes seen in cutaneous capillaries are large gaps between endothelial cells. Within these gaps are noted single-membrane vesicles and myelin structures that appear to be in transit. Somewhat later, endothelial cells show vascularization of cytoplasm and the nucleus show-linear rearrangement of chromation. The basil lamina is thickened by several layers but is not invaded by collagen. Endothelial cells, pericytes, and perivascular fibroblasts show prominent rough endoplasmic reticulum. Late changes include capillary destruction characterized by the appearance of a granular and homogenous nucleus, disruption of cellular membranes, and organelles existing free in the extracellular matrix. An increase in thymidine labeling of "endothelial" cells can also be demonstrated. Other findings that suggest vascular injury is of some significance in the etiology and pathogenesis of PSS are increased factor VIII-von Willebrand factor antigen and von Willebrand factor activity (51), and elevated levels of circulating platelet aggregates and B thromboglobulin (52). These are abnormalities that are characteristically associated with vascular injury and repair. Several studies have reported the presence of a circulating serum factor cytotoxic to human endothelial cells in some of the rheumatic diseases including PSS (53,54).

Cellular and humoral abnormalities in scleroderma are abundant. Specifically, serum immune complexes have been reported in 82% of patients with scleroderma and internal organ involvement (55,56). Antibodies to type I (interstitial) and type IV (basement membrane) collagen have been reported in the sera of patients with scleroderma (57).

Immune system dysfunction is also demonstrated by the presence of hypergammaglobulinemia, cryoglobulinemia, and antinuclear, anticentromere, and antinucleolar antibodies in the sera of patients with PSS. Racial differences and disease severity appear to correlate with the frequency of occurrence of certain scleroderma-related antibodies (58). In a study of 156 white, black, and Hispanic patients anticentromere antibodies were found more often in white than black patients, 36% versus 4%. Antitopoisomerase I (SCL-70) antibodies were found more often in black than white patients, 37% versus 17%. Antinucleolar and anti-U-1 RNP antibodies were found with equal frequency in both groups. It is well to recall that anticentromere antibodies are characteristically found in patients with the CREST, or purportedly benign, variant of PSS, whereas anti-SCL-70 antibodies are generally associated with widespread and severe cutaneous and systemic diseases.

A variety of cellular immune abnormalities have been described in patients with PSS (59–61), although a number of discrepancies in reporting have occurred. Total circulating T-lymphocyte numbers appear to be decreased. It has been suggested that these numbers are low because most T lymphocytes are consumed in cellular infiltrates in skin and other organ systems. Circulating peripheral blood mononuclear cells in patients with PSS have been shown to have a markedly reduced propensity to adhere to endothelial cells in vitro (62). This observation has led some investigators to conclude that vascular changes in PSS are begun with an unknown process in which a subpopulation of peripheral blood mononuclear cells are activated. Activation of this subpopulation leads to an enhanced adhesiveness of some mononuclear cells to vascular endothelium in vivo and migration of activated cells to the extracellular space. Migration of this subpopulation of mononuclear cells to the extravascular spaces increases mononuclear cells in the perivascular region. Perivascular mononuclear cell infiltrates are thus formed, and the vascular adherent cell population is eliminated from the peripheral blood. T-helper and T-suppressor cell ratios appear to be normal; however, there are some reports that describe changing ratios depending on disease stage. In spite of depressed T-cell numbers in the serum of patients with scleroderma there appears to be an excess of T-helper cell function in scleroderma and an impairment of suppressor cell function.

Dermal mast cell populations have been evaluated in patients with PSS (63,64). Mast cell numbers appear to be greater in clinically involved versus uninvolved skin of the same patients, as well as greater than in normal controls. The increase appears to be larger in the reticular than in the papillary dermis, 152% versus 85%. It also appears that mast cell numbers return to normal in late-stage disease. Mast cell numbers are known to increase in chronic inflammatory and allergic disease states such as fibrotic lung disease, keloids, and healing wounds. They appear to decrease in number in acute inflammatory states; however, this apparent decrease is believed to be related to mast cell degranulation and an inability to recognize the characteristic morphological features of the degranulated cell.

The finding of increased numbers of mast cells in early sclerodermatous disease has led to numerous discussions of the role of mast cells in the production of fibrosis, particularly fibrosis in scleroderma. Dermal mast cells contain heparin proteoglycan which is capable of binding to a variety of extracellular matrix proteins as fibronectin, laminin, and thrombospondin and is capable of stimulating capillary endothelial cell migration. Dermal mast cells also contain a number of proteolytic enzymes that degrade extracellular matrix components such as type IV collagen, elastin, proteoglycan, and fibronectin. Histamine and a variety of vasoactive materials comprise major components of dermal mast cells. Each, such as prostaglandin D_2, leukotrienes, and platelet activating factor, possess a variety of properties that may in someway aid in the development of fibrosis.

Among these are stimulation of growth in cultured fibroblasts, increase in local blood flow and vascular permeability, and promotion of the influx of plasma proteases and fibroblast mitogens to inflamed tissues.

Needleman has measured cytokine levels in the sera of patients with PSS and in a control population (65). IL-2, IL-4, and IL-6 were detected more frequently in the sera of scleroderma patients. TNF-α and IL-1 α were not detected. Among its many activities, IL-2 rapidly induces natural killer cell adhesion to human endothelial cells. The presence of IL-2, IL-4, and IL-6 in the sera of patients with scleroderma may imply these cytokines are among a group that contribute to the disease process in scleroderma. There is also evidence that IL-8 and autoantibodies to IL-8 are present in the sera of patients with PSS (66).

Defects in collagen synthesis appear to occur secondary to vascular damage and immune system-somatic cell interactions. Leroy and Uitto et al. have shown that scleroderma fibroblasts in vitro synthesize large quantities of collagen (67,68). Borstein et al. subsequently demonstrated that there is heterogeneity in the ability of human skin fibroblasts to produce collagen and that clones of fibroblasts exposed to sera of patients with scleroderma showed selective groups of high collagen-producing fibroblasts (69). These observations led to a hypothesis that the high level of collagen production observed in scleroderma-derived fibroblast cultures is the result of in vivo selection of high collagen-producing fibroblasts from a heterogeneous fibroblast population.

Perlish et al., Buckingham et al., and Tajima and Pinnell (70–72) have described heterogeneity of fibroblast populations found in normal and sclerodermatous skin. Fibroblasts from the reticular and lower layers of dermis in normal individuals and in scleroderma synthesize more collagen that those from the papillary and upper dermis. Fleischmajer et al., using cultured fibroblasts from the papillary, reticular, reticular-fat, and fat layers of skin of patients with scleroderma, showed variability of synthesis of total and collagenous protein, fibronectin, and type III collagen (73). Increased synthesis varying from 10 to 20 times normal were noted principally in the reticular and reticular-fat layers rather than the papillary and fat layers. Additionally, when procollagen mRNA was measured in scleroderma fibroblasts, a correlation appeared to exist between levels of usable procollagen mRNA and increased collagen synthesis (74). Increased levels of procollagen mRNA were found in scleroderma skin fibroblasts. The increased levels of collagen synthesis in scleroderma can thus be explained by the increased levels of procollagen mRNA. Increased levels of collagen can be related to a defect in the regulation of collagen synthesis by the amino-propeptide of procollagen I and III. Normally, amino-propeptide inhibits translation of procollagen of mRNA. A reduced inhibition of translation leads to an increased synthesis of mRNA and thus of collagen. Increased serum levels of amino-propeptide of type III procollagen have been detected in patients with diffuse cutaneous systemic sclerosis and in patients with more limited disease (75). Increased levels appear to correlate with the extent of the disease and the rapidity of progression and extension of lesions.

Numerous other somatic cell-immune system interactions have been described that can account for increased collagen synthesis and accumulation in scleroderma. Fibronectin, a product of activated tissue macrophages and dermal mast cells, is a potent chemoattractant of tissue fibroblasts (76). Likewise, human lymphocytes are capable of producing a substance that is chemotactic for fibroblasts (77). There are other substances produced by lymphocytes and macrophages that stimulate fibroblast replication (78,79), increase collagen production (80), and inhibit fibroblast migration (81), collagen production (82,83), and fibroblast replication (84). In scleroderma the implications are that fibronectin, assisted by at least one other cytokine, is capable of recruiting active fibroblasts to an area of damaged tissue where fibroblasts can be stimulated to proliferate and produce collagen in abundance. The process of repair ends after a predetermined period with the end of collagen synthesis and the production of normal scar tissue. In PSS the control mechanism appears to go astray, and therefore inhibition of cell replication and collagen production go astray.

A number of hypotheses for the pathogenesis of PSS have been advanced. Two have emerged as the most plausible: the vascular and the immune, and/or a combined hypothesis. In each, the initial event or the primary causative agent that acts as a stimulus for the earliest reaction in scleroderma remains unknown. A very plausible hypothesis begins with the development of Raynaud's phenomenon. At some point in the course of PSS 95% or more of patients experiencing this disease will describe signs and symptoms that are indicative of Raynaud's phenomenon. Raynaud's phenomenon, as described previously, is caused by overstimulation of the cutaneous vascular system and possibly the small blood vessels of other organs by the sympathetic nervous system (85). Even in the absence of any measurable abnormalities of the immune system, in this syndrome somatic injury occurs within small blood vessels, probably by mechanisms akin to those that cause vascular injury in large blood vessels in patients with chronic hypertension.

Endothelial cell damage is one of the first morphological abnormalities detected in patients with Raynaud's phenomenon and scleroderma (42–46,49). The presence of endothelial cell damage in scleroderma is supported by the finding of increased von Willebrand factor activity and factor VIII-von Willebrand factor antigen in the serum (51). Injury to the endothelial lining of the walls of small blood vessels or any other vessel is associated with platelet aggregation and platelet deposition at the injured site. Increased circulating platelet aggregates and serum levels of B thrombogobulin have been described in PSS (52). Platelet aggregation stimulates the early process of inflammation and microvascular permeability through the release of a variety of platelet-derived vasoactive amines. Lymphocytes, macrophages, and mast cells are recruited to the site of injury and through the release of a variety of cytokines cause a further increase in local tissue injury. Subsequent to local vascular injury inflammatory cells, serum, water, electrolytes, and other substances in sera infuse into the surrounding tissue, thereby initiating the early edematous stage of PSS. Interstitial (type I) and basement membrane (type IV) collagens become exposed to the wide variety of inflammatory cells recruited to the area. In the genetically susceptible host, antibodies to type I and type IV collagen other cellular and nuclear constituents are produced (55–57), and antigen-antibody complexing further intensifies local injury, thereby increasing the number of inflammatory cells at the site.

Some of the cells that are recruited to the site of injury after activation are programmed to begin the process of repair. Mast cells and macrophages at the repair site secrete fibronectin (76) and lymphocytes secrete a factor that attracts high-productivity fibroblasts (77). Other lymphocytes and macrophages produce a fibroblast migration inhibitory factor that forces recruited fibroblasts to remain "fixed" in the injury area (81). Fixed fibroblasts are stimulated to proliferate and begin the process of collagen synthesis (80) and the synthesis of other substances as matrix glycoproteins (86–88). In genetically susceptible individuals fibroblasts, once activated, continue to proliferate and produce collagen unabated. Normal control mechanisms for growth (84) and collagen synthesis (74,82,83) become ineffective. Fibrous tissue is then produced in abundance and sclerosis of organs and organ systems is the end result (Figure 1).

C. Indications for Use of Immunomodulatory and Cytotoxic Agents

Treatment of PSS, like other rheumatic diseases, remains controversial. It is generally agreed that intensive physical therapy should be made part of any therapeutic program. The introduction of calcium channel blockers into cardiovascular medicine has revolutionized the treatment of Raynaud's phenomenon; the use of angiotensin-converting enzyme inhibitors has improved the management of patients with renal disease and hypertension; and a number of new prokinetic agents are considered promising in the treatment of gastrointestinal disease in PSS. However, in the treatment of debilitating cutaneous and pulmonary disease, controversy reigns. Treatment suffers principally from the lack of a true understanding of disease etiology, the lack of a set of standards establishing markers of disease activity, and the unnecessary entrenchment of a variety of camps championing either the use of penicillamine, extracorporeal photochemotherapy, or immunosuppressive agents. Even worse is the nonactivities of a group of therapeutic anhialists. As more and more data accumulates, it becomes clearer that treatment with various modalities and medications can alleviate morbidity and possibly mortality in early disease or disease in the early edematous or inflammatory stage. It appears that whether one uses D-penicillamine, azathioprine/cyclophosphamide, or extracorporeal photochemotherapy in early

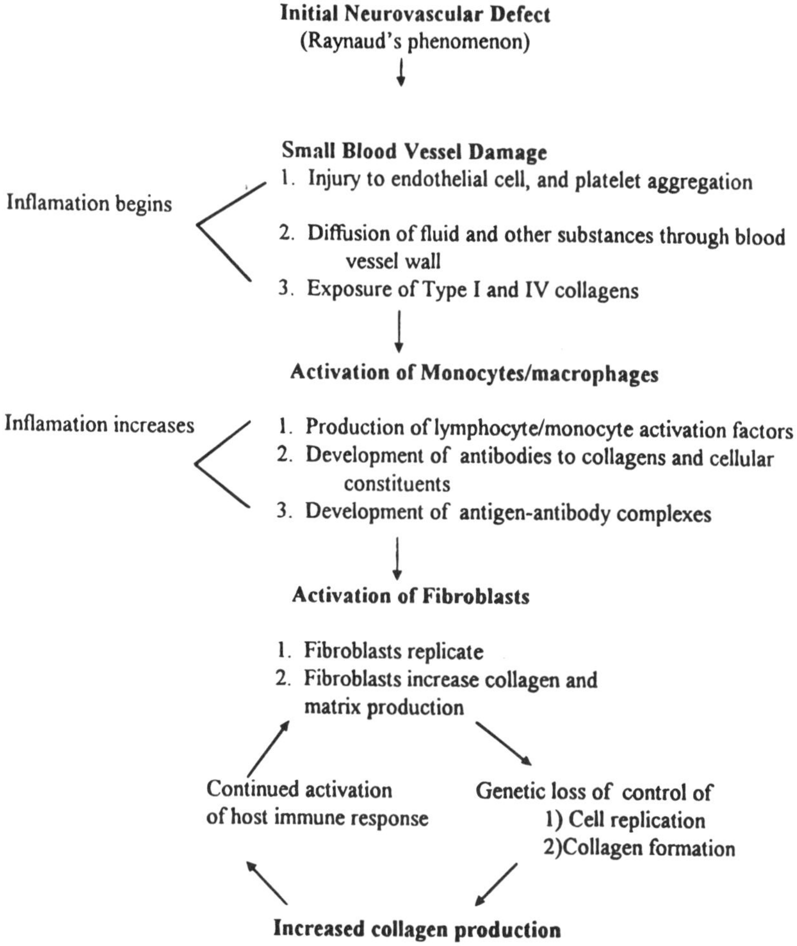

Figure 1 Postulated pathogenesis of scleroderma.

stage disease—because these agents interfere with protein, nucleic acid, cytokine, and proteoglycan synthesis—or substances that are necessary for macrophage, mast cell, lymphocyte and fibroblast proliferation and production of cytokines, collagen, and matrix proteins, improvement occurs.

There is no useful immunomodulatory or cytotoxic treatment for late stage sclerotic disease.

D. Method and Rationale for Treatment

The authors greatest experience has been in the use of systemic chemotherapeutic agents in the treatment of PSS. A summary of this experience is outlined below.

In the late 1960s and early 1970s the author, among others, initiated investigations on the use of cytotoxic drugs, as well as D-penicillamine, in the treatment of rheumatic diseases. Ironically, the vast majority of patients recruited for these studies were patients with "end-stage" scleroderma. The fibrotic rather than inflammatory stage of the disease predominated. As a result disease response to treatment was practically nonexistent. The inexperience of many investigators in the use of cytotoxic drugs, and an overwhelming ignorance of the methods used and the real need to monitor patients for adverse effects, led to a series of patient disasters and ultimately disdain for the use of cytotoxic agents in PSS and a variety of responsive diseases. It was fortuitous that somewhat later colleagues in oncology and I noted complete disappearance of all signs and symptoms of scleroderma in a patient with early PSS and breast cancer. This patient was being treated with a combination of cytotoxic agents. Similar experience has recently been reported (89).

During the next two decades an open study was begun on the use of cytotoxic drugs in patients with early PSS. A total of 16 patients were entered into the study. Each patient was submitted to the following examinations: a) Laboratory: complete SMA-12 to include BUN and creatinine, complete serologic studies, CBC, sedimentation rate, and urinalysis; b) Systemic evaluation: skin and joints—ring size of all digits, degree of digital flexion and extension, large and small joint mobility, and x-rays of the hands and feet; pulmonary—chest x-ray, lung capacity, lung compliance, and gas diffusion; gastrointestinal—esophageal manometrics, barium swallow with cinefluoroscopy and small bowel follow-through; cardiovascular—blood pressure and electrocardiogram.

All laboratory studies were repeated at monthly intervals. Pulmonary studies and cardiovascular studies were repeated at 6 mo intervals and gastrointestinal studies were repeated at yearly intervals. The acute phase of the study lasted 5 y. All patients were started on azathioprine at 90 mg/m^2 or a maximum of 150 mg/d. Patients unable to tolerate azathioprine-5 were given cyclophosphamide-4 or chlorambucil-1. A number of patients continue to be monitored in a chronic toxicity study. The results of the study are summarized in Table 1. In terms of response and time to response there were three very impressive changes noted. Reduction in swelling of the digits and extremities occurred in 14 of 14 patients within 3 mo. Increased hair growth in areas previously devoid of hair was noted in 7 of 16 patients in an average of 6–12 mo. Large terminal-type hair often replaced fine lanugo-type hair on the extremities. An increase in gas perfusion was noted in 9 of 13 patients. Early improvement in diffusion was noted within 6 mo. Maximum changes were noted after 12–18 mo. Raynaud's phenomenon and gastrointestinal signs and symptoms were changed the least after therapy with cytotoxic drugs. The addition of vasodilators and other gastrointestinal manipulations and medications were required in most patients with Raynaud's phenomenon and gastrointestinal disease.

Table 1 Clinical Response of 16 Patients with Progressive Systemic Sclerosis

Clinical abnormality	Degree of response				Total number responding	Average time to response
	+	++	+++	++++		
Skin swelling		1*	3	10	14/14**	3 mo
Skin tightness	1	2	7	3	13/16	3 mo
Skin appendages						
Sweating				5	5/5	6 mo
Hair growth			2	5	7/16	6–12 mo
Pigmentation			2	2	4/4	6–7 mo
Ulceration			1	5	6/6	
Range of motion		2	7	5	13/16	6 mo
Raynaud's syndrome		2	2		4/16	12 mo
GI symptoms		3	1	1	5/8	12–18 mo
Pulmonary						
DLCO			4	5	9/13	6–12 mo

\+ = 25% response or return to normal
++ = 50% response
+++ = 75% response
++++ = 100% response
* Number responding
** Number of total responding

Adverse reactions were mostly confined to the peripheral blood, with intermittent low white counts and platelets occurring in several patients. Two patients experienced the development of two different solid tumors. One patient, a 60+-year-old male, former smoker, developed a fatal lung cancer 2 y after discontinuing treatment with azathioprine. The second patient, a 70-year-old female, developed transitional cell cancer of the bladder while on chronic treatment with cyclophosphamide. Repeated urinalysis while taking cyclophosphamide did not show hematuria. Instead hematuria began instantaneously and in a substantial amount.

To summarize, an open study of the use of cytotoxic agents in early systemic scleroderma has shown that a substantial number of patients can receive some benefit from these drugs. This is particularly true of patients with pulmonary and cutaneous disease. Adverse reactions in properly managed patients are few, and in the majority are reversible. This is essentially the experience of a number of investigators (76,90–93). Other treatments that have been reported as successful in correcting disease in patients with PSS include plasma exchange (94) and extracorporeal photophoresis (95). The effect of extracorporeal photochemotherapy most nearly approaches that attributable to the cytotoxic agents, that is, depletion of activated lymphocyte populations.

IV. DERMATOMYOSITIS

Dermatomyositis and polymyositis are among the least common of the rheumatic/connective tissue diseases. The two diseases are primarily associated with inflammation of skeletal muscle. Skeletal muscle is damaged by infiltrates of lymphocytes. Symmetry and proximal muscle weakness are characteristic, occasionally pain is associated with muscle weakness. Dermatomyositis and polymyositis are often classified into six categories: a) primary idiopathic dermatomyositis; b) primary idiopathic polymyositis; c) polymyositis and dermatomyositis associated with malignant neoplasms; d) juvenile dermatomyositis or polymyositis; e) dermatomyositis or polymyositis associated with other rheumatic/connective tissue diseases; and f) myopathic dermatomyositis.

There has been some disagreement among dermatologists and rheumatologists regarding the existence of myositis associated with malignant neoplasms. Experience has shown that dermatitis followed by myositis is most often the presenting manifestation of disease in patients with malignancy and myopathy. Thus, this combination of signs and symptoms is often encountered by dermatologists rather than rheumatologists. Nevertheless, myositis, dermatitis, and malignancy are now well recognized as a specific disease state. Retrospective studies have shown that malignancy will occur in approximately 15% of patients with myositis. Malignancies associated with myositis are found most often in the lungs, ovaries, breasts and gastrointestinal tract.

Primary idiopathic dermatomyositis and polymyositis can occur at any age. The mean age of presentation is 50 years. Each disease is seen more often in women than men. The initial presentation in the two diseases is the same, except there is no skin disease evident in polymyositis. Muscle weakness begins insidiously in proximal muscle groups of the upper and lower extremities. Early on, patients complain of difficulty raising the head from the supine position or exhaustion while combing the hair. Later they may experience great difficulty upon arising from a chair or while climbing stairs. In late disease patients complain of difficulty initiating a swallowing motion. This compliant may be confused with that of the patient with advanced scleroderma. Scleroderma patients also complain of difficulty swallowing solid foods, but the mechanisms are different. In dermatomyositis striated muscle of the cricopharyngeal area is severely inflamed, resulting in difficulty initiating the swallowing reflex; whereas in scleroderma, smooth muscle surrounding the esophagus is affected. The act of swallowing can be initiated but solid food cannot be propelled through the esophagus. It is most important to be cognizant of this phenomenon during diagnostic evaluation of the patient in whom one wishes to establish a diagnosis of scleroderma or dermatomyositis/polymyositis using dynamic x-rays of the gastrointestinal tract.

The skin lesions of dermatomyositis are fairly unique. In some situations they may mimic the cutaneous lesions of lupus erythematosus. The facial rash is often quite subtle consisting of a faint purple to red discoloration of the upper eyelids, often described as heliotropic in color. Severe disease may be associated with blister formation and erosions and scars on the upper eyelids. The lower eyelids may be edematous and quite puffy. Over proximal muscle groups an eruption may be seen that varies from morbilliform to "lupus-like." This eruption is often associated with intense pruritus. Over the interphalangeal joints one may find one or more polygonal-shaped papules. These are Gotron's papules and are a pathognomonic finding in dermatomyositis.

Childhood dermatomyositis is rarely, if ever, associated with malignancy. It is found more often in boys than girls. The gastrointestinal tract is found to be involved more often than in adult disease. Arthritis and Raynaud's phenomenon are quite frequently associated, and deposition of calcium in the skin causing large, often painful, nodules occurs with considerable frequency. Many of the differences between adult and childhood disease may be accounted for by the presence of a vasculitis involving muscle groups in children.

A. Etiology and Pathogenesis

The autoimmune nature of dermatomyositis/polymyositis is suggested by the presence of a variety of circulating antibodies. Antibodies to nuclear antigen often give a positive ANA. Antibodies to Jo-1 (directed to the enzymehistidyl RNA synthetase) occur in patients with myositis and pulmonary disease, and antibodies to n-RNP are seen in patients with myositis and other rheumatic/connective tissue diseases. Antibodies to SSA and SSB may also be observed. Yet to date there have been no specific antibodies found that are directed against striated muscle fibers. Other findings that suggest autoimmunity include the detection of a polymyositis syndrome that can be produced in rats and guinea pigs immunized with skeletal muscle. A similar syndrome has been induced in laboratory animals through the transfer of sensitized lymphocytes. The implication is that some form of cellar immunity is involved in the pathogenesis of the disease. Lymphocytes from muscle obtained from patients with polymyositis produce a toxic lymphokine that is injurious to monolayers of human fetal muscle cells.

The association of dermatomyositis/polymyositis with malignant neoplasms and with other rheumatic/connective tissue disease also suggests autoimmunity.

B. Pathology

Histopathologically the skin lesions of dermatomyositis may vary from that of a mild nonspecific dermatitis to the classical appearance of lupus erythematosus, thereby giving little clue to the true nature of the disease. The lesions in muscle contain an infiltrate consisting predominantly of perivascular accumulations of lymphocytes, plasma cells, histiocytes, eosinophils, and neutrophils. Similar infiltrates may be noted among muscle fibers. There is evidence that even as necrosis of muscle fibers is taking place, regeneration of striated muscle is occurring. Laboratory findings, in addition to the array of autoantibodies, include increased levels of creatine phosphokinase (CPK), aldolase, and transaminase (SGOT, SGPT) and an increased sedimentation rate. The technique of electromyography is often helpful in detecting muscle groups that are inflamed. Care must be taken to assure that muscle biopsy is not done in a site that has been previously used for the placement of electrical probes during electromyography.

C. Indications for Use of Cytotoxic Agents

Corticosteroids, particularly prednisone at 60–80 mg/d, have been used as the agents of choice in the treatment of dermatomyositis/polymyositis (96). The response rate is highly, yielding remission rates on the order of 90–95%. Tuffanelli and Lavole (97) state that 20% of all patients either do not respond to corticosteroids or are unable to tolerate them. There is some evidence that high-dose corticosteroid therapy is preferential to low-dose therapy. In that patient population with corticosteroid nonresponsiveness who continue to develop destructive muscle disease, the use of cytotoxic agents is clearly indicated. Cytotoxic drugs are also indicated in that population of patients who require continuous moderate- to high-dose prednisone as maintenance therapy.

Caution is to be exercised in making the diagnosis of a corticosteroid nonresponsive patient or in the treatment of a patient who requires moderate- to high-dose maintenance therapy. Patients with muscle disease and malignancy often require two to three times the normal dosage of systemic corticosteroids. Patients who do not respond immediately to adequate dosages of corticosteroids, 60–80 mg/d of prednisone, or who require moderate- to high-dose maintenance therapy should be subjected to an appropriate array of diagnostic examinations to rule in or out malignant neoplasms or inapparent infection.

D. Method of Treatment and Rationale

Once it has been decided to use cytotoxic drugs, one must decide upon a specific agent or agents. Azathioprine, cyclophosphamide, methotrexate, chlorambucil, mercaptopurine, and cyclosporine have all been found useful in treating patients with polymyositis/dermatomyositis. To date, azathioprine, principally because of its ease of use, and cyclophosphamide, because of theoretical efficacy, have been selected most frequently for use in the two diseases.

Azathioprine or any other cytotoxic may be introduced into the therapeutic regimen as soon as it has been determined the drug may be safely used in an individual patient. It may be started on day 1 of a treatment regimen rather than waiting until the patient has experienced a steroid response. This is particularly true when azathioprine has been selected. Azathioprine's effect on the immune system is rather slow in occurring and will not occur for 2–3 wk after the initial drug starting date. The dosage of azathioprine found most effect is 90 $mg/m^2/d$ not to exceed a total dose of 200 mg/d. The daily dose of drug may be divided into three or four parts.

Acute toxicity using azathioprine consists of a flu-like syndrome of fever, chills, lethargy, and malaise, sometimes associated with jaundice and an acute elevation of liver enzymes. This reaction occurs fairly early in the treatment period and requires that treatment with azathioprine be terminated. Azathioprine's effect on the peripheral blood occurs late in the course of treatment and is slow in onset and progression. Recovery from azathioprine bone marrow toxicity may also be slow. Platelets and white cells are more commonly affected by this agent.

Cyclophosphamide, probably the most potent immunosuppressive drug of the group except cyclosporine, is considered by some to be the agent of choice in adult and childhood disease (96,97). It has a fairly rapid onset of action and is tolerated very well in either the oral or parenteral route. Just as the onset of action occurs rather rapidly using cyclophosphamide, the onset of toxicity occurs as rapidly. Therefore, frequent monitoring of blood and urine is extremely important as long as a patient is being administered this agent. Thrombocytopenia and leukopenia may occur fairly rapidly after drug administration. Hemorrhagic cystitis followed by malignant neoplasms in the bladder is of great concern. We have observed the development of bladder malignancy in a patient who never experienced hematuria. Therefore, we suggest that the urine be scanned fairly often for the presence of malignant cells in any patients on long-term treatment with cyclophosphamide.

Cyclophosphamide is administered in a dosage of 150 mg/d, preferably divided into three doses when given orally. It may also be given by continuous infusion or by pulse dosing. Severe sequelae may occur after pulse dosing regimens. Therefore, it is recommended that pulse dosing regimens be used by individuals experienced in the use of chemotherapeutic agents who have available all of the necessary support systems that are required should expected and unforeseen adverse reactions arise.

Methotrexate is the third most commonly used agent in this disease (98). It is favored by dermatologists, probably because of their experience in using the drug in psoriasis. When used by the intravenous or oral route, this drug *should not* be given in a cycle of less than every 5–7 d. Toxicity to the bone marrow and gastrointestinal tract are certain to occur, particularly in debilitated patients with dermatomyositis/polymyositis within days to weeks. The toxicity of methotrexate is directly related to the period of time the target cell is exposed to drug. A small daily dosage of 0.15 mg infused over a 24 h period each day is more toxic than a 50 mg bolus of methotrexate.

Although chlorambucil (99) and cyclosporin (100) have been experimented with in the treatment of dermatomyositis, there is little experience other than anecdotal using these agents, therefore their use will not be covered.

REFERENCES

1. Hochberg MC, Boyd RE, Ahern JM, et al. Systemic lupus erythematosus: a review of clinical laboratory features and immunogenetic markers in 150 patients with emphasis on demographic subsets. Medicine 1985; 64:285–295.
2. Lawrence RC, Hochberg MC, Kelsey JL, et al. Estimate of the prevalence of selected arthritic and musculoskeletal diseases in the U.S. J Rheum 1989; 16:427–441.
3. Sontheimer D, Madison PJ, Reichlin M, et al. Serological and HLA association of subacute cutaneous lupus erythematosus. Ann Intern Med 1982; 97:664–671.
4. Provost TT, Talal N, Harley JB. The relationship between anti-RO antibody positive Sjogren's syndrome and anti-RO antibody positive lupus erythematosus. Arch Dermat 1988; 124:63–71.
5. Arnett FC, Bias WB, Reveille JD. Genetic studies on Sjogren's syndrome and systemic lupus erythematosus. J Autoimm 1989; 2:403–413.
6. Frank MD, McArthur R, Harley JB. Anti-Ro antibodies are associated with T-cell receptor beta genes in systemic lupus erythematosus patients. J Clin Invest 1990; 85:33–39.
7. Fowler JF, Callen JP, Stelzer GT, et al. Human histocompatibility antigen associations in patients with chronic cutaneous lupus erythematosus. J Am Acad Dermat 1985; 12:73–77.
8. Lahita RE. Sex steroids in the rheumatic diseases. Arthr Rheum 1985; 28:121–126.
9. Roubinian JR, Paporan R, Talal N. Androgenic hormones modulate autoantibody response and improve survival in marine lupus. J Clin Invest 1977; 59:1066–1070.
10. Kochever I. Action spectrum and mechanism of UV radiation-induced injury in lupus erythematosus. J Invest Dermat 1985; 85:140–143.
11. Davis TL, Lyde CB, Davis BM, Sontheimer RD. Pertubation of experimental UVB induced erythema by positive transfer of serum from subacute cutaneous lupus erythematosus patients. J Invest Dermat 1989; 92:573–577.
12. Lehman P, Holzle E, Kind P, et al. Experimental reproduction of skin lesions in lupus erythematosus by UVA and UVB radiation. J Acad Dermat 1990; 22:181–187.
13. Kupper TS, Chau AO, Flood P, et al. Interleukin-1 gene expression in cultured human keratinocytes is augmented by UV irradiation. J Clin Invest 1987; 80:430–436.
14. Urbanski A, Schwartz T, Neuner P, et al. Ultraviolet light induces increased circulating interleukin-6 in humans. J Invest Dermat 1990; 94:808–811.

15. Sauder DN, Monick MM, Hunninghake GW. Epidermal cell-derived thymocyte-activating factor (ETAF) is a potent T-cell chemoattractant. J Invest Dermat 1985; 85:431–433.
16. Norris DA, Bennion SD, Middleton MH. Further definition of the effects of ultraviolet light on ICAm-1 (CD54) expression by human keratinocytes. Clin Res 1990; 538:285a.
17. Velthius PJ, Kater L, van der Tweel I, et al. Immunofluorescence microscopy of healthy skin from patients with systemic lupus erythematosus: more than just the lupus band. Ann Rheum Dis 1992; 51:720–725.
18. Davis BM, Gilliam JN. Prognostic significance of subepidermal immune deposits in uninvolved skin of patients with systemic lupus erythematosus: a ten year longitudinal study. J Invest Dermat 1984; 83:242–247.
19. Smith CD, Marino C, Rothfield NF. The clinical utility of the lupus band test. Arthr Rheum 1984; 27:382–387.
20. Donadio JV. Cytotoxic-drug treatment in lupus nephritis (editorial). N Eng J Med 1984; 311:528–529.
21. Felson DT, Anderson J. Evidence of the superiority of immunosuppressive drugs and prednisone over prednisone dose alone in lupus nephritis. Results of a pooled analysis. N Eng J Med 1984; 311(24):1528–1533.
22. Steinberg AD. The treatment of lupus nephritis. Kidney Int 1986; 30:769–787.
23. McClure WJ, Golburn J, Zeldes W, et al. Clinical and immunologic effects of monthly administration of intravenous cyclophosphamide in severe systemic lupus erythematosus. N Eng J Med 1988; 318:1423–1431.
24. Stratta P, Canavese C, Dogliani M, Thea A, Ferrero S, et al. Intravenous cyclophosphamide pulse therapy in the treatment of systemic lupus erythematosus long-term results. In: Sessa A, Meroni M, Battini G (eds.), Systemic lupus erythematosus: renal vasculitis. Contrib Nephrol (vol. 99) Basel: Karger 1992; 126–128.
25. Brun DT, Barex S, Klippel JH, Balow JE. Intermittent cyclophosphamide for the treatment of autoimmune thrombocytopenia in systemic lupus erythematosus. Ann Intern Med 1990; 112:672–674.
26. Godeau B, Cormier C, Menkes CJ. Bronchiolitis obliterans in systemic lupus erythematosus: beneficial effect of cyclophosphamide. Ann Rheum Dis 1991; 50:956–958.
27. Boumpas DT, Yamata H, Patronus NJ, et al. Pulse cyclophosphamide for severe neuropsychiatric lupus. Q J Med New Ser 1991; 81:975–984.
28. Simeon-Aznar CP, Tolosa-Vilella C, Cuenca-Luque R, et al. Transverse myelitis in systemic lupus erythematosus: two cases with magnetic resonance imaging. Br J Rheum 1992; 31:555–558.
29. Klaiman MD, Miller SD. Transverse myelitis complicating systemic lupus erythematosus: treatment including hydroxychloroquine. Am J Physic Med Rehabil 1993; 72:158–161.
30. Esdaile, JM. The efficacy of antimalarials in systemic lupus erythematosus. Lupus 1993; 2(suppl):S3–8.
31. Canadian Hydroxychloroquine Study Group. A randomized study of the effect of withdrawing hydroxychloroquine sulfate in systemic lupus erythematosus. N Engl J Med 1991; 324:150–154.

32. Kahn, MF. The treatment of lupus in the 1990's. Clin Exp Rheum 1990; 8(supp 5):45–49.
33. Austin AH, Klippel JH, Balow JE, et al. Therapy of lupus nephritis. Controlled trial of prednisone and cytotoxic drugs. N Engl J Med 1986; 314:614–669.
34. Levly AS, Lam S, Corwin HL, et al. Progression and remission of renal disease in the lupus nephritis collaborative study group. Ann Intern Med 1992; 116:114–123.
35. McInnes PM, Schuttinga J, Sanslone WR, et al. The economic impact of treatment of severe lupus nephritis with prednisone and intravenous cyclophosphamide. Arthr Rheum 1994; 37:1000–1006.
36. Lehman TJ. Aggressive therapy for childhood rheumatic diseases. When are immunosuppressives appropriate? Arthr Rheum 1993; 36:71–74.
37. Goronzy JJ, Weyand CM. Persistent suppression of virus-specific cytotoxic T-cell responses after transient depletion of $CD4^+$ T cells in vivo. J Immunol 1989; 142:4435–4442.
38. Takeno M, Suzuki H, Nagafuchi Y, et al. Selective suppression of resting B cell function in patients with systemic lupus erythematosus treated with cyclophosphamide. Clin Exp Rheum 1993; 11:263–270.
39. Olsen N, Neilson SL. Prevalence of primary Raynaud's phenomenon in young females. Scand J Clin Lab Invest 1978; 37:761–764.
40. Medsger TA, Masi AT. Epidemiology of systemic sclerosis. Ann Intern Med 1971; 74:714–718.
41. Medsger TA, Masi AT, Rodnan GP, et al. Survival with systemic sclerosis: a life-table analysis of clinical and demographic factors in 309 patients. Ann Intern Med 1971; 75:369–376.
42. Burch GE, Harb JM, Sun LS. Fine structure of digital vascular lesions in Raynaud's phenomenon and disease. Angiology 1979; 30:361–376.
43. Lewis T, Lundis EM. Further observations upon a variety of Raynaud's disease: with special reference to arteriolar disease and scleroderma. Heart 1931; 15:329–350.
44. Lewis T. The pathologic changes in the arteries supplying the fingers in warm-handed people and in cases of so-called "Raynaud's Disease." Clin Sci 1938; 3:287–313.
45. Harper FE, Marica HR, Turner RE, et al. A prospective study of Raynaud's phenomenon and early connective tissue disease. A five year report. Am J Med 1982; 72:883–888.
46. Maricq HR, LeRoy EC. Correlation of capillary morphology and flow during cold exposure in Raynaud's syndrome. Biblio Anat 1979; 18:382–384.
47. Dowd PM, Kirby JD, Holborow EJ, et al. Detection of immune complexes in systemic sclerosis and Raynaud's phenomenon. Br J Dermat 1981; 105:179–188.
48. van der Maulen J, Wouda AA, Maydema AE, et al. Immune complexes in peripheral blood polymorphonuclear leukocytes of patients with Raynaud's phenomenon. Clin Exp Immunol 1979; 35:62–66.
49. Fleischmajer R, Perlish JS. Capillary alterations in scleroderma. J Am Acad Dermat 1980; 2:161–170.
50. Fleischmajer R, Perlish JS. ^{3}H-thymidine labeling of dermal endothelial cells in scleroderma. J Invest Dermatol 1977; 69:379–382.

51. Kahaleh MB, Osborn I, LeRoy EG. Increased factor VIII/von Willebrand factor antigen and von Willebrand factor activity in scleroderma and in Raynaud's phenomenon. Ann Intern Med 1981; 94:482–484.
52. Kahaleh MB, Osboran I, LeRoy EG. Elevated levels of circulating platelet aggregates and beta thromboglobulin in scleroderma. Ann Intern Med 1982; 96:610–613.
53. Kahaleh MB, Sherer GK, LeRoy EC. Endothelial injury in scleroderma. J Exp Med 1979; 149:1326–1335.
54. Shanahan WR Jr, Korn JH. Cytotoxic activity of sera from scleroderma and other connective tissue diseases. Arthr Rheum 1982; 25:1391–1396.
55. Siminovitch K, Klein M, Pruzawski W, et al. Circulating immune complexes in patients with progressive systemic sclerosis. Arthr Rheum 1982; 25:1174–1178.
56. Siebold JR, Medsger RA Jr, Winkelstein A, et al. Immune complexes in progressive systemic sclerosis (scleroderma). Arthr Rheum 1982; 25:1162–1173.
57. Mockel AM, DeLustro F, Harper FE, LeRoy EL. Antibodies to collagen in scleroderma. Arthr Rheum 1982; 25:522–531.
58. Reveille JD, Durban E, Goldstein R, et al. Racial differences in the frequency of scleroderma related antibodies. Arthr Rheum 1992; 35:216–218.
59. Horwitz DA, Garrett MA, Craig AH. Lymphocyte reactivity to mitogens in subjects with systemic lupus erythematosus, rheumatoid arthritis and scleroderma. Clin Exp Immunol 1977; 27:92–95.
60. Baron M, Keystone EC, Glicksman DD, et al. Lymphocyte sub-population and reactivity to mitogens in patients with scleroderma. Clin Exp Immunol 1981; 46:70–76.
61. Gupta S, Malaviya AN, Rajagopalan P, et al. Subsets of human T lymphocytes: imbalance of T cell population in patients with progressive systemic sclerosis. Clin Exp Immunol 1979; 38:342–347.
62. Rudnicka L, Majewski S, Blaszczyk M, Skiendzielewska A, Mukida B, Skopinska M, Jablonska S. Adhesion of peripheral blood mononuclear cells to vascular endothelium in patients with systemic sclerosis. Arthr Rheum 1992; 35:771–775.
63. Hawkins RA, Claman HN, Clark RAF, et al. Increased dermal mast cell populations in progressive systemic sclerosis: a link in chronic fibrosis? Ann Intern Med 1985; 102:182–186.
64. Nishioka K, Kobayashi L, Katayoana I, et al. Mast cell numbers in diffuse scleroderma. Arch Dermat 1987; 123:205–208.
65. Needleman BW. IL-1, IL-2, IL-6, TNF alpha, IFN gamma levels in sera from patients with scleroderma. Arthr Rheum 1992; 35:67–72.
66. Reitamo S, Remitz A, Varga J, et al. Demonstration of interleukin 8 and antibodies to interleukin 8 in the serum of patients with systemic sclerosis and related disorders. Arch Dermat 1993; 129:189–193.
67. LeRoy EC. Increased collagen synthesis by scleroderma skin fibroblasts in vitro: a possible defect in the regulation or activation of the scleroderma fibroblast. J Clin Invest 1974; 54:880–889.
68. Uitto J, Bauer EA, Eisen AZ. Increased biosynthesis of triple-helical type I and type III procollagens associated with unaltered expression of collagenase by skin fibroblast in culture. J Clin Invest 1979; 64:921–930.

69. Borstein GR, Sherer GK, LeRoy EC. Fibroblast selection in scleroderma. Arthr Rheum 1982; 25:189–195.
70. Perlish JS, Bashey RI, Stephens RE, et al. Connective tissue synthesis by cultured scleroderma fibroblasts: in vitro collagen synthesis by normal and scleroderma fibroblasts. Arthr Rheum 1976; 19:891–901.
71. Buckingham RB, Prinle RK, Rodnan GP, et al. Increased collagen accumulation in dermal fibroblasts cultures from patients with progressive systemic sclerosis. J Lab Clin Med 1978; 92:5–21.
72. Tajima S, Pinnell S. Collagen synthesis by human skin fibroblasts in culture: studies of fibroblasts explanted from papillary and reticular dermis. J Invest Dermat 1981; 72:410–412.
73. Fleishmajer R, Perlish JS, Krieg T, et al. Variability in collagen and fibronectin synthesis by scleroderma fibroblasts in primary culture. J Invest Dermat 1981; 76:400–405.
74. Perlish JS, Bashey RI, Stephens RE, et al. Collagen synthesis regulation by the aminopropeptide of procollagen I in normal and scleroderma fibroblasts. Arthr Rheum 1985; 28:647–651.
75. Heickendorff L, Parvez A, Bjerring P, Halkier S, Sorensen L, Zachariae H. Serum aminoterminal propeptide of type III collagen in systemic sclerosis. A follow-up investigations in subclasses and during pro-therapy. Acta Derm Vener (Stockh) 1991; 71:185–188.
76. Tsukamoto Y, Helsel WE, Wahl SM. Macrophage production of fibronectin, a chemoattractant for fibroblasts. J Immunol 1981; 127:673–678.
77. Postlethwaite AE, Snyderman R, Kang AH. The chemotactic attraction of human fibroblasts to a lymphocyte-derived factor. J Exp Med 1976; 144:1188–1203.
78. DeLustro F, Sherer G, LeRoy EC. Human monocyte stimulation by fibroblast growth by a soluble mediator. J Retic Soc 1980; 28:519–532.
79. Schmidt JA, Mizel SB, Cohen D, Green I. Interleukin l, a potential regulator of fibroblast proliferation. J Immunol 1982; 128:2177–2182.
80. Cathcart MK, Karkauer RS. Immunologic enhancement of collagen accumulation in progressive systemic sclerosis (PSS). Clin Immunol Immunopathol 1981; 21:128–133.
81. Rola-Pleszczynski M, Lieu H, Hamel J, Lemaire I. Stimulated human lymphocytes produce a soluble factor which inhibits fibroblast migration. Cell Immunol 1982; 74:104–110.
82. McArthur W, Derr K, Dixon M, Jimenez SA, Rosenbloom J. Immune modulation of connective tissue functions: studies on the production of collagen synthesis inhibitory factor by populations of human peripheral blood mononuclear cells. Cell Immunol 1982; 74:126–139.
83. Jimenez SA, et al. Selective inhibition of excessive scleroderma fibroblast collagen production by lymphokines from normal human mononuclear cells. Arthr Rheum 1985; 28:502–510.
84. Korotzer TI, Page RC, Grauger GA, Rabinovitch PS. Regulation of growth of human diploid fibroblasts by factors elaborated by activated lymphoid cells. J Cell Physiol 1982; 111:247–254.

85. McDonald, CJ. Raynaud's syndrome. Dermat Clin 1983; 1:493–504.
86. Uitto J, Heling-Helin P, et al. Connective tissue in scleroderma. Acta Dermat Vener 1971; 51:401–406.
87. Fleischmajer R, Perlish JS. Glycosamino glycans in scleroderma and scleredema. J Invest Dermat 1972; 58:129–132.
88. Ninomya Y, Hota RI, Najai Y, et al. Glycosaminoglycan metabolism by scleroderma fibroblasts in culture. Biomed Res 1982; 3:70–72.
89. Comer M, Harvey AR. Remission of scleroderma during chemotherapy for lymphoma. Ann Rheum Dis 1992; 51:998–1000.
90. Clements PJ. Cyclosporine in systemic sclerosis (SSC): analysis of 48-week open safety study in 10 patients. Arthr Rheum 1993; 36:75–83.
91. Silver RM. Cyclophosphamide and low dose prednisone therapy in patients with systemic sclerosis (scleroderma) in patients with interstitial lung disease. J Rheum 1993; 20:838–844.
92. Medsger TA Jr. Treatment of systemic sclerosis. Ann Rheum Dis 1991; 50(suppl 4):877–886.
93. Dau PC, Kahaleh MB, Sagebiel RW. Plasmapheresis and immunosuppressive drug therapy in scleroderma. Arthr Rheum 1981; 24:1128–1136.
94. Tamura K, Akiyama J, Dono K, Kadowaki S, Shimada T. A successful therapy with plasma exchanges for interstitial pneumonia of progressive systemic sclerosis. Intern Med 1992; 31:649–654.
95. Rook AH, Freundlich B, Jegasothy BV, et al. Treatment of systemic sclerosis with extracorporeal photochemotherapy. Results of a multi-center trial. Arch Dermat 1992; 128:337–346.
96. Boyd AS, Nelder KH. Therapeutic options in dermatomyositis/polymyositis. Int J Dermat 1994; 33:240–250.
97. Tuffanelli DL, Lavole PE. Prognosis and therapy of polymyositis dermatomyositis. Clin Dermat 1988; 6:93–104.
98. Miller LC, Sisson BA, Tucker BA, et al. Methotrexate treatment of recalcitrant childhood dermatomyositis. Arthr Rheum 1992; 35:1143–1149.
99. Sinoway PA, Callen JP. Chlorambucil. An effective corticosteroid-sparing agent for patients with recalcitrant dermatomyositis. Arthr Rheum 1993; 36:319–324.
100. Casato M, Bonomo L, Caccavo D, Giorgi A. Clinical effects of cyclosporin in dermatomyositis. Clin Exp Dermat 1990; 15:121–123.

15

Evaluation and Treatment of Mycosis Fungoides and the Sezary Syndrome

Timothy M. Kuzel and Joan Guitart
Northwestern University Medical School, Chicago, Illinois

I. INTRODUCTION

The term "cutaneous T-cell lymphoma" is a misnomer; it has been used to suggest a discrete pathological entity. It is now clear, however, that a number of different disease states, all within the broad category of non-Hodgkin's lymphoma, may be included within this category by virtue of involvement of the skin by neoplastic T lymphocytes. Examples include mycosis fungoides (MF) and the Sezary syndrome (SS), the adult T-cell lymphoma/leukemia associated with the human T-cell lymphotropic virus I (HTLV-I), peripheral non-Hodgkin's large cell T-cell lymphoma, lymphomatoid papulosis, lymphomatoid granulomatosis, angioimmunoblastic lymphadenopathy, and T-gamma lymphoproliferative disorders. This chapter will briefly address issues central to the diagnosis and evaluation of MF and SS and review the current state-of-the-art treatment alternatives.

The T lymphocyte is a central participant in the body's ability to mount an immune response and is the neoplastic cell in these disorders. The diversity of the immune system is in part due to the rearrangement of the T-cell gene receptor loci (1), which encode the T-cell receptor, a structure analagous to the immunoglobulin molecule on B lymphocytes. This T-cell receptor is a surface glycoprotein and lies in close approximation with another surface antigen, CD-3. Most mature T lymphocytes have receptors composed of an α and β chain; these subunits form the binding site for antigens through a random matching process through their variable regions and the major histocompatibility complex. The CD-3 subunit is thought to serve a signal transduction function. Each homodimer chain consists of a variable, diverse, joining, and constant portion. Thus, through recombination, a limited number of distinct genes of each portion can generate a multitude of receptors. Southern analysis of DNA can be used to identify a distinct clone of T cells due to the presence of a detectable rearrangement (2). Polymerase chain reaction (PCR) technology has greatly increased the sensitivity of these molecular techniques and should allow earlier detection of residual or recurrent disease in the future (3).

II. EPIDEMIOLOGY AND ETIOLOGY

The most common of the cutaneous lymphomas is MF and the related SS (4). For unclear reasons, the incidence of this disease has nearly doubled over the last several decades to approximately 0.4 per 100,000 population. The incidence increases with increasing age and is slightly more common in African Americans and males. The average age at presentation is 50 y, although many young adults with the disease have been described.

No single entity has been found to be implicated in the development of MF or SS. Genetics, retroviral infectious agents, or exposure to one or multiple environmental toxins may be significant. A number of case reports of familial clustering (5) and the association of cases with certain histocompatibility antigens (AW31, AW32, B8, and BW35) are suggestive of genetic factors, but by no means are the results all inclusive (6–8). Cytogenetic studies have demonstrated no single specific chromosomal abnormality associated with these diseases, but this does not rule out more subtle genetic disturbances that may predispose to the development of MF or SS. Indeed, alterations in the levels of mRNA encoding a number of cellular components has been recognized in T-helper disorders, such as increased levels of transferrin receptor, α-tubulin, and interferon-α (9).

Environmental and occupational exposures to chemicals, heavy metals or their salts, pesticides or herbicides, and organic solvents are frequently linked to human neoplasms. However, several case-control studies have found no evidence of such a link in the case of MF/SS (10,11).

Other investigators, noting the presence of infiltrating nonneoplastic T lymphocytes in the patch/plaques lesions of MF, have postulated that prolonged immune stimulation (perhaps through contact allergens) might be an inciting feature in the disease (12,13). Again, case-control studies were unable to identify significant differences in skin allergy to plants, metals, cosmetics, topical or nontopical medications, food, or insect bites between the cases and the controls (11). Additionally, fewer cases than controls tested positively to scratch or prick tests for inhalants or ingestants despite similar responses to tests for systemic anergy (e.g., tuberculin skin tests or patch tests for contact allergens).

Of most interest recently is the finding of retroviral elements within the neoplastic lymphocytes or evidence of prior infection to retroviruses in patients with MF/SS (14–16). Retroviruses implicated to date include HTLV-I and HTLV-V. A recent preliminary report found 46 of 50 SS patients positive for retroviral sequences using PCR/Southern analysis (17). Given the spectrum of clinical and histopathological findings associated with MF/SS, however, several viral agents or combinations of viral infection and environmental exposure may be responsible for these syndromes.

III. CLINICAL PRESENTATION

The diagnosis of MF is often suspected when a long-lasting, poorly classified dermatosis eventually becomes recalcitrant to topical steroids. This so-called premycotic stage may resemble atopic eczema, seborrheic dermatitis, or psoriasis. The histological examination of early lesions is also nonspecific, showing chronic inflammatory changes only without significant numbers of atypical lymphocytes. Occasionally the premycotic (significant risk of transformation into MF) nature of the lesions can be recognized early in the disease course. These identifiable conditions are termed large plaque parapsoriasis or poikiloderma atrophicans vasculare. The large plaque form of parapsoriasis presents with erythematous plaques of more than 10 cm in diameter and characteristically afflicts the buttocks. This lesion may be considered an early manifestation of MF. Poikiloderma implies atrophic patches with mottled pigmentation and telangiectasia and can be observed in dermatoses other than premycotic lesions. The initial patches can resolve spontaneously, sometimes after sun exposure, but eventually lesions reappear although not necessarily in the same location.

After a variable length of time and often several inconclusive skin biopsies, the diagnosis of MF is reached. The initial stage or patch stage MF is sometimes only a retrospective consideration after the patient has entered a more advanced stage. The early patches have distinct borders and the intensity of the erythema often correlates with the density of the lymphocytic infiltrate. Hypopigmented MF can be seen among black patients (18).

The natural progression of the disease is accompanied by an increase in the density of the neoplastic cell infiltrate resulting in indurated plaques (Figure 1). The plaques are red to purple with a smooth surface and may arise de novo or within old patches. The size and shape is variable, although arcuate plaques are particularly characteristic. When the neoplastic infiltrate causes significant destruction of the dermal-epidermal junction the lesions may have a liquid appearance. Scaliness may reflect a marked epidermotropism of the tumor cells, a superimposed inflammatory condition (i.e., hypersensitivity dermatitis), or superficial infection. In advanced cases, tumors develop from preexistent plaques or previously uninvolved skin (Figure 2). During the tumor stage, patches, plaques, and tumors may manifest a rapid growth rate. Necrosis with superficial ulceration

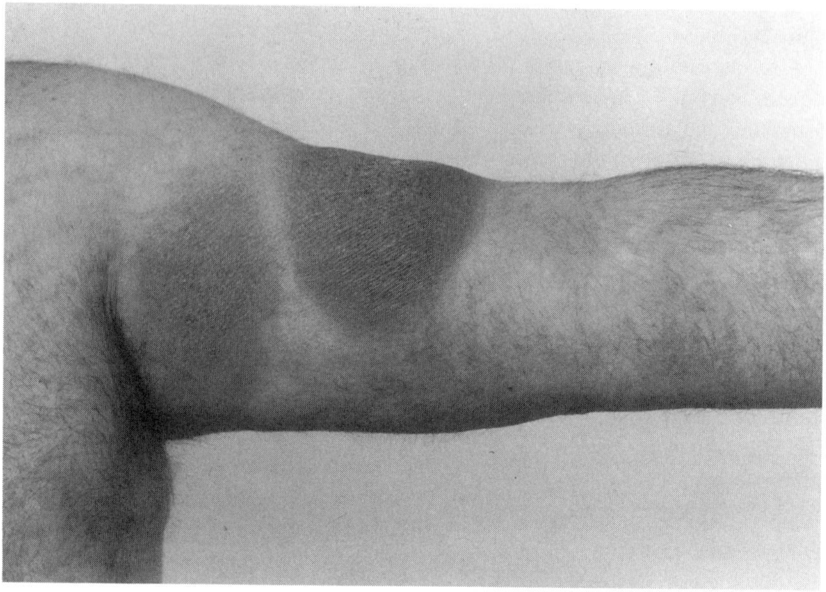

Figure 1 Plaque stage mycosis fungoides. Well-demarcated red tan plaques with slight scaliness.

is a frequent complication of the tumors. This may be a source of infection which may lead to the demise of the patient. On rare occasions the tumors arise de novo, sparing the initial stages. This so-called "d'emblee" presentation is observed in about 10% of CTCL patients (19).

The erythrodermic form of MF (or SS if leukemic neoplastic lymphocytes are present) can evolve from a preexisting MF or can arise de novo (Figure 3). The circulating hyperconvoluted T lymphocytes are refered to as Sezary cells. The patient presents with generalized erythema and scaliness, often with associated thick scaly palms and soles, dystrophic nails, ectropion, and alopecia. The patient may be very debilitated with malaise, intense pruritus, and poor regulation of body temperature. High-output cardiac failure can further complicate the picture.

Although more common in patients with cutaneous tumors or generalized erythroderma, lymphadenopathy can develop at any time during the course of the disease (19). Regardless of the pathological findings, the detection of lymphadenopathy indicates a poor prognosis (20). Sausville et al. developed a scale reflecting involvement of lymph nodes ranging from an occasional neoplastic lymphocyte to complete effacement of normal architecture (20), termed LN-1 to LN-4 nodes, respectively. Finally, autopsy evaluation of patients with MF has

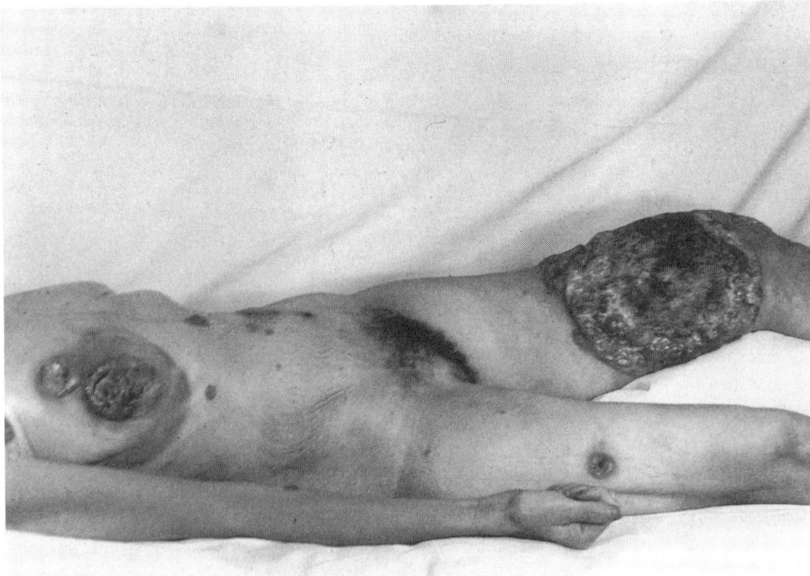

Figure 2 Tumor stage mycosis fungoides. Large ulcerated tumors with central necrosis in a patient with advanced mycosis fungoides.

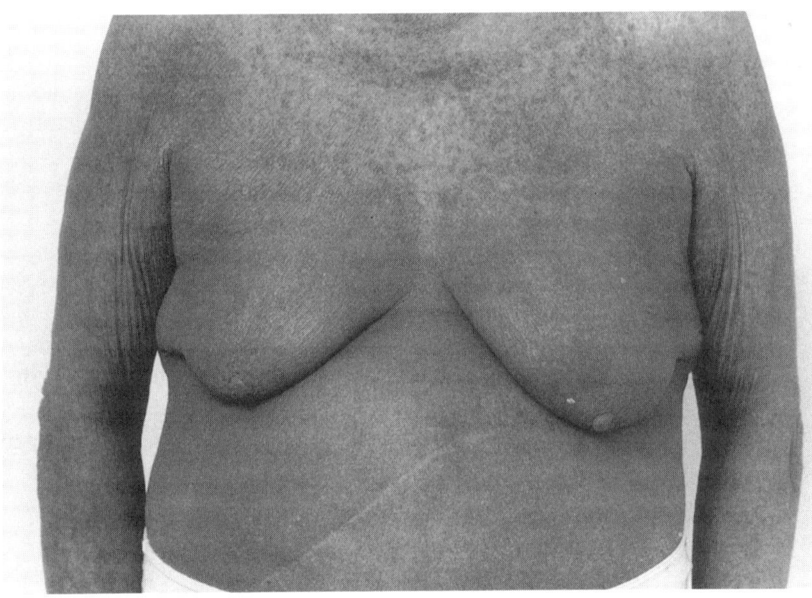

Figure 3 Generalized erythema and mild scaliness in a patient with Sezary syndrome.

demonstrated a high incidence of visceral involvement in advance stages of the disease (21), although the disease was rarely evident clinically antemortem. Clinically apparent hepatomegaly, splenomegaly, and bone marrow involvement are usually only seen in advanced cases.

IV. HISTOPATHOLOGY

The histological diagnosis of MF is often reached after many nonspecific skin biopsies. The distinction between a benign reactive infiltrate and a malignant lymphoma of the skin is often a judgment call by the pathologist, who may be influenced by several objective and subjective parameters. Inflammatory epidermal changes, like acanthosis, hyperkeratosis, and spongiosis are common in the premycotic stages (22). A predominantly reactive infiltrate often masks the neoplastic T cells in early MF. But even if able to isolate the clonal population, the cytological atypia of early MF cells is subtle. The defining cytological features as outlined by electron microscopy studies are the large size and the hyperconvolution of the nuclei (23). The biopsies show a mononuclear cell infiltrate involving the papillary dermis with variable exocytosis of the lymphocytes (Figure 4A). Epidermotropism of the atypical lymphocytes with microabscess formation, the pathognomonic feature, is not always present (Figure 4B). More often single lymphocytes infiltrate the basal and suprabasal layers. The epidermotropism can also involve the epithelium of the hair follicles. Follicular mucinosis is the degeneration of the follicular epithelium, which may eventually cause focal alopecia. In the papillary dermis, fibroplasia in a wiry pattern can be found. A variable infiltrate of eosinophils and plasma cells can also be found in some patients.

As the disease advances, the pathological findings become more obvious. This transformation is primarily due to an increase in the tumor burden accompanied by a decrease in the reactive lymphocytic infiltrate. Therefore, nuclear atypia and epidermotropism become more noticeable. The thickness and density of the infiltrate also increase in plaques and tumors. The lymphocytes in the late tumor stage are more anaplastic and less hyperconvoluted and epidermotropic. In the erythrodermic presentation, the histological findings are variable. Even advanced cases of SS may not show diagnostic histological features. The more consistent finding is a perivascular collection of lymphocytes with variable atypia and epidermotropism. Biopsies of palpable lymph nodes may show dermatopathic changes with paracortical hyperplasia of reactive histiocytes with focal melanin deposition. Large numbers of cerebriform lymphocytes are often found. Although the same pathological features can be seen in extensive inflammatory dermatoses, gene rearrangement studies have demonstrated the frequent presence of clonal

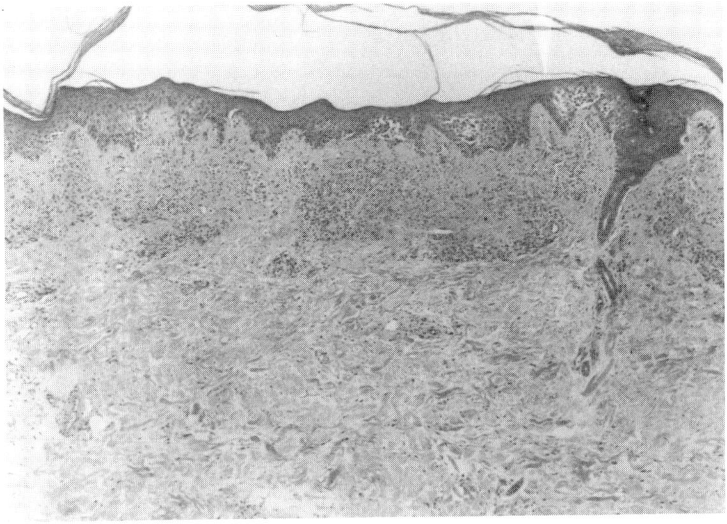

(A)

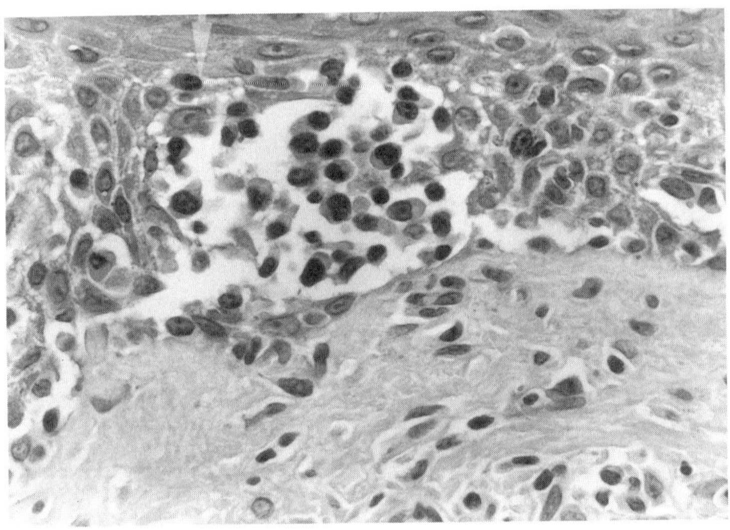

(B)

Figure 4 Histopathology of mycosis fungoides. A) Low-power view showing an upper dermal mononuclear infiltrate with marked epidermotropism. B) High-power view showing hyperchromatic and hyperconvoluted lymphocytes with marked eipidermotropism and Pautrier microabscess formation.

lymphocytes (24). This finding supports the clinical observation that lymphadenopathy has a poor prognosis regardless of the biopsy results (25).

V. IMMUNOPATHOLOGY

The frustrations associated with the imprecise diagnosis rendered by routine biopsies of initial lesions has prompted an intense search for a more specific diagnostic tool for MF. Numerous studies have evaluated the immunophenotype of the neoplastic lymphocyte in this disorder. The masking effect of the predominantly reactive population of T lymphocytes in early lesions has hampered the efforts in this area also. Therefore, immunohistochemistry is of limited help in patch stage MF.

Information gathered by immunohistochemistry may be relevant in the following circumstances:

Identification of the mononuclear cell population. Pan T-cell, pan B-cell, and monocyte/macrophage markers will define the infiltrate in broad terms. CD4 and CD8 are particularly helpful when the malignant CD4+ population outgrows the reactive CD8+ cells. A CD4/CD8 ratio higher than 5/1 is rarely encountered in benign infiltrates, suggesting MF. Conversely, a predominant CD8+ population may be seen in the rare cases of CD8 MF.

Detection of an aberrant phenotype. CD7 has consistently proved to be the most consistent antigen deleted in MF. Other markers, such as the pan T-cell markers CD3 and CD5, can be deleted, but only in advanced cases when the lymphocytes become dedifferentiated. We consider a deletion significant when more than two-thirds of the T cells do not express the marker. Nonetheless, less obvious deletions restricted to the epidermotropic population can be important, especially in early stages when a pure neoplastic population can be found only among the epidermotropic cells.

Detection of clonality. A new commercially available panel of monoclonal antibodies to different subfamilies of the V region of the T-cell receptor may suggest clonality (26). Unfortunately, the panel only covers 7 of the more than 20 subfamilies of the V region; strong expression of one of the markers is suggestive of clonality.

Proliferation rate of the tumor cells. PCNA or Ki-67 can provide information regarding the mitotic activity of the tumor which may have prognostic significance.

VI. STAGING EVALUATION

In 1979 the staging committee at an international consensus conference on MF devised the staging classification based on the international TNM system that is currently used (27). Factors included in the system include extent of skin disease at diagnosis (T), type of lymph node involvement (N), presence or absence of peripheral blood disease (PB), and the presence or absence of visceral disease (M). A number of staging procedures are recommended for routine clinical evaluation of patients with MF or SS. These should include a complete medical history and physical examination, mapping of skin lesions at diagnosis, complete blood count with differential, a Sezary cell count, serum chemistries [with careful attention to liver function tests and level of lactate dehydrogenase (LDH)], chest roentgenogram, and lymph node biopsy if significant palpable adenopathy is present. Computed tomography scans are not routinely recommended outside the setting of a clinical trial if the above tests are within normal limits and the pathology suggests classic MF without question of a variant cutaneous T-cell lymphoma (28). Lymphangiograms and bone marrow aspiration or biopsy are not generally useful.

VII. TREATMENT

Multiple modalities now exist for the treatment of MF/SS. The approaches with the most clinical experience include the use of psoralens with ultraviolet A (UVA) light exposure (PUVA or photophoresis), radiation therapy (external beam or total-skin electron beam), topical chemotherapy, and systemic chemotherapy. In addition, combination approaches have been utilized. Experimental approaches focus on the development of new active agents including biological response modifiers, cytotoxic agents, differentiation agents, or novel combinations of the above. The goals of any treatment program, however, should remain control of skin disease for symptomatic relief. The curability of these diseases remains to be proven.

A. Phototherapy

8-Methoxypsoralen (8-MOP) is a member of a family of photoactivated compounds that interfere with DNA and RNA synthesis in the presence of various wavelengths of light. These drugs are inactive in tissues not exposed to light. PUVA treatments rely on the administration of these agents several hours prior to external application of UVA light (penetration limited to the epidermis and upper dermis). Photophoresis treatments rely on administration of 8-MOP prior to removal, irradiation with UVA light of mononuclear cells in an extracorporeal device, and subsequent reinfusion.

A number of trials have demonstrated benefit for PUVA in patients with MF/SS (29–33). A large review of 82 patients treated with PUVA at our institution demonstrated complete clearing in 59% of patients. Results were stage dependent.

Eighty-eight percent of patients with limited patch/plaque disease, and 52% of those with more extensive plaque disease cleared. Only 46% of erythrodermic patients responded completely, with 75% relapsing during maintenance therapy. No patient with tumor stage disease achieved a complete response. The lack of even a single complete response in thick tumor lesions would suggest that PUVA is a topical therapy and that immunological changes or exposure of the blood pool in superficial capillaries may not play a role in the benefit derived from PUVA. However, research into the biology of these responses is needed.

We initiate PUVA three times per week at a UVA dose of 1.5–3.0 joule/cm^2, and this can be increased by approximately 0.5 joule/cm^2 per treatment as tolerated. The frequency of treatments is reduced once complete clearing has occurred, but we feel that maintenance treatment (every 2–4 wk) prolongs the duration of remission.

In contrast to PUVA, the results with photophoresis suggest that systemic or immune mechanisms may be operative in the benefits achieved with psoralens and UVA light. The original article reported preliminary results of therapy in 37 patients (34). Twelve of 29 patients with generalized erythroderma achieved complete or partial responses. Three of 8 patients with extensive plaque or tumor lesions responded. In an update, Heald et al. reported long-term follow-up data on the erythrodermic patients (35). Median survival times of 60.33 mo from diagnosis and 48 mo from treatment initiation were achieved.

Zic et al. have reported on their results in 20 patients with CTCL (36). In contrast to the above results, they observed an objective response rate of 71% in patients with patch/plaque stage disease and 33% in erythrodermic patients. Again, no patients with tumor stage disease responded. Duration of remission is impossible to assess as 10 of the 11 responding patients received adjunctive PUVA, chemotherapy, steroids, or radiation.

Most investigators initiate the extracorporeal phototherapy at every 2–5 wk depending upon the extent and severity of the disease. The mechanism by which photophoresis benefits patients is not clear. Investigators at Yale University have reported that photophoresis alters the neoplastic cells in a fashion which makes them more immunogenic, and the resulting host immune response is responsible for the beneficial effects. A number of investigators have suggested that patients with greater levels of T-suppressor cells are the best candidates for therapy, also suggesting a host immune response to therapy.

Toxicity with either PUVA or photophoresis is relatively minor. Psoralen administration may be complicated by nausea, vomiting, or diarrhea. PUVA results in some chronic dryness and erythema of skin, or pruritus. Occasional PUVA "burns" may mimic a disease flare. Long-term PUVA exposure is associated with abnormal amyloid depositions in the skin (37) and an increased incidence of cutaneous carcinomas, especially squamous cell carcinomas of the skin and male genitalia (38). Photophoresis toxicity is mild and related to the phoresis process; occasional fevers and mild hypotension may be witnessed, neither of which typically requires inpatient therapy.

B. Radiation Therapy

The non-Hodgkin's lymphomas in general, and MF/SS in particular, are quite radiosensitive. External beam radiotherapy has been demonstrated to control local areas of resistant MF or provide palliation to large tumor lesions or troublesome adenopathy. The cumulative dosage of radiation therapy that can be delivered is limited, however, by the radiation tolerance of neighboring normal organs. In addition, chronic cytopenias can limit the ability to deliver subsequent therapeutics. Still newer techniques involving total nodal irradiation, fractionated total body irradiation, or hemibody irradiation are being investigated.

Given the limitations noted above, the development of protocols to deliver total skin electron beam radiation therapy was an important advance. Linear accelerator-generated electron beams are scattered by a penetrable plate placed at the collimator site. The energy of the electrons is reduced to 4–7 meV, and adequate field distribution is assured. The low energy level limits penetrance to the superficial tissues (depth approximately 1 cm). Most patients tolerate total doses of approximately 3000–3600 cGy over an 8–10 wk period (39).

A number of investigators have reported their experience with total skin electron beam radiation therapy (40–42). Approximately 80% of patients will achieve a complete remission with therapy, although overall response rates and durability of response is stage dependent. Complete responses of 95% have been cited for limited patch/plaque disease, but responses of only 50% are common for patients with generalized erythroderma or nodal involvement. Long-term remissions (longer than 3 y) have been observed in 50% of patients with limited stage disease, but have been observed in only 25% of patients with more generalized disease.

Side effects of chronic dryness and scaling of the skin, telangiectasia formation, skin ulceration, and hair or sweat gland loss can be distressing to patients. Careful radiation dosimetric techniques are important to minimize toxicity and maximize benefit. Administration of this therapy should be limited to centers with substantial experience. Given the difficulty and potential toxicity of this treatment, as well as the number of alternative topical therapies currently available, we have observed total skin electron beam radiotherapy being utilized less commonly.

C. Topical Chemotherapy

Since much of the symptomatology of MF relates to the skin, applications of chemotherapy directly to lesions represented one the earliest therapeutic approaches. Mechlorethamine hydrochloride was the first agent to demonstrate efficacy (43). The solution used for topical application contains 10–20 mg of mechlorethamine dissolved in 50–100 ml of tap water (no vesicant activity at this low concentration). Self-administration to the entire skin surface at home is the preferred method of application. Time to response is usually short, approximately 1–2 wk, but long-term administration may be necessary to achieve durable, maximal remissions.

Vonderheid et al. reported their experience with topical mechlorethamine and found that it compared favorably to total skin electron beam radiotherapy with 80%, 68%, and 61% of patients achieving complete clearing for limited plaque, extensive plaque, and tumor lesions, respectively (44). Some patients have achieved durable remissions, but others have relapsed as long as 8 y after completion of therapy, illustrating the chronic, indolent nature of this disease.

Side effects mainly consist of hypersensitivity in approximately 35% of patients. The concentration of the solution can be varied depending upon the degree of sensitivity seen. Once true hypersensitivity develops, patients can be desensitized by injecting minute daily doses of mechlorethamine over a period of several weeks (45). This should be done only in a carefully supervised medical setting. Hoppe et al. demonstrated that ointment-based (aquaphor or polyethylene glycol) topical mechlorethamine may offer lower rates of sensitivity and maintain similar response rates (46). In addition, there have been reports of an increased incidence of other skin cancers in patients exposed to long-term topical mechlorethamine.

A number of other agents have been tested topically in MF and SS, including corticosteroids, cytarabine, dianhydrogalactitol, dacarbazine, guanazole, teniposide, hydroxyurea, thiotepa, and methotrexate. However, topical carmustine is the only other agent that has demonstrated clinical benefit (47). Side effects of contact dermatitis are less frequent with this agent, but systemic side effects can be greater. This agent may be most helpful for the treatment of patients who do not tolerate topical mechlorethamine due to cutaneous sensitivity.

D. Systemic Chemotherapy

Systemic chemotherapy should be reserved for those patients with relapsed or refractory disease after topical interventions, or for those patients with nodal/visceral disease at presentation. Single-agent chemotherapy with alkylating agents, cisplatin, etoposide, bleomycin, doxorubicin, vincristine, vinblastine, or oral corticosteroids have all been utilized. Complete response has ranged from 20–50% in most trials, but the duration of remission is usually short.

McDonald and Bertino reported particularly good results with a regimen of intravenous methotrexate followed by oral citrovorum factor (48). Patients received 1–5 mg/kg of intravenous methotrexate every 5 d. If a patient tolerated the lowest dose well, each subsequent dose was escalated. After five intravenous doses, patients were switched to oral methotrexate (25–50 mg) with oral citrovorum as weekly maintenance. All 11 patients achieved "good" or better clearing (greater than 60%) for a median duration of 24 mo. Mucousitis and skin ulcerations were the most significant toxicity witnessed. Myelosuppression was mild in general.

Combinations of chemotherapeutic agents have been extensively studied as well. Most commonly used are combinations of an alkylating agent (oral or intravenous) with corticosteroids, and perhaps a vinca alkaloid and doxorubicin (49,50). These regimens yield complete remissions of 80–100%, with longer durations of remission compared to single agents. Unfortunately there is no survival benefit associated with early utilization of such aggressive regimens, and toxicity is certainly greater than observed with other palliative approaches. Severe myelosuppression associated with infection can be fatal in some patients, and thus very close follow-up is needed in patients treated in this fashion.

E. Interferons

The α interferons (IFN) are now recognized as one of the most potent agents for the treatment of MF/SS (51–56). Unfortunately the dosage and schedule that provide the most benefit have yet to be identified. High-dose ($36–50 \times 10^6$ IU) therapy provided complete response rates of 10–27% in trials by Bunn et al. (51,52) and Olsen et al. (53) respectively, in heavily pretreated patients. The median duration of the remissions was relatively short (5.5 mo) and toxicity was substantial, including constitutional symptoms and cytopenias. In less heavily pretreated patients and with lower doses (3×10^6 IU), overall response rates of 76% were been observed with much less toxicity (Olsen et al., unpublished data). Supporting the use of low and moderate-dose IFN, Covelli et al. treated 15 previously untreated MF patients with daily subcutaneous IFN-α in doses escalated from 3×10^6 IU to 18×10^6 IU (54). Of 12 assessable patients, 5 achieved a complete response and 6 achieved a partial response (overall response rate was 92%). Independently, Tura et al. achieved an 80% response rate with 3 complete responses and 9 partial responses among 15 patients treated with a similar IFN regimen (55). The dose of IFN-α that seems to be tolerable when administered daily or three times weekly appears to be approximately 12×10^6 IU.

Alternative IFNs or routes of administration have also been tested. Vonderheid et al. demonstrated that IFN-α-2b injected intralesionally (three times weekly for 4 wk) resulted in lesion regression (56). Interestingly, when given systemically, this agent did not have activity. This may relate to the dosage schedule or timing used in this study.

One trial evaluated IFN-γ in patients with MF. Kaplan et al. administered recombinant human IFN-γ to 16 patients with heavily pretreated MF or SS (57).

No complete responses were seen, but 31% of patients achieved a partial response, including some patients who had failed on IFN-α. The median duration of remission was 10 mo, and toxicities were similar to those witnessed in trials of IFN-α.

VIII. INVESTIGATIONAL APPROACHES

It is apparent that multiple modalities currently exist to palliate the symptoms of MF and SS. Unfortunately it is not currently thought that these modalities can result in long-term survival in more than a few patients. Thus, a major focus of research in these disorders continues to be the development of new agents or approaches to impact on the survival of patients.

A. Combined Modality Therapy

A number of investigators have attempted to combine the active modalities mentioned above, with the goal being improvement of response rates and survival. Hallahan et al. compared local radiation therapy, total-skin electron beam radiation therapy, and total-skin electron beam followed by combination chemotherapy in a nonrandomized pilot study (58). Although they demonstrated an early difference between response rates and a disease-free survival advantage for the combination arm, the limitations of the study design, with small numbers of patients not randomly assigned, prevent firm conclusions from being established.

Braverman et al. treated 40 newly diagnosed patients with stage I or II MF with 3600 cGy of total-skin electron beam radiation followed by six monthly cycles of combination chemotherapy (59). Compared with a historical control group treated with total-skin electron beam radiation only, patients receiving combined modality therapy were more likely to remain in a clinical complete remission. This study suffers from the lack of a randomized control group and unclear response classifications.

The most definitive trial with combined modality therapy was performed at the National Cancer Institute. Kaye et al. compared aggressive combination chemotherapy and total-skin electron beam radiation therapy with a series of palliative topical interventions applied sequentially as needed (60). Patients with all stages of disease and levels of performance status were eligible to be randomized. After a median follow-up time of 75 mo they were able to demonstrate significant differences between the treatment groups in rates of complete remission induction (combined > conservative) but not in disease-free or overall survival. In addition, the combined therapy treatment was associated with considerable toxicity.

In light of the considerable activity of interferons in these diseases and the low acute toxicity associated with PUVA, our group has conducted a series of trials combining these modalities. In a phase I trial, 12 of 15 patients achieved a complete response (61). The maximum tolerated dosage of IFN-α-2a was 12×10^6 IU/m^2 when administered three times weekly, with PUVA initially administered three times weekly also. Twenty-four more patients were treated at those doses in a phase II trial. Long-term data (median follow-up 28 mo) for the whole group is now available. Despite being heavily pretreated, 62% of patients achieved a complete remission and 28% a partial remission. The median duration of response was 28 mo (62). In general, patients with large cell variants of MF or SS, and those with significant antigen deletions from the neoplastic cell surface, did less well with the IFN-based treatments (63).

Since the original reports of IFN and PUVA benefit, several reports have appeared that support this approach. One patient with SS received combined therapy with IFN and photophoresis and achieved a complete remission (documented clearing by Southern blot of peripheral blood), ongoing for at least 22 mo (64). Another report demonstrated that patients refractory initially to PUVA therapy alone could achieve complete remissions when IFN was added to their regimen (65). These exciting observations are the basis for a proposed national clinical trial of topical therapies alone or in combination with IFN to determine if significant benefits are observed with combined therapy. Proven benefits will be important given the increased toxicity and cost associated with combined therapy.

B. New Agents

A variety of new agents have been developed or evaluated for use in patients with MF and SS. Antithymocyte globulin has been administered to patients with advanced MF with transient improvement. Murine monoclonal antibodies alone, or conjugated to radioisotopes or toxins, have also been tested. Transient improvement in skin lesions and clearance of malignant circulating cells have been documented. Several studies with cyclosporin A have suggested a partial benefit in patients with MF, although these responses required continued therapy to be maintained (66,67). Renal toxicity was substantial in these reports. A synthetic thymic hormone analog, thymopentin (a pentapeptide), when administered intravenously, has demonstrated objective antineoplastic effects in 50–75% of SS patients with low circulating cell numbers (68,69).

A variety of retinoid derivatives have been tested in this disease. Kessler et al. treted 25 patients with isotretinoin and observed a 44% objective response rate, including 4 patients with a clinical complete response (but biopsies still showed disease) (70). We have demonstrated a response rate of approximately 30% in patients with MF utilizing all-trans retinoic acid (71). Interestingly, most of our responses were also more impressive clinically than apparent histologically.

Autologous bone marrow transplantation has now been recognized as a potentially curable therapy for certain subsets of the non-Hodgkin's lymphomas. A number of institutions internationally are performing pilot studies of the efficacy and toxicity of various approaches.

Recently, new agents with novel mechanisms of action, such as the purine analogs and recombinant protein fusion toxins, have been found to have significant activity for the treatment of MF and SS. In general, the purine analogs deoxycoformycin, fludarabine monophosphate, and 2-chlorodeoxyadenosine can effectively treat MF and SS. These agents either inhibit or are resistant to degradation by adenosine deaminase and result in nucleoside pool imbalances which T cells tolerate exceptionally poorly. As single agents, deoxycoformycin was associated with a 50% response rate (72), fludarabine monophosphate with a 19% response rate (73), and 2-chlorodeoxyadenosine with a 30% response rate (74,75). Myelosuppression can be significant with these agents, although 2-chlorodeoxyadenosine is least myelosuppressive unless multiple cycles are utilized. Trials exploring the combinations of 2-chlorodeoxyadenosine and IFN-α are now under way.

Finally, recombinant fusion proteins have manifested activity against MF. DAB_{389}IL-2, a molecule consisting of the enzymatic and translocation portions of diphtheria toxin and the ligand binding portions of human interleukin-2, has been developed and entered into clinical trials. In phase I trials remarkable activity against MF has been noted, including 5 responses out of 11 patients treated with the most recent construct (76). These agents, with differential toxicity spectra and new mechanisms of action, able to escape recognized drug resistance pathways, should allow for better palliation or curability of MF and SS either alone or in combination with other active modalities.

REFERENCES

1. Royer HD, Reinherz EL. Ontogeny, function, and relevance to clinical disorders. N Eng J Med 1987; 317:1136.
2. Aisenberg AC, Krontiris TC, Mak TW, et al. Rearrangement of the gene for the beta chain of the T-cell receptor in T-cell chronic lymphocytic leukemia and related disorders. N Eng J Med 1985; 313:529.
3. Staib G, Sterry W. Detection of clonal T-cell population in peripheral blood of patients with cutaneous T-cell lymphoma. Proc Am Assoc Cancer Res 1994:238.
4. Weinstock MA, Horm JW. Mycosis fungoides in the United States—increasing incidence and descriptive epidemiology. JAMA 1988; 260:42.
5. Sandbank M, Katzenellenbogen I. Mycosis fungoides of prolonged duration in siblings. Arch Dermat 1968; 98:620.
6. MacKie R, Dick HM, DeSousa MB. HLA and mycosis fungoides. Lancet 1976; 1:1179.
7. Safai B, Myskowski PL, Dupont B, et al. Association of HLA-DR5 with mycosis fungoides. J Invest Dermat 1983; 80:395.

8. Rosen ST, Radvany R, Roenigk HH Jr, et al. Human leukocyte antigens in cutaneous T-cell lymphoma. J Am Acad Dermat 1985; 12:531.
9. Woloschak GE, Hooper WC, Doerge MJ. Oncogene expression in T-cell lymphoproliferative disorders. Cancer Res 1988; 48:856.
10. Tuyp E, Burgoyne A, Aitchison T, et al. A case-control study of possible causative factors in mycosis fungoides. Arch Dermat 1987; 123:196.
11. Whittemore AS, Holly EA, Lee IM, et al. Mycosis fungoides in relation to environmental exposures and immune response: a case-control study. J Natl Cancer Inst 1989; 81:1560.
12. Tan RS, Butterworth CM, McLaughlin H, et al. Mycosis fungoides—a disease of antigen persistence. Br J Dermat 1974; 91:607.
13. Rowden G, Lewis MG. Langerhans cells: involvement in the pathogenesis of mycosis fungoides. Br J Dermat 1976; 95:665.
14. Manzari V, Gismondi A, Barillari E, et al. A new human retrovirus isolated in a tac-negative T-cell lymphoma/leukemia. Science 1987; 238:1581.
15. Knobler RM, Rehle T, Grossman M, et al. Clinical evolution of cutaneous T-cell lymphoma in a patient with antibodies to human T-lymphotropic virus type I. J Am Acad Dermat 1987; 17:903.
16. Wantzin GL, Thomsen K, Nissen NI, et al. Occurrence of human T-cell lymphotropic virus (type I) antibodies in cutaneous T-cell lymphoma. J Am Acad Dermat 1986; 15:598.
17. Zucker-Franklin D, Pancake BA. Cutaneous T-cell lymphoma is another HTLV-associated disease: a study of 65 patients. Proc Am Fed Clin Res 1994; 42:127a.
18. Whitmore SE, Simmons-O'Brien E, Rotter FS. Hypopigmented mycosis fungoides. Arch Dermat 1994; 130:476.
19. Kuzet TM, Roenigk HH Jr, Rosen ST. Mycosis fungoides and the Sezary syndrome: a review of pathogenesis, diagnosis and therapy. J Clin Oncol 1991; 9:1298.
20. Sausville EA, Worsham GF, Matthews MJ, et al. Histologic assessment of lymph nodes in mycosis fungoides/Sezary syndrome (CTCL): clinical correlations and prognostic import of a new classification system. Hum Pathol 1985; 16:1098.
21. Rappaport H, Thomas LB. Mycosis fungoides: the pathology of extracutaneous involvement. Cancer 1974; 34:1198.
22. Nikoloff BJ. Light microscopic assessment of 100 patients with patch/plaque stage mycosis fungoides. Am J Dermatopathol 1988; 10:469.
23. McNutt NS, Heilbron DC, Crain WR. Mycosis fungoides: diagnostic criteria based on quantitative electron microscopy. Lab Invest 1981; 44:466.
24. Weiss LM, Hu E, Wood GS, et al. Clonal rearrangement of T-cell receptor genes in mycosis fungoides and dermatopathic lymphadenopathy. N Engl J Med 1985; 313:539.
25. Burke JS, Colby TV. Dermatopathic lymphadenopathy: comparison of cases associated and unassociated with mycosis fungoides. Am J Surg Pathol 1981; 5:343.
26. Hunt SJ, Charley MR, Jegasothy BV, et al. Cutaneous T-cell lymphoma; utility of antibodies to the variable region of the human T-cell antigen receptor. J Am Acad Dermat 1992; 26:552.
27. Bunn PA, Lamberg SI. Report of the committee on staging and classification of cutaneous T-cell lymphomas. Cancer Treat Rep 1979; 63:725.

28. Rosen ST, Gore R, Brennan J, et al. Evaluation of computed tomography in the staging of cutaneous T-cell lymphomas. Arch Dermat 1986; 122:884.
29. Gilchrest BA. Methoxsalen photochemotherpay for mycosis fungoides. Cancer Treat Rep 1979; 63:663.
30. Roenigk HH Jr. Photochemotherapy for mycosis fungoides: long term follow-up study. Cancer Treat Rep 1979; 63:669.
31. Lowe NJ, Cripps DJ, Dufton PA, et al. Photochemotherapy for mycosis fungoides. A clinical and histological study. Arch Dermat 1979; 115:50.
32. Minna JD, Roenigk HH Jr, Glatstein E. Report of the committee on therapy for mycosis fungoides and Sezary syndrome. Cancer Treat Rep 1979; 63:729.
33. Roenigk HH Jr, Kuzel TM, Skoutelis AP, et al. Photochemotherapy alone or combined with interferon alfa-2a in the treatment of cutaneous T-cell lymphoma. J Invest Dermat 1990; 95(suppl):198s.
34. Edelson RL, Berger C, Gasparro F, et al. Treatment of cutaneous T-cell lymphoma by extracorporeal photochemotherapy. N Engl J Med 1987; 316:297.
35. Heald P, Rook A, Perez M, et al. Treatment of erythrodermic cutaneous T-cell lymphoma with extracorporeal photochemotherapy. J Am Acad Dermat 1992; 27:427.
36. Zic J, Arzubiaga C, Salhany KE, et al. Extracorporeal photopheresis for the treatment of cutaneous T-cell lymphoma. J Am Acad Dermat 1992; 27:729.
37. Greene I, Cox AJ. Amyloid deposition after psoriasis therapy with psoralen and long wave ultraviolet light. Arch Dermat 1979; 115:1200.
38. Stern RS. Members of the photochemotherapy follow-up study: genital tumors among men with psoriasis exposed to psoralens and ultraviolet A radiation (PUVA) and ultraviolet B radiation. N Engl J Med 1990; 322:1093.
39. Hoppe RT, Cox RS, Fuks Z, et al. Electron beam therapy for mycosis fungoides: the Stanford University experience. Cancer Treat Rep 1979; 63:691.
40. Fuks ZY, Hoppe RT, Bagshaw MA. The role of total skin irradiation with electrons in the management of mycosis fungoides. Bull Cancer 1977; 64:291.
41. Nisce LZ, Safai B. Once weekly total skin electron beam therapy for mycosis fungoides: 7 years experience. Cancer Treat Rep 1979; 63:633.
42. Freeman CR, Suissa S, Shenouda G, et al. Clinical experience with a single field rotational total skin electron irradiation technique for cutaneous T-cell lymphoma. Radiother Oncol 1992; 24:155.
43. Kierland RR, Watkins CH, Schullenberger CC. The use of nitrogen mustard in the treatment of mycosis fungoides. J Invest Dermat 1947; 9:195.
44. Vonderheid EC, Tan ET, Kantor AF, et al. Long-term efficacy, curative potential and carcinogenicity of topical mechlorethamine chemotherapy in cutaneous T-cell lymphoma. J Am Acad Dermat 1989; 20:416.
45. Van Scott EJ, Kalmanson JD. Complete remissions of mycosis fungoides lymphoma induced by topical nitrogen mustard. Cancer 1973; 32:18.
46. Hoppe RT, Abel EA, Deneau DG, et al. Mycosis fungoides: management with topical nitrogen mustard. J Clin Oncol 1987; 5:1796.
47. Zackheim HS, Epstein EH Jr, Crain WR. Topical carmustine (BCNU) for cutaneous T-cell lymphoma: a 15-year experience in 143 patients. J Am Acad Dermat 1990; 22:802.

48. McDonald CJ, Bertino JR. Treatment of mycosis fungoides lymphoma: effectiveness of infusions of methotrexate followed by oral citrovorum factor. Cancer Treat Rep 1978; 62:1009.
49. Winkelmann RK, Buechner SA, Diaz-Perez JL. Pre-Sezary syndrome. J Am Acad Dermat 1984; 10:992.
50. Grozea PN, Jones SE, McKelvey EM, et al. Combination chemotherapy for mycosis fungoides: a southwest oncology group study. Cancer Treat Rep 1979; 63:647.
51. Bunn PA Jr, Foon KA, Ihde DC, et al. Recombinant leukocyte A interferon: an active agent in advanced cutaneous T-cell lymphomas. Ann Intern Med 1984; 101:484.
52. Bunn PA Jr, Ihde DC, Foon KA. The role of recombinant interferon alfa-2a in the therapy of cutaneous T-cell lymphomas. Cancer 1986; 57:1689.
53. Olsen EA, Rosen ST, Vollmer RT, et al. Interfeorn alfa-2a in the treatment of cutaneous T-cell lymphoma. J Am Acad Dermat 1989; 20:395.
54. Covelli A, Cavalieri R, Coppla G, et al. Recombinant leukocyte A interferon (IFN-rA) as initial therapy in mycosis fungoides and the Sezary syndrome. Proc Am Soc Clin Oncol 1987; 6:189.
55. Tura S, Mazza P, Ainzani PL, et al. Alpha recombinant interferon in the treatment of mycosis fungoides. Haematological 1980; 72:337.
56. Vonderheid EC, Thompson R, Smiles KA, et al. Recombinant interferon alpha-2b in plaque mycosis fungoides. Arch Dermat 1987; 123:757.
57. Kaplan EH, Rosen ST, Norris DB, et al. Phase I study of recombinant human interferon gamma for treatment of cutaneous T-cell lymphoma. J Natl Cancer Inst 1990; 82:208.
58. Hallahan DE, Griem ML, Griem SF, et al. Combined modality therapy for tumor stage mycosis fungoides: results of a 10-year follow-up. J Clin Oncol 1988; 6:1177.
59. Braverman IM, Yager NB, Chen M, et al. Combined total body electron beam irradiation and chemotherapy for mycosis fungoides. J Am Acad Dermat 1987; 16:45.
60. Kaye FJ, Bunn PA Jr, Steinberg SM, et al. A randomized trial comparing combination electron-beam radiation and chemotherapy with topical therapy in the initial treatment of mycosis fungoides. N Engl J Med 1989; 321:1784.
61. Kuzel TM, Gilyon K, Springer E, et al. Interferon alfa-2a combined with phototherapy in the treatment of cutaneous T-cell lymphoma. J Natl Cancer Inst 1990; 82:203.
62. Kuzel TM, Roenigk HH Jr, Samuelson E, et al. Effectiveness of interferon alfa-2a combined with phototherapy for mycosis fungoides and the Sezary syndrome. J Clin Oncol 1995; 13:257.
63. Springer EA, Kuzel TM, Variakojis D, et al. Correlation of clinical responses with immunologic and morphologic characteristics in patients with cutaneous T-cell lymphoma treated with interferon alfa-2a. J Am Acad Dermat 1993; 29:42.
64. Rook AH, Prystowsky MB, Cassin M, Boufal M, Lessin SR. Combined therapy for Sezary syndrome with extracorporeal photochemotherapy and low-dose interferon alfa therapy. Arch Dermat 1991; 127:1535.
65. Mostow EN, Neckel SL, Oberhelman L, Anderson TF, Cooper KD. Complete remissions in psoralen and UV-A (PUVA)-refractory mycosis fungoides-type cutaneous T-cell lymphoma with combined interferon alfa and PUVA. Arch Dermat 1993; 129:747.

66. Cooper DL, Braverman IM, Sarris AH, et al. Cyclosporine treatment of refractory T-cell lymphomas. Cancer 1993; 71:2335.
67. Kreis W, Budman DR, Shapiro PE. Cyclosporin A in the treatment of cutaneous T-cell lymphoma (mycosis fungoides). J Am Acad Dermat 1988; 18:1138.
68. Bernengo MG, Appino A, Bertero M, et al. Thymopentin in Sezary syndrome. J Natl Cancer Inst. 1992; 84:1341.
69. Foss F, Snozl M, Urba W, et al. Biological activity of thymopentin in cutaneous T-cell lymphomas. Proc Am Assoc Cancer Res, 1994: 237.
70. Kessler JF, Jones SE, Levine N, et al. Isotretinoin and cutaneous helper T-cell lymphoma (mycosis fungoides). Arch Dermat 1987; 123:201.
71. T. Kuzel, Roenigk HH Jr, Samuelson E, Rosen ST, The treatment of mycosis fungoides with all-trans retinoic acid. Proc Am Soc Hematol 1993:570a.
72. Cummings FJ, Kim Kyungmann K, Neiman RS, et al. Phase II trial for pentostatin in refractory lymphomas and cutaneous T-cell disease. J Clin Oncol 1991; 9:565.
73. Von Hoff DD, Dahlberg S, Harstock RJ, Eyre HJ. Activity of fludarabine monophosphate in patients with advanced mycosis fungoides: a southwest oncology group study. J Natl Cancer Inst 1990; 82:1353.
74. Saven A, Carrera CJ, Carson DA, Beutler E, Piro LD. 2-chlorodeoxyadenosine: an active agent in the treatment of cutaneous T-cell lymphoma. Blood 1992; 80:587.
75. Kuzel TM, Hurria A, Samuelson E, et al. Phase II trial of 2-chlorodeoxyadenosine for the treatment of cutaneous T-cell lymphomas. Blood 1996; 87:906.
76. Kuzel T, Foss F, LeMaistre C, et al. Phase I trial of a diptheria toxin fusion protein DAB_{389}IL-2 for the treatment of interleukin-2 receptor expressing hematologic neoplasms. Blood 1995; 86(Suppl 1):274a.

16
Immunomodulatory and Cytotoxic Therapy of Vasculitis

Jeffrey P. Callen
University of Louisville School of Medicine, Louisville, Kentucky

Joseph L. Jorizzo
Bowman Gray School of Medicine of Wake Forest University, Winston-Salem, North Carolina

I. INTRODUCTION

A. Vasculitis

Vasculitis is a general term that refers to inflammation and damage to blood vessel walls (1). The term does not specify the type of inflammation nor the size of the vessel involved (2). Often the skin serves as the initial organ upon which vasculitis is manifest, with involvement of the small- to medium-sized vessels that supply nutrients to the skin. Although there are times when the only recognizable organ system involved is the skin, vasculitis represents a systemic disease process which in many cases is linked to the presence of circulating immune complexes, but which may also occur through direct vessel-based immunological mechanisms or nonimmunological mechanisms.

Vasculitis is not a distinct clinical syndrome but may manifest in a wide variety of clinical signs and symptoms dependent on the localization and size of the vessels involved, the nature of the inflammatory process, and the presence of an underlying or associated condition. Classification, generally, is based on the size of the involved vessels (3), the histopathological and clinical findings, and the mechanisms or inciting agents that may underly the disease process (Tables 1 and 2). For a number of idiopathic vasculitides, criteria for classification have been developed by the American College of Rheumatology (ACR) (4). In this chapter, therapy for a variety of vasculitides are discussed with an emphasis

Table 1 A Traditional Classification of Necrotizing Vasculitis

1. Leukocytoclastic hypersensitivity or allergic vasculitis
    - A. Henoch-Schönlein purpura
    - B. Hypocomplementemic (urticarial) vasculitis
    - C. Vasculitis associated with a paraprotein
    - D. Special forms of dermal vasculitides
2. Vasculitis associated with rheumatic diseases
    - A. Systemic lupus erythematosus
    - B. Rheumatoid arthritis
    - C. Scleroderma
    - D. Sjögren's syndrome
    - E. Dermatomyositis
3. Granulomatous vasculitis
    - A. Allergic granulomatous angiitis of Churg-Strauss
    - B. Wegener's granulomatosis
    - C. Lymphomatoid granulomatosis
4. Polyarteritis nodosa (medium-sized vessel)
    - A. Classic type
    - B. Cutaneous disease
    - C. Associated with hepatitis B antigen
    - D. Vasculitis in drug addicts
5. Large vessel vasculitis (giant-cell arteritis)
    - A. Temporal arteritis
    - B. Polymyalgia rheumatica
    - C. Takayasu's disease

on the use of immunomodulatory (immunosuppressive) and cytotoxic agents. The discussion focuses on the selection of appropriate patients as well as appropriate agents.

B. Leukocytoclastic Vasculitis

The term leukocytoclastic vasculitis (LCV) is used to describe a process that is recognized within a biopsy specimen (5). The features that are observed include fibrinoid necrosis of the vessel walls with infiltration of polymorphonuclear neutrophils (PMNs), some of which are disrupted, resulting in the presence of nuclear debris within the tissue. This pathological process is not specific and can be observed in a variety of vasculitic syndromes, including those that have severe associated systemic disease, as well as those processes in the skin which are not vasculitic in their nature, such as insect bites.

Table 2 A Proposed Working Classification of Vasculitis

1. Small-vessel necrotizing vasculitis
   A. Necrotizing venulitis (hypersensitivity vasculitis)
   B. Henoch-Schönlein purpura
   C. Paraprotein associated (cryoglobulinemia, hyperglobulinemia)
   D. Collagen-vascular disease associated
   E. Urticarial vasculitis
   F. Erythema elevatum diutinum
   G. Rheumatoid nodulosis
   H. Septic vasculitis
2. Larger-vessel necrotizing vasculitis
   A. Polyarteritis nodosa
      1. Benign cutaneous form
      2. Classic systemic PAN
      3. Microscopic PAN
   B. Granulomatous vasculitis
      1. Wegener's granulomatosis: limited or classical forms
      2. Allergic granulomatous angiitis of Churg-Strauss
   C. Giant cell arteritis
   D. Association with collagen-vascular disease
   E. Nodular vasculitis

C. Hypersensitivity Vasculitis

Hypersensitivity vasculitis (HSV) (necrotizing venulitis, allergic angiitis, leukocytoclastic vasculitis, small vessel vasculitis) is a term that was introduced by Pearl M. Zeek, a pathologist, in the late 1940s. Zeek and her coworkers were struggling with the many overlapping features that they observed in patients with vasculitis (6). Their work provided the first classification system and began the separation of hypersensitivity vasculitis (angiitis) from rheumatic vasculitis, polyarteritis (periarteritis) nodosa, granulomatous vasculitis, and large vessel vasculitis, a modification of which is presented in Tables 1 and 2. The definition of HSV in general refers to a clinicopathological process that is manifest as leukocytoclastic vasculitis of the postcapillary venule and often includes the observation that the condition was precipitated by a drug or other substance. However, this term has also been used to describe those patients in whom the disease is an idiopathic small-vessel cutaneous LCV (7). As such, some authors have used this term to include patients with palpable purpura associated with abnormal proteins (e.g., cryoglobulinemia, hyperglobulinemia, etc.), with a variety of infections, with a variety of autoimmune disorders, or with malignancy (paraneoplastic vasculitis).

Hypersensitivity vasculitis is generally manifest by the appearance of palpable purpura, most commonly on the lower extremities below the knees (Figure 1). The disease is usually symmetrical and may be exacerbated by prolonged dependency of the legs. In addition, patients who are confined to bed will manifest their lesions on dependent surfaces such as the buttocks and back. Lesions may also occur in areas of trauma (pathergy) or under tight-fitting clothing. Intertriginous areas may be spared, perhaps due to a warmer environment. While the lesions are most frequent on dependent surfaces, at times the disease may be generalized and may even involve the mucosal surfaces.

The lesions of HSV are usually asymptomatic, but occasionally patients may have burning or itching. The lesions often occur in crops and usually begin as a macular erythema, macular purpura, or as urticarial papules that progress over hours to palpable purpura. Sams et al. (5) suggested that the development of the clinical lesion is dynamic, often beginning as nonpalpable purpura that eventually becomes palpable. Further, they suggested that in "later stages, some lesions become nodular, bullous, infarctive, and ulcerative." Most often the patient has only one type of lesion which fades as reparative processes begin. There are patients who have nodules, bullae, ulcers, necrosis, and/or livedo reticularis in combination with palpable purpura or as a sole manifestation of small-vessel

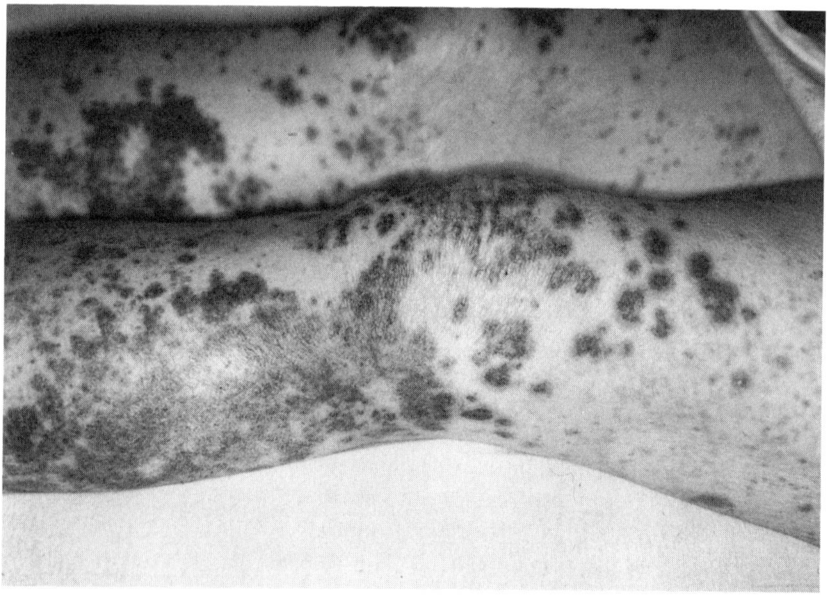

Figure 1 Palpable purpura of hypersensitivity vasculitis. This patient developed vasculitis following the administration of a cephalosporin antibiotic.

vasculitis. Most patients with these additional findings will be classified with another vasculitic syndrome despite finding leukocytoclastic vasculitis on histopathological examination of biopsy specimens.

Systemic involvement in patients with HSV is not uncommon, but its frequency has not been clearly determined. In a recent review of 58 patients with HSV by Liss and Wolverton (personal communication, 1991), 19 of 44 (43%) had renal involvement as defined by an abnormal urinary sediment (renal failure was not documented in this group of patients), 13 of 44 (32%) had arthralgias, 9% had liver or lung involvement, 5% had gastrointestinal involvement, and only 2% had central nervous system or cardiac involvement. Further, constitutional symptoms such as fever or myalgias were present in 20% and 11%, respectively. Rechallenge resulted in confirmation that a drug was involved in 13 of their patients.

The course of HSV is highly variable. The disease duration ranges from 1 d to up to 10 mo. The duration of the disease is usually short (less than 1 mo) in patients in whom the skin is the sole clinical manifestation of the disease process, and in whom there is an easily identified and removable antigen. In patients in whom the source of the antigen is not known or cannot be altered, the disease may be prolonged. When there is evidence of systemic involvement, widespread cutaneous lesions are commonly observed. The course of systemic HSV is often prolonged, and death may occur in up to one-third of patients.

D. Henoch-Schönlein Purpura

Henoch-Schönlein purpura (HSP) (anaphylactoid purpura, purpura urticans) was first described by Schönlein (8) in 1837 and then by Henoch (9) in 1868. Heroch-Schönlein purpura was defined as a syndrome that combines the tetrad of palpable purpura, arthritis, gastrointestinal involvement, and nephritis (10). It is recognized that not all patients will manifest involvement of all four of the organ systems. It also appears that HSP is much more common in childhood, but can occur during adulthood (11). During recent years it has also been recognized that these patients, whether adults or children, frequently have IgA immune complexes in circulation and/or deposited within the skin or kidneys (12). However, depending on the definition used, it may not be necessary that the patient possess these immune complexes in order to diagnose HSP.

The disease is usually acute in its onset and often follows an upper respiratory tract infection, particularly streptococcal pharyngitis. By definition, children are more frequently affected than adults, and HSP is more frequent in men. Also, the disease appears to have a seasonal variation with a peak during the winter.

Skin lesions are one of the defining features of HSP. The cutaneous eruption may begin as macular erythema or urticaria, but over a very short time period the eruption becomes purpuric. The lower extremities and buttocks are the most common sites for skin lesions. Recently, Piette and Stone (13) have attempted to distinguish IgA-related palpable purpura from other forms of leukocytoclastic vasculitis. They described a distinct pattern of IgA-associated cutaneous vasculitis in which the lesions were superficial purpuric plaques with multifocal areas of hemorrhage and necrosis arranged in a retiform pattern. The importance of recognizing this form of cutaneous small-vessel vasculitis is because of the association of IgA cutaneous vasculitis with IgA nephropathy.

The joints are involved in 60–90% of patients with HSP. Perhaps joint involvement is less frequent in adults than in children. Arthritis and/or arthralgias occur most often in the knees and ankles, but the wrists and elbows may also be involved. The joints of the pelvic and shoulder girdle and the small joints of the hands and feet are rarely affected. Physical examination of the joints reveals periarticular edema, without joint effusions; warmth or tenderness are not usually found. With resolution of the process there is no permanent damage to the affected joints.

Gastrointestinal involvement occurs in about 50–70% of patients. The most common symptom is colicky abdominal pain which may be accompanied by vomiting. Bloody diarrhea or melena occur in about 50% of affected individuals. In some patients the symptoms are so severe that they mimic an acute abdomen. Bowel involvement may be complicated by perforation or intussusception. The involvement of the bowel is due to a vasculitis of the small vessels in the submucosa with resultant edema and hemorrhage of the bowel wall.

Renal involvement in HSP occurs in 20–100% of the patients. The manifestations of renal involvement include hematuria, proteinuria, hypertension, and impaired renal function. The involvement may be transient and minor or may result in progressive renal insufficiency. In HSP, notably in adults, the whole clinical spectrum of glomerulonephritis can be found. The histopathological patterns can vary from minor abnormalities to severe lesions. In mild cases there is only mesangial proliferation. In more severe cases, focal and segmental intracapillary and extracapillary proliferation with adhesions and small crescents are seen. The most severe lesion is characterized by diffuse proliferation with influx of polymorphonuclear leukocytes and crescents and interstitial infiltration (14).

Despite complete resolution of the acute process in most patients with HSP, long-term follow-up studies have demonstrated that subsequent pregnancies are more frequently complicated by hypertension, and that the frequency of hypertension or renal insufficiency is higher than that for the general population (15).

Manifestations of HSP may also occur in other organ systems. Individual reports of associated asthma, hemoptysis, myocarditis, hepatomegaly, seizures, hemiparesis, subarachnoid hemorrhage, parotitis, orchitis, adrenal necrosis with resultant Addison's disease, and pancreatitis have been published.

E. Urticarial Vasculitis

Urticarial vasculitis (UV) is a disease characterized clinically by urticarial lesions and histopathologically by leukocytoclastic vasculitis. This disorder was perhaps first clearly distinguished as an entity by McDuffie et al. (16) when they reported "four patients with recurrent attacks of erythematous urticarial and hemorrhagic skin lesions associated with synovitis and sometimes abdominal distress." Two of their four patients also had glomerulonephritis and all four had hypocomplementemia. For this entity they coined the term "hypocomplementemic urticarial vasculitis." Since the original description, it has become recognized that a) some patients with urticaria have vasculitis in the absence of hypocomplementemia, b) about one-fifth of the patients with urticarial vasculitis will have significant pulmonary disease (17,18), c) when urticaria occurs in patients with collagen vascular diseases, leukocytoclastic vasculitis is the usual histopathological correlate and the urticarial vasculitic lesions usually correlate with active systemic inflammatory disease (19,20), d) urticarial vasculitis also may occur in patients with hepatitis-associated vasculitis, paraneoplastic vasculitis, and paraprotein-associated vasculitis (21), and e) almost all of the patients have long-standing chronic urticarial lesions.

Clinically urticarial vasculitis is distinguished from routine urticaria by lesions that are painful or burning rather than pruritic, by lesions that last more than 24 h, and by lesions that resolve with purpura or bruising (22). Histopathologically, the lesions are represented by leukocytoclastic vasculitis with fibrinoid necrosis and leukocytoclasis. These changes should be distinguished from the nonvasculitic processes of neutrophilic urticaria and urticaria with diffuse dermal neutrophilia. Both of these conditions have been described by Winkelmann and his colleagues at the Mayo Clinic (23). These two conditions do not seem to be associated with the risk of systemic disease or hypocomplementemia that may occur in some patients with urticarial vasculitis.

Laboratory evaluation is usually unremarkable, with the exception of an increased erythrocyte sedimentation rate, abnormalities that would be found with an associated disease process, and possibly depressed complement levels (CH100, C3, and/or C4). In a recent analysis of 72 patients with urticarial vasculitis, Mehregan et al. (24) found that only 23 of the 68 tested patients had an elevated sedimentation rate. Thus, while an elevated sedimentation rate is more often present in patients with urticaria who have vasculitis, a normal rate does not rule out the presence of this type of vasculitis. Likewise only 23 of 65 patients had a depressed total hemolytic complement (CH100), only 18 had a decreased C3 level, and only 6 had a decreased C4 level. Abnormal urinary sediment correlated with the presence of nephritis, usually associated with an accompanying disease such as lupus erythematosus (see below). Tests of lung function reveal abnormalities in those with associated chronic obstructive pulmonary disease. Mehregan et al. (24) also analyzed the differences between those patients with hypocomplementemia and those with normocomplementemia. They found that those with hypocomplementemia had a significantly higher frequency of residual purpura, arthralgias, abdominal pain, chronic obstructive pulmonary disease, and deposition of immunoglobulin or C3 in blood vessels or the basement membrane zone.

F. Cutaneous Vasculitis as Part of Another Rheumatic Disease Process

Cutaneous vasculitis may be a feature of the group of disorders often referred to as "collagen-vascular diseases" (25). Vasculitis is a common occurrence in patients with rheumatoid arthritis, systemic lupus erythematosus, and Sjögren's syndrome. Vasculitis may also occur in some patients with mixed connective tissue disease, scleroderma, relapsing polychondritis, and juvenile dermatomyositis.

G. Cutaneous Vasculitis as a Manifestation of Paraproteinemia

Abnormal immunoglobulins either arising from a monoclonal proliferation (e.g., paraprotein and cryoglobulinemia type I or II) or from polyclonal proliferation as in hyperglobulinemic purpura and cryoglobulinemia type III may be associated with vasculitis. Diseases associated with various types of paraproteins include lymphoproliferative disorders, collagen-vascular diseases, and infectious diseases (26). The cutaneous manifestations of patients with abnormal proteins includes purpura, livedo reticularis, urticaria, and/or ulceration. Histopathological evaluation of skin biopsy specimens from patients with abnormal proteins most commonly reveals either a vasculitis or a noninflammatory hyaline thrombosis within the vessel.

H. Polyarteritis Nodosa

Polyarteritis nodosa (PAN) is an inflammatory necrotizing vasculopathy involving small- and medium-sized arteries in multiple organs and as such it is associated with a wide variety of manifestations. It has recently been proposed to restrict the diagnosis of PAN to patients with involvement of medium-sized arteries only and to diagnose patients with small-vessel vasculitis in conjunction with involvement of larger vessels as microscopic polyangiitis or -arteritis (27). There are patients who develop a disease that involves only the cutaneous surface, yet histopathological specimens demonstrate inflammation of the small-or medium-sized arteries with polymorphonuclear leukocytes (28). In these patients the designation, cutaneous polyarteritis (CPAN) seems reasonable.

Classic PAN is a multisystem disease that has significant associated morbidity and potential mortality if untreated. Classic PAN occurs in middle age and is more common in men (2:1). Patients frequently have constitutional symptoms at the onset including fever, malaise, and weight loss. Neuropathy, headache, or other neurological symptoms are common at the onset of the disease, with mononeuritis multiplex being the characteristic neurological finding. Abdominal pain is also a common presenting manifestation. The etiology of PAN is not known, but it may occur in conjunction with a variety of other disorders including infections, collagen-vascular diseases, and others.

Cutaneous lesions are actually a rare presenting manifestation (4%), however, 40–50% of patients with PAN will eventually have cutaneous disease. Since the disease is one that affects small arteries, the characteristic cutaneous lesions are nodules, ulcers, and livedo reticularis (Figure 2). However, palpable purpura and urticarial lesions may occur in patients with PAN. Digital necrosis may also occur in PAN (Figure 3).

Systemic features of PAN are common. The kidney is involved in 70% of patients, and renal failure or its complications are the cause of death in 50% of patients who succumb to PAN. Hypertension is common and can be related to renal disease or to involvement of the renal arteries. Peripheral neuropathy occurs in 50% of patients, and nerve biopsy may serve as a good source of tissue to confirm the diagnosis. Gastrointestinal vasculitis with infarction of the bowel occurs in about 40% of patients and is another major cause of death (29). Cardiac involvement occurs in about 30% of the patients with PAN, but lung involvement is uncommon. If lung involvement is seen, the alternative diagnoses of Wegener's granulomatosis, allergic granulomatosis, or microscopic polyangiitis should be strongly considered.

The diagnosis of PAN is suspected in patients with multisystem disease in whom necrotizing vasculitis of small- or medium-sized arteries or typical radiographic demonstration of abnormalities such as arterial aneurysms are observed. There is no diagnostic serologic test available for classic PAN, but some patients will have a positive ANCA (about 30%) with specificity for myeloperoxidase (p-ANCA). Patients with this antibody generally have more widespread systemic involvement (30). Tissue for diagnosis can be obtained from the skin, muscle, testis, sural nerve, or rectum. Another useful diagnostic procedure is an arteriogram, which can demonstrate multiple fusiform aneurysms or occlusions, particularly in the mesenteric or renal arteries.

Microscopic PAN or microscopic polyangiitis (mPAN) is a systemic vasculitis affecting small vessels with an associated focal and segmental necrotizing glomerulonephritis (31). Other recognized vasculitic syndromes must be excluded. The distinction from classic PAN is facilitated by the lack of aneurysms and the propensity in mPAN to involve smaller vessels. The skin is involved in

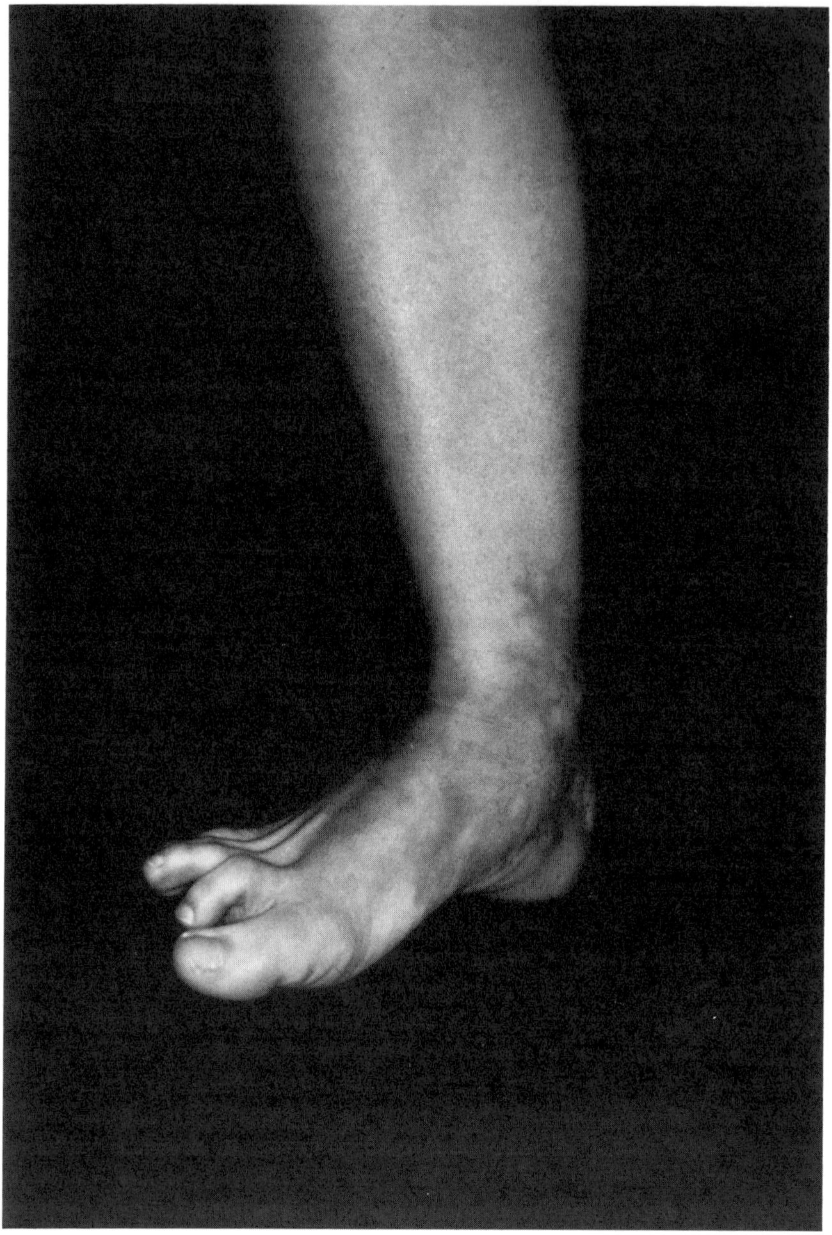

Figure 2 Cutaneous polyarteritis nodosa.

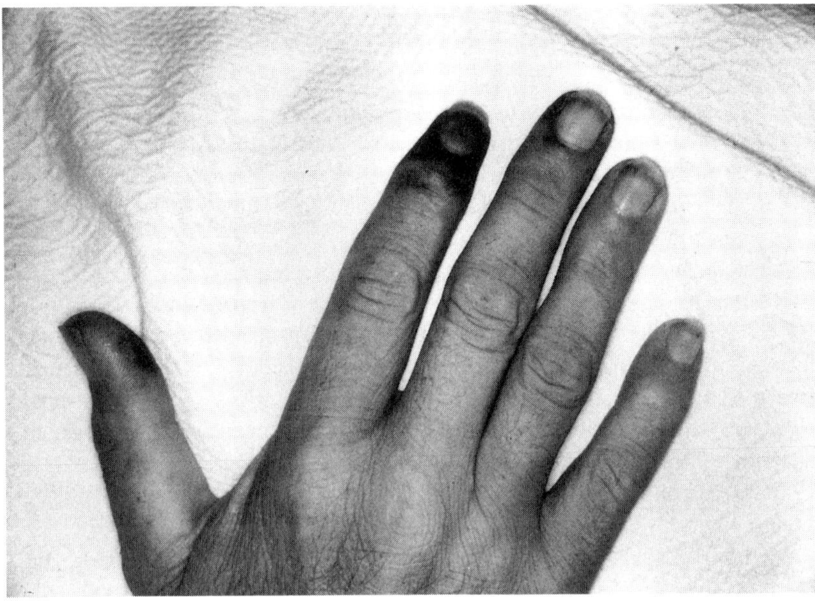

Figure 3 Digital necrosis in a patient with systemic necrotizing vasculitis.

30–40% of patients with microscopic PAN and it is similar in its manifestations to that observed in classic PAN.

Cutaneous PAN differs from classic PAN by the absence of severe systemic disease (32,33). Although cutaneous PAN is thought to represent a localized vasculitic process, systemic features such as fever, neuropathy, myalgias, arthralgias, and arthritis occur in up to half of the patients (34,35). In addition, some patients have associated systemic diseases including inflammatory bowel disease (both Crohn's and ulcerative colitis), hepatitis B infection, and paraproteinemia. The prognosis for patients with cutaneous PAN is good, but a chronic course with associated disability is common.

I. Granulomatous Vasculitis

Granulomatous vasculitis takes at least two forms: Wegener's granulomatosis (WG) and Churg-Strauss syndrome (CSS). Wegener's granulomatosis is characterized by a triad in which the upper airway, the lower airway, and the kidneys are affected by granulomatous inflammation and/or vasculitis. The diagnosis is confirmed when four criteria are present: nasal or oral inflammation, abnormal chest roentgenographic findings (nodules, fixed infiltrate, or cavitating lesions), abnormal urinary sediment (hematuria or red blood cell casts), and granulomatous inflammation (demonstrated on biopsy specimens) (36). Limited WG occurs when only the respiratory tract is affected. In 1985 a report from van der Woude et al. (37) described the high sensitivity of the antineutrophil cytoplasmic autoantibodies (ANCAs) for WG and correlated the titer of the ANCA with disease activity. The antibodies produce a cytoplasmic fluorescence pattern (c-ANCA) in most patients with WG (30). Titers of antibodies follow disease activity and may be used to guide treatment (38).

Cutaneous disease occurs in about half of patients with WG (39). The lesions can be palpable purpuric papules, nodules, necrotic patches, or ulcers (40–42). Histopathological examination of biopsy specimens from the skin demonstrate either small vessel vasculitis or granulomatous vasculitis. Cutaneous disease is a rare presenting manifestation and does not usually correlate with disease activity. However, in a recent report of three patients with WG, Mangold and Callen found that the cutaneous disease was a key factor in the recognition of the disease in one patient, and in the other two it was associated with disease exacerbation (43). Without treatment, death is common.

Churg-Strauss syndrome, also known as allergic granulomatosis with angiitis, is a disorder characterized by hypereosinophilia and systemic vasculitis occurring in patients with asthma and/or allergic rhinitis. The 1990 ACR classification criteria for CSS require the presence of at least four of the following six criteria for diagnosis: asthma, eosinophilia ($>$ 10%), mono- or polyneuropathy, nonfixed pulmonary infiltrates, paranasal sinus abnormality, and extravascular eosinophils (44). Antibodies to myeloperoxidase (p-ANCA) are frequently present (45).

Churg-Strauss syndrome is a disorder characterized by systemic vasculitis that occurs in association with hypereosinophilia, asthma, and allergic rhinitis (46). Pulmonary involvement is almost always present in CSS and is usually represented by asthma and/or transient pulmonary infiltrates. The other systemic findings are similar to those observed in PAN. Cutaneous lesions occur in about half of the patients with CSS and are similar to those described in patients with WG (47).

II. PATHOGENESIS

Current evidence suggests that leukocytoclastic vasculitis, whether of the small- or medium-sized vessels, usually represents an immune complex-mediated disorder (48–51). It is presumed that antibodies are formed to some antigen and that these either bind in situ or form circulating immune complexes. Most vasculitides are associated with IgG or IgM immune complexes, but Henoch-Schönlein purpura is associated with IgA immune complexes. Soluble immune complexes that are not removed by the mononuclear/phagocytic system and granulocytes can become lodged between the endothelial cells of the vessel wall. This process can be exacerbated by vasoactive amines, specifically histamine, which can dilate the vessel, creating spaces between endothelial cells within which the circulating immune complexes can lodge. This observation can be exploited clinically to reproduce lesions. Once lodged, the circulating immune complexes can activate complement via the classical pathway. This eventuates in the release of chemotactic factors, in particular C5a, which both attracts neutrophils and results in the formation of the membrane attack complex which may damage the endothelial cells directly. The cytokine C5a specifically attracts polymorphonuclear leukocytes that release their lysosomal enzymes and cause tissue destruction with resultant edema and hemorrhage (i.e., "innocent bystander injury"). The destroyed tissue is eventually cleared by the recruitment of mononuclear cells. Thus in this dynamic process, the polymorphonuclear leukocyte precedes the mononuclear cell in the inflammatory tissue infiltrate.

While there is evidence supportive of the immune complex theory, there are also data that suggest that vasculitis is a more complex process and that immune complexes may not be the primary pathogenetic factor. Savage (52), in a recent review, discussed the role of not only immune complexes, but direct damage from cells involved in inflammation, the role of the endothelial cell both as a target for injury and a contributor to injury, the interaction of the coagulation pathway (53), the role of platelet and platelet-derived factors, and the role of cytokines in the immunopathogenesis of vasculitic syndromes.

In many instances of vasculitis, autoantibodies to endothelial cells (54) have been described. The diagnostic as well as pathophysiological significance of these autoantibodies is a matter of debate. The close association between ANCA with specificity for proteinase-3 (c-ANCA) or myeloperoxidase (p-ANCA) and the occurrence of necrotizing vascuilitis without immune deposition suggests that autoantibodies are involved in the pathogenesis of these disorders (55). It has been demonstrated that ANCA can stimulate primed neutrophils in vitro to produce reactive oxygen species and to release lytic enzymes (56). In a recently described animal model the significance of the autoimmune response to myeloperoxidase in the induction of pauci-immune necrotizing glomerulonephritis has been demonstrated (57). However, the pathophysiological role of ANCA has not been definitely established.

There may also be a central role for the mast cell and for basophils which are located in close proximity to postcapillary venules (one of the presumed targets of vessel damage) (58). At a minimum mast cells may be involved in the production of cytokines which serve as chemoattractants for other inflammatory cells. Mast cells release factors that cause vasodilation which in vivo have been linked to trapping of immune complexes within the vessel walls. Similarly, monocytes, macrophages, and lymphocytes may have a role in the pathogenesis of lesions via the release of cytokines.

In recent years the role of adhesion molecules in the pathophysiology of vasculitis has begun to be elaborated. Cytokine (e.g., tumor necrosis factor) stimulation of endothelial cells results in their expression of E-selectin and the up-regulation of other adhesion molecules such as intercellular adhesion molecule-1 (ICAM-1) and vascular adhesion molecule-1 (VCAM-1). These molecules have their ligands on polymorphonuclear leukocytes (the so-called β_2-integrins CD 11 and CD 18 for ICAM-1) and on mononuclear cells (e.g., the very late antigen VLA-4 for VCAM-1). The cytokine-induced expression and up-regulation of these molecules is an essential initial step in the adherence and invasion of inflammatory cells in the vessel wall (59, 60). Modification of the expression of these molecules may in the future constitue a target for treatment.

In addition to immunopathological factors, several nonimmunological factors are involved in disease expression. Increased hydrostatic pressure predisposes certain areas to involvement, explaining the observation that vasculitis is more common on the legs and buttocks. Fibrinolytic activity may also be abnormal in some patients.

III. PATIENT EVALUATION

Since significant morbidity can result from systemic involvement in patients who present with cutaneous vasculitis, an exacting evaluation (Table 3) of the patient should be done to rule out or define the type and severity of systemic involvement (Table 4). Evaluation of a patient suspected of having cutaneous small-vessel vasculitis should be guided by knowledge of possible etiological agents, underlying disease associations, and the differential diagnosis of the most common clinical manifestations, that is, palpable purpura, urticaria, and leg ulceration. Evaluation should include a thorough history and physical examination with attention to possible etiological agents, ingestants, infections, and associated symptomatology. Once a skin biopsy has been obtained to confirm the diagnosis of leukocytoclastic vasculitis, laboratory studies should include a complete blood count, urinalysis, cryoglobulins, serum protein electrophoresis, hepatitis profile (B and C), antinuclear antibodies, complement, chest roentgenogram, and an assessment of renal function. Some of this testing is waived in the patient with an obvious cause for acute vasculitis, for example, a drug-related case. Also, in patients in whom systemic vasculitic syndromes are being considered, tests such as ANCA may be diagnostically helpful. In addition, in patients in whom the diagnosis of IgA-associated vasculitis is being considered, direct immunofluorescence biopsy of an early lesion can aid in confirmation of this immunopathological entity.

Table 3 An Approach to Evaluation of the Patient with Vasculitis

1. History
   - Infections?
   - Drug ingestion?
   - Prior history of one of the "associated" disorders?
   - Are there systemic symptoms?
2. Physical examination
   - General appearance
   - Type of skin lesion
   - Complete physical examination
3. Histopathologic evaluation(s)
   - Skin biopsy
     - Routine histopathology of an appropriate specimen—deeper incisional biopsy is needed for larger vessel vasculitis
     - Immunofluorescence is optional, perhaps useful when considering IgA disease
   - Renal biopsy: light microscopy and direct immunofluorescence, in case of abnormal urine sediment and/or proteinuria
   - Sural nerve biopsy: see text
   - Muscle biopsy: see text
   - Nasal biopsy: when granulomatous vasculitis is suspected
   - Lung biopsy: when granulomatous vasculitis is suspected, and other biopsies are negative.
4. Laboratory studies
   - Strongly suggested
     - Complete blood count
     - Urinalysis, tests of renal function
     - Chest x-ray
     - Tests for collagen vascular diseases—ANA, rheumatoid factor, etc.
     - Hepatitis B surface antigen, hepatitis C antibody
     - Tests for paraproteins, cryoglobulins, cryofibrinogens, rheumatoid factor, etc.
     - Antineutrophil cytoplasmic antibody (p-ANCA and/or c-ANCA) followed by antigen-specific assay (i.e. antiproteinase-3 and antimyeloperoxidase if the test is positive)
   - When appropriate or under special circumstances
     - Other autoantibodies, depending on the above test results
     - Total hemolytic complement
     - Circulating immune complexes
     - Sedimentation rate
     - Anticardiolipin antibody
     - von Willebrand (factor VIII) antigen
     - Blood cultures

Table 4 Examples of Systemic Involvement in Vasculitis

Cutaneous involvement	Palpable pupura Urticarial lesions Vesiculobullous lesions Necrosis Ulceration Livedo reticularis
Musculoskeletal involvement	Arthralgias Arthritis Myalgias Myositis
Renal involvement	Hematuria Proteinuria (nephrotic syndrome) Renal insufficiency Hypertension
Gastrointestinal involvement	Colicky pain Hemorrhage (bloody diarrhea, melena) Ulceration Perforation
Pulmonary involvement	Infiltrates Pleuritis and/or pleural effusions Nodules (solid or cavitating) Asthma
Neurologic involvement	Motor or sensory neuropathy Cephalalgia Diplopia Stroke Mononeuritis multiplex
Cardiac involvement	Myocarditis Pericarditis Coronary artery vasculitis
Eye involvement	Retinal vasculitis Conjunctivitis/keratitis Psuedotumor cerebri
Ear, nose, and throat involvement	Particularly in granulomatous vasculitis
Miscellaneous	Fever/constitutional symptoms Pancreatitis

The recommended battery of laboratory studies, roentgenograms, serologic tests, and cutaneous biopsy all serve as a guide to exclude systemic vasculitis. If the laboratory testing is normal, further invasive studies to uncover systemic involvement are probably unwarranted. In a recent study, 40 consecutive patients with suspected systemic necrotizing vasculitis (polyarteritis) were assessed by sequential testing (61). First, screening laboratory tests were obtained, and depending on the results, the investigation progressed to "safe" tests (e.g., skin, muscle, rectal biopsies). These were followed by "invasive" tests such as arteriography and kidney or lung biopsy, if indicated. No single laboratory test was found to adequately predict systemic involvement. Skin biopsy, rectal biopsy, and arteriography were found to be insensitive, nonspecific, and of poor predictive value. Muscle biopsy was the most valuable "safe" procedure to predict the presence of systemic involvement.

Based on their findings, the authors offer the following diagnostic approach to the patient with possible systemic necrotizing vasculitis. If the diagnosis of systemic disease is still being considered after the initial screening tests, three options are available: a) sural nerve electrophysiology followed by biopsy if abnormal; b) muscle biopsy; and c) open lung biopsy if pulmonary disease is prominent. If the diagnosis remains unconfirmed after these studies and the patient has an abnormal "active" urinary sediment, percutaneous renal biopsy should be considered. If the urine sediment is negative, other studies such as testicular biopsy and/or visceral angiography can be considered.

In another recent study, the association of a variety of autoantibodies and factors released by damaged endothelial cells were analyzed for their predictive value in the diagnosis of systemic vasculitides including PAN and WG (62). Of the four tests that were analyzed (ANCA, anticardiolipin antibody, von Willebrand factor antigen, and fibronectin), only ANCA was specific. While the other tests were often abnormal (highly sensitive), they were not specific.

IV. THERAPY

The therapy for a patient with vasculitis depends on whether or not there is clinical evidence of systemic disease and on the severity of the cutaneous and/or systemic disease. The patient with severe systemic necrotizing vasculitis should be treated rapidly and aggressively with systemic corticosteroids and an immunosuppressive agent (63, 64). Pulse therapy with either methylprednisolone or cyclophosphamide can result in rapid control of the disease. Also, plasma exchange and cryofiltration have been beneficial for individual patients, but these need to be accompanied by a plan for long-term therapy with corticosteroids and/or an immunosuppressive agent (65, 66). However, in the patient with chronic cutaneous vasculitis (small-vessel vasculitis) without clinically apparent systemic involvement, each therapeutic agent should be evaluated for the possible risks versus benefits (67).

A. Therapy for Patients Without Severe Systemic Disease

The patient with chronic cutaneous (small vessel) vasculitis may become frustrated and desire therapy for symptomatic relief or for cosmetic reasons. In some patients, recurrent purpuric lesions with superficial ulceration can compromise the patient's ability to work, and in this instance effective therapy that can allow the patient to again become functional is warranted. In patients with acute disease such as occurs in Henoch-Schönlein purpura, it may not be necessary to treat the patient other than symptomatically. In a recent report, Saulsbury documented that the use of systemic corticosteroids did not prevent the delayed development of nephritis in children with HSP (68).

It is important to identify and remove any offending antigen that may be present. In addition, underlying diseases that have specific therapies should be treated. Some examples are the identification of an ingestant, such as a drug, food, or food additive, which can be removed. Lunardi et al. (69) reported successful use of a elimination diet in five patients with hypersensitivity vasculitis. Patients were given a 1 wk elimination diet followed by open and blind food and food-additive challenges. They identified benzoates, tartrazines (2), eggs (2), beans, potatoes, and chicken as the precipitants of vasculitis in these patients. Interestingly, three of their patients had a documented lowering of the level of circulating immune complexes following the diet. Some patients with "paraneoplastic" vasculitis experience resolution of their manifestations of vasculitis upon removal of their tumor (70,71). Patients with paraproteinemia may be good candidates for treatment with an immunomodulatory agent to suppress the formation of the abnormal protein.

Patients with chronic cutaneous (small vessel) vasculitis who require therapy can be treated with a variety of agents. Therapeuticians must realize that no double-blind, prospective, controlled clinical trials exist for the therapy of chronic cutaenous vasculitis. A therapeutic "ladder" can be designed from which therapy can be sequentially selected until an appropriate and effective agent is identified. Since the postulated mechanism for cutaneous vasculitis involves immune complex-mediated vessel damage, complement activation, chemotaxis of polymorphonuclear leukocytes, lysosomal enzyme release and resultant cell destruction, and modulation of the process by vasoactive substances, agents that interfere with any of these processes may be beneficial. While systemic agents such as antihistamines, nonsteroidal antiinflammatory agents, antimalarials, oral potassium iodide, and sulfones have been reported to be effective in individual cases, they have not been uniformly effective. Corticosteroids, if given in a high enough dosage, are almost always effective (1 mg/kg/d). Colchicine is effective for cutaneous lesions in 75–80% of patients with cutaneous vasculitis (72).

Patients with urticarial vasculitis are most often bothered by the burning or itching of the lesions. They may also have angioedema and more typical urticarial lesions. These patients should first be treated with around-the-clock antihistamine therapy. More than one H1 antagonists can be combined, but it is often noted that the doses required cause drowsiness. In some cases, the use of doxepin HCl, which has effects on both H1 and H2 receptors, is effective. Newer, nonsedating agents such as terbenifine, astemizole, or loratidine can be used during waking hours and a soporific agent can be given before retiring.

In patients with chronic cutaneous (small vessel) vasculitis, oral colchicine given at a dose of 0.6 mg two to three times daily is often selected as an initial therapy (72). Colchicine is an alkaloid that is known to inhibit neutrophil chemotaxis, block lysosomal formation, and stabilize lysosomal membranes. These factors are believed to be involved in the pathogenesis of leukocytoclastic vasculitis, and thus perhaps this agent blocks the end response of immune-complex directed, neutrophil-induced vessel damage. About 80% of patients treated with colchicine will respond, as judged by the disappearance of lesions and the lack of appearance of new lesions (72). In most cases where response occurs, if the colchicine is stopped, the disease returns, and with reinstitution of the therapy the clinical signs are again suppressed. The onset of action is rapid, usually occurring within the first 4–7 d, and if no response is noted by 2 wk the therapy should be considered a failure.

In addition to the cutaneous benefits, arthralgias and/or arthritis may respond. However, no changes are noted in CIC levels or abnormalities of immunoglobulin levels (72). This therapy is reserved for those patients who lack severe systemic involvement. Colchicine is generally well tolerated and can be used over long periods of time. Toxicity is most frequently gastrointestinal, but long-term use should not be undertaken in potentially pregnant women, and blood counts should be monitored periodically because of reports of neutropenia in elderly patients.

While corticosteroids can be used to stop progression of the disease when it is acute, or can be used to treat severe systemic involvement, their use in chronic, non-life-threatening small-vessel necrotizing vasculitis is often complicated by multiple side effects. For this reason, immunosuppressive agents can be used in conjunction with corticosteroids or as steroid-sparing agents. Immunosuppressive or cytotoxic therapy is indicated when the patient fails less toxic therapy, when the patient is disabled physically or psychologically, and/or when steroid-related side effects are present. Cyclophosphamide, which is used for severe necrotizing vasculitis, polyarteritis nodosa, or Wegener's granulomatosis, may be used, but we prefer to avoid daily dose therapy in patients with small-vessel vasculitis because of its side effects. Azathioprine has been reported to be effective in patients with a variety of vasculitic syndromes. In a recent report, five of six patients with chronic recalcitrant cutaneous leukocytoclastic vasculitis responded to oral azathioprine in a dose of 150 mg/d (73). The onset of action is delayed, often not taking effect for 4–8 wk (Figures 4 and 5). Corticosteroid doses in our patients were lowered and/or stopped. Side effects in these patients are usually minimal, but several patients developed verrucae. Heurkens et al. (74) used azathioprine for the treatment of patients with rheumatoid arthritis complicated by vasculitis. They reported that this therapy was effective for their patients with severe systemic vasculitis. They divided their patients with cutaneous vasculitis into two groups. One group received prednisone plus azathioprine and the other group continued the existing antirheumatic therapy without the addition of prednisone or azathioprine. While both groups improved over 18 mo, there was little statistical difference between them. They concluded that the addition of prednisone and azathioprine was not indicated for patients with rheumatoid arthritis who had only cutaneous vasculitis. However, when one carefully reviews their data, it is evident that of the 8 treated patients only 1 had active disease at 18 mo, whereas of the 11 "untreated" patients 5 had active cutaneous disease. Furthermore, the issue of morbidity is not addressed in their report. Therapy for

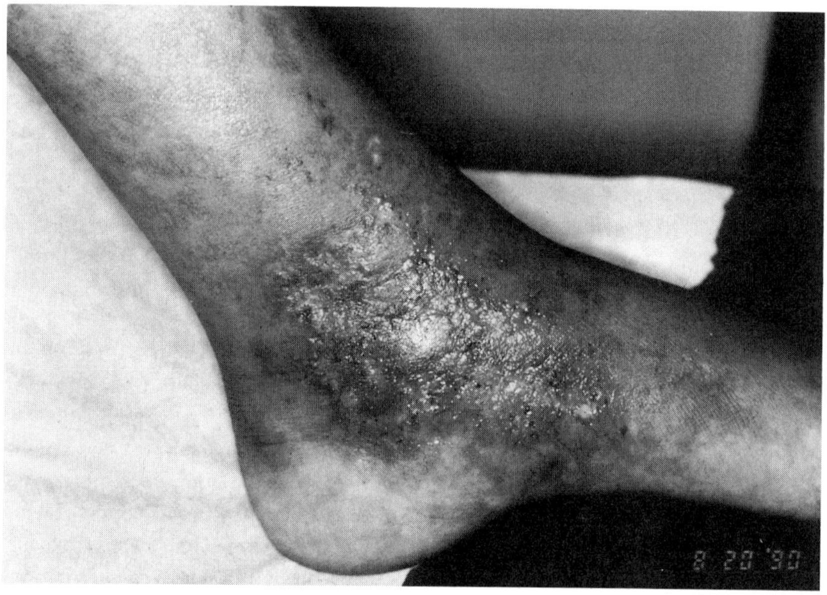

Figure 4 Cutaneous small-vessel vasculitis with palpable purpura and superficial ulceration before azathioprine therapy. At the time of this photograph the patient was on oral prednisone at 60 mg/d.

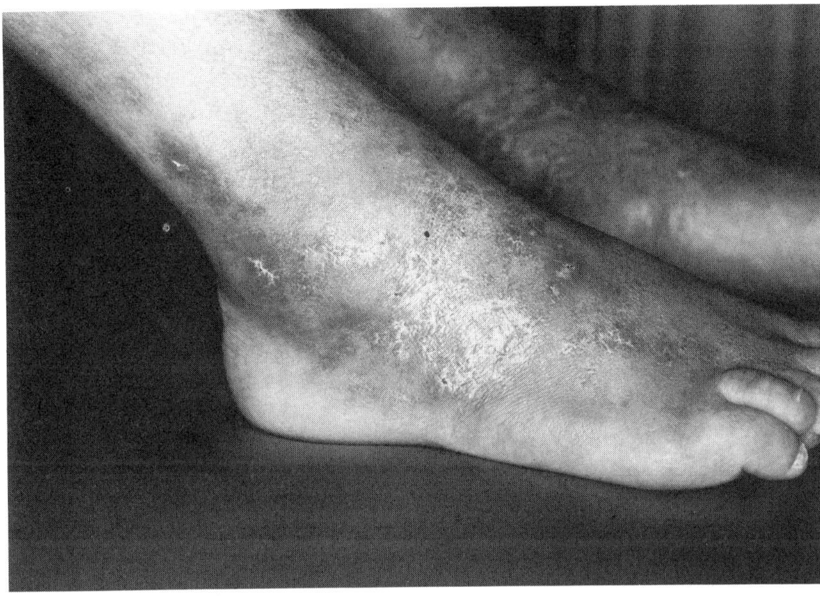

Figure 5 Same patient as seen in Figure 4, 4 wk after beginning azathioprine at 150 mg/d.

the underlying rheumatoid arthritis also obscures how generalizable this data is to all patients with small-vessel necrotizing vasculitis. Often, healing of even small ulcerations results in an improved quality of life for the patient with cutaneous vasculitis. Thus the benefits versus the risks of azathioprine therapy must be carefully assessed in each individual patient.

Cutaneous polyarteritis while by definition not a life-threatening process, it is frequently disabling. The patient may continue to develop painful nodules or ulcerations. Moreland and Ball reported six patients with CPAN and emphasized their view that patients be treated conservatively (33). However, five of their six patients required prednisone therapy, with most being on short-term or low-dose therapy. Our experience has differed in that we have seen that most patients require higher doses of prednisone to control their disease, and in most instances the prednisone cannot be discontinued. In this setting Jorizzo et al. have successfully utilized low-dose weekly methotrexate as a corticosteroid-sparing agent (75). In their three patients, 7.5–15 mg given orally once weekly led to control of the disease and gradual elimination of oral corticosteroids.

Patients with cryoglobulinemia or other paraproteinemia-associated vasculitis may be treated with an immunosuppressive or cytotoxic agent. It is our belief that these patients, regardless of their disease manifestations, should be treated more aggressively since removal of the paraprotein and suppression of its continued formation can lead to a prolonged remission of the disease. Geltner et al. combined prednisone and plasmapheresis therapy in three patients and prednisone, plasmapheresis, and chlorambucil therapy in two patients with vascular involvement secondary to mixed cryoglobulinemia (76). Healing of cutaneous ulcers occurred in three of three patients and control of the purpuric eruption occurred in two of two patients. Recently it has been recognized that patients with essential mixed cryoglobulinemia frequently have hepatitis C virus infection (77,78). Patients with this association have been successfully treated with interferon-α-2a (79).

B. Therapy for Patients with Severe Systemic Disease or with the Potential for Severe Systemic Disease

1. Wegener's Granulomatosis

While some patients with WG, may have an indolent course, most untreated patients with generalized disease experience a rapidly progressive and often fatal disease course. In 1971 Novack and Pearson (80), then Fauci et al. (81), clearly documented the benefit of cyclophosphamide therapy in patients with WG. These results have been extended to larger numbers of patients such that in 1992 Hoffman et al. reported the benefits of low-dose daily cyclophosphamide (2 mg/kg/d) and prednisone (1 mg/kg/d) in 158 patients with WG (40). However, this form of therapy was not curative, with relapse being frequently observed with lowering of the doses of medication. Furthermore, during phases of therapy with both cyclophosphamide and prednisone the risk of opportunistic infection was high. Many of the patients developed corticosteroid-related complications. Long-term cyclophosphamide therapy was frequently associated with hemorrhagic cystitis (43%) and higher frequencies of bladder cancer (2.8%) and myelodysplasia (2%) than would be expected in the normal population.

Because of these complications, investigators including those at the National Institutes of Health (NIH) have explored alternate therapies. Anecdotes purporting the usefulness of trimethoprim-sulfamethoxazole (82) have not been replicated by the NIH group. However, a recent study suggesting that nasal carriage of *Staphylococcus aureus* is associated with a poorer prognosis in WG may allow selection of a group who might better respond to the trimethoprim-sulfamethoxazole therapy (83). Hoffman et al. (84) have recently reported their results with methotrexate in 29 patients with WG. They administered weekly methotrexate either orally or intramuscularly in doses of 15–25 mg in combination with oral prednisone at 1 mg/kg/d. Remission was induced in 76% of their patients, a comparable rate to that observed in cyclophosphamide-treated patients.

Another form of delivery of cyclophosphamide has also been evaluated in WG. High-dose monthly intravenous (pulse) therapy has been used to limit the long-term toxicity of cyclophosphamide. Pulse therapy may result in a lower total dose of cyclophosphamide and is associated with a shorter time of exposure. Patients may be induced with weekly, biweekly, or monthly therapy. During the initial phases of therapy prednisone is also administered in "standard" doses (1 mg/kg/d). Eventually some patients may be maintained with only quarterly cyclophosphamide pulses. Concomitant administration of mesna can prevent acute bladder toxicity, and in animal studies it has been shown to reduce the risk of bladder cancer.

Patients with WG have also been treated with systemic azathioprine or chlorambucil. Clearly, azathioprine appears to be a less effective agent than cyclophosphamide, and therefore it is relegated to therapy of the less severely affected patient who is steroid dependent. Chlorambucil therapy may also be less effective than cyclophosphamide therapy, although this is based on one early study. Since chlorambucil is not associated with the risk of bladder toxicity, it might be reasonable to evaluate it as a part of other regimens and in larger numbers of patients.

2. Severe Necrotizing Vasculitis and Polyarteritis Nodosa

These entities are often treated with systemic corticosteroids plus an immunosuppressive or cytotoxic agent. The choice of agent depends upon the severity of the disease: mild to moderate disease may be controlled with prednisone plus azathioprine, whereas severe disease warrants the use of prednisone plus cyclophosphamide (63).

In a recent report from England, it was clear that although aggressive therapy can lead to remission, with tapering of the therapy relapse was common (85). Relapse occurred in 41.7% of patients with classical PAN, 25.4% of patients with microscopic PAN, 44% of patients with WG, and 52% of patients with limited WG. In many instances the relapse was more severe than the initial disease, but relapse could not be predicted accurately by ANCA testing or other laboratory testing. These authors stress the importance of long-term follow-up in patients with systemic vasculitis.

In acute phases plasmapheresis (65) or intravenous immunoglobulin have been successfully utilized. Intravenous immunoglobulin contains primarily IgG. The mechanism of effect is not understood, but may involve binding to Fc receptors, inhibition of antibody synthesis, modulation of cytokine production and/or secretion, and production of anti-idiotype antibodies. Intravenous immunoglobulin is useful in Kawasaki's syndrome and has been used in small numbers of patients with systemic vasculitis. Jayne et al. (86) were able to obtain sustained improvement in six of seven patients. In addition, they noted a fall in the ANCA levels with therapy. Jayne and colleagues (87) have extended these observations to patients with WG and microscopic polyarteritis and have suggested that the mechanism of effect is through ANCA anti-idiotype antibody regulation. Most trials have been open label observations, thus this work will need replication in carefully controlled clinical trials before widespread use can be recommended.

REFERENCES

1. Callen JP. Cutaneous vasculitis: relationship to systemic disease and therapy. Curr Probl Dermat 1993; 5:45–80.
2. Churg A, Churg J (eds.). Systemic vasculitis. New York: Igaku-Shoin Medical Publishers, 1991.
3. Jennette CJ, Milling DM, Falk RJ. Vasculitis affecting the skin. Arch Dermat 1994; 130:899–906.
4. Hunder GG. The American College of Rheumatology 1990 criteria for the classification of vasculitis. Arth Rheum 1990; 33:1065–1144.
5. Sams WM Jr, Thorne EG, Small P, et al. Leukocytoclastic vasculitis. Arch Dermat 1976; 112:219–226.
6. Zeek PM, Smith LC, Wector JC. Studies on perivasculitis nodosa. III. The differentiation between the vascular lesions of periarteritis nodosa and hypersensitivity. Am J Pathol 1948; 24:889–917.
7. Swerlick RA, Lawley TJ. Small-vessel vasculitis and cutaneous vasculitis. In: Churg A, Churg J (eds.), Systemic vasculitis. New York: Igaku-Shoin Medical Publishers, 1991: 193–201.
8. Schönlein JL. Allegemeine and specielle pathologie und therapie. ed 3. aol 2. Herisau, Germany: Literatur-Comptoir, 1837:48.
9. Henoch EH. Ueber eine eigenthumliche form von purpura. Berl Klin Wochenschr 1874; 11:641–643.
10. Saulsbury F. Henoch-Schönlein purpura. Pediatr Dermat 1984; 1:195–201.
11. Ilan Y, Naparstek Y. Schönlein-Henoch purpura in adults and children. Sem Arthr Rheum 1991; 21:103–109.
12. Kauffmann RH, Herrmann WA, Meÿyer CJLM, et al. Circulating IgA-immune complexes in Henoch-Schönlein purpura. Am J Med 1980; 69:859–866.
13. Piette WW, Stone MS. A cutaneous sign of IgA-associated small dermal vessel leukocytoclastic vasculitis in adults (Henoch-Schönlein purpura). Arch Dermat 1989; 125:53–56.
14. Levy M, et al. Adv Nephrol 1976; 6:183–186.
15. Goldstein AR, White RHR, Akuse R, Chantler C. Long-term follow-up of childhood Henoch-Schönlein nephritis. Lancet 1992; 339:280–282.
16. McDuffie FC, Sams WM Jr, Maldonado JE, et al. Hypocomplementemia with cutaneous vasculitis and arthritis. Mayo Clin Proc 1973; 48:340–348.
17. Schwartz HR, McDuffie FC, Black LF, et al. Hypocomplementemic urticarial vasculitis: association with chronic obstructive pulmonary disease. Mayo Clin Proc 1982; 57:231–238.
18. Wisnieski JJ, Baer AN, Christensen J, et al. Hypocomplementemic urticarial vasculitis syndrome. Medicine 1995; 74:24–41.

19. Provost TT, Zone JJ, Synkowski D, et al. Unusual cutaneous manifestations of systemic lupus erythematosus: I. Urticaria-like lesions. Correlation with clinical and serological abnormalities. J Invest Dermat 1980; 75:495–499.
20. Asherson RA, D'Cruz D, Stephens CJM, et al. Urticarial vasculitis in a connective tissue disease clinic: patterns, presentations and treatment. Semin Arthr Rheum 1991; 20:285–296.
21. Yasue T, Yasue A. Urticarial vasculitis with circulating immune complexes and mixed cryoglobulins: studies of pathogenesis. J Dermat 1987; 14:597–603.
22. Callen JP, Kalbfleisch S. Urticarial vasculitis: a report of nine cases and review of the literature. Br J Dermat 1982; 107:87–94.
23. Winkelman RK, Wilson-Jones E, Smith NP, et al. Neutrophilic urticaria. Acta Dermat Venereol 1988; 68:129–133.
24. Mehregan DR, Hall MJ, Gibson LE. Urticarial vasculitis: a histopathologic and clinical review of 72 cases. J Am Acad Dermat 1992; 26:441–448.
25. Lakhanpal S, Conn DL, Lie JT. Clinical and prognostic significance of vasculitis as an early manifestation of connective tissue disease syndromes. Ann Intern Med 1984; 101:743–748.
26. Churg J. Cryoglobulinemic vasculitis. In: Churg A, Churg J (eds), New York: Systemic vasculitis, Igaku-Shoin Medical Publishers, 1991:293–304.
27. Jennette JC, Falk RJ, Andrassy K, et al. Nomenclature of systemic vasculitides: Proposal of an international consensus conference. Arthr Rheum 1994; 37:187–192.
28. Diaz-Perez JL, Winkelmann RK. Cutaneous periarteritis nodosa. Arch Dermat 1974; 110:407–414.
29. Lopez LR, Schocket AL, Stanford RE, et al. Gastrointestinal innvolvement in leukocytoclastic vasculitis and polyarsteritis nodosa. J Rheum 1980; 7:677–684.
30. Cohen TJW, Goldschmeding R, Elema JD, et al. Association of autoantibodies to myeloperoxidase with different forms of vasculitis. Arthr Rheum 1990; 33:1264–1270.
31. Kallenberg CGM, Mulder AHL, Cohen TWJ. Anti-neutrophil cytoplasmic antibodies: a still growing class of autoantibodies in inflammatory disorders. Am J Med 1992; 93:675–682.
32. Chen KR. Cutaneous polyarteritis nodosa: a clinical and histopathological study of 20 cases. J Dermat 1989; 16:429–442.
33. Moreland LW, Ball GV. Cutaneous polyarteritis nodosa. Am J Med 1990; 88:426–430.
34. Mekori YA, Awai LE, Weidel JD, Kohler PF. Cutaneous polyarteritis nodosa associated with rapidly progressive arthritis. Arthr Rheum 1984; 27:574–578.
35. Dewar CL, Bellamy N. Necrotizing mesmeteric vasculitis after longstanding cutaneous polyarteritis nodosa. J Rheum 1992; 19:1308–1311.
36. Leavitt RY, Fauci AS, Bloch DA, et al. The American College of Rheumatology 1990 criteria for the classification of Wegener's granulomatosis. Arthr Rheum 1990; 33:1101–1107.
37. van der Woude TJ, Rasmussen N, Lobatto S, et al. Autoantibodies against neutrophils and monocytes: tool for diagnosis and marker of disease activity in Wegener's granulomatosis. Lancet 1985; 1:425–429.

38. Cohen TJW, Huitema MG, Hené RJ, et al. Prevention of relapses in Wegener's granulomatosis by treatment based on antineutrophil cytoplasmic antibody titre. Lancet 1990; 336:709–711.
39. Frances C, Du LTH, Piette J-C, et al. Wegener's granulomatosis. Arch Dermat 1994; 130:801–807.
40. Hoffman GS, Kerr GS, Leavitt RY, et al. Wegener granulomatosis: an analysis of 158 patients. Ann Intern Med 1992; 116:488–498.
41. Hu CH, O'Loughlin S, Winkelmann RK. Cutaneous manifestations of Wegener granulomatosis. Arch Dermat 1977; 113:175–182.
42. Francés C, Huong DLT, Piette JC, et al. Dermatological manifestations of Wegener's granulomatosis. Arthr Rheum 1992; 35:S165.
43. Mangold MC, Callen JP. Cutaneous leukocytoclastic vasculitis associated with active Wegener's granulomatosis. J Am Acad Dermat 1992; 26:579–84.
44. Masi AT, Hunder GG, Lie JT, et al. The American College of Rheumatology 1990 criteria for the classification of Churg-Strauss syndrome (allergic granulomatosis and angiitis). Arthr Rheum 1990; 33:1094–1100.
45. Cohen TJW, Goldschmeding, von dem Borne AEGK, Kallenberg CGM. Anti-myeloperoxidase antibodies in the Churg-Strauss syndrome. Thorax 1991; 46:70–71.
46. Lanham JG, Elkon KB, Pusey CD, Hughes GR. Systemic vasculitis with asthma and eosinophilia: a clinical approach to the Churg-Strauss syndrome. Medicine 1984; 63:65–81.
47. Finan MC, Winkelmann RK. The cutaneous extravascular necrotizing granuloma (Churg-Strauss granuloma) and systemic disease: a review of 27 cases. Medicine 1983; 62:142–158.
48. Mackel SE, Jordon RE. Leukocytoclastic vasculitis. Arch Dermat 1982; 118:296–301.
49. Giangiacomo J, Tsai CC. Dermal and glomerular deposition of IgA an anaphylactoid purpura. Am J Dis Child 1977; 131:981–983.
50. Kammer GM, Soter NA, Schur PH. Circulating immune complexes in patients with necrotizing vasculitis. Clin Immunol Immunopathol 1980; 15:658–670.
51. Braverman IM, Yen A. Demonstration of immune complexes in spontaneous and histamine-induced lesions and in normal skin of patients with leukocytoclastic angiitis. J Invest Dermat 1975; 64:105–112.
52. Savage COS. Pathogenesis of systemic vasculitis. In: Churg A, Churg J (eds), Systemic vasculitis. New York: Igaku-Shoin Medical Publishers, 1991:7–30.
53. Jordan JM, Allen NB, Pizo SV. Defective release of tissue plasminogen activator in systemic and cutaneous vasculitis. Am J Med 1987; 82:397–400.
54. Kallenberg CGM. Autoantibodies in vasculitis: current perspectives. Clin Exp Rheum 1993; 11:355–360.
55. Kallenberg CGM, Cohen TJW, van der Woude FY, et al. Autoimmunity to lysozomal enzymes: new clues to vasculitis and glomerulonephritis? Immunol Today 1991; 12:61–64.
56. Falk RJ, Terrell RS, Charles LA, Jennette JC. Anti-neutrophil cytoplasmic autoantibodies induce neutrophils to degranulate and produce oxygen radicals in vitro. Proc Natl Acad Sci USA 1990; 87:4115–4119.

57. Brouwer E, Huitema MG, Klok PA, et al. Anti-myeloperoxidase associated proliferative glomerulonephritis: an animal model. J Exp Med 1993; 177:905–914.
58. Tosca N, Stratigos JD. Possible pathogenic mechanisms in allergic cutaneous vasculitis. Int J Dermat 1988; 27:291–296.
59. Pober JS, Cotran RS. Cytokines and endothelial cell biology. Physiol Rev 1990; 76:427–451.
60. Springer TA. Adhesion receptors of the immune system. Nature 1990; 346:425–432.
61. Dahlberg PJ, Lockhart JM, Overholt EL. Diagnostic studies for systemic necrotizing vasculitis. Arch Intern Med 1989; 149:161–165.
62. Bliel L, Manger B, Winkler TH, et al. The role of antineutrophil cytoplasm antibodies, anticardiolipin antibodies, von Willebrand factor antigen, and fibronectin for the diagnosis of systemic vasculitis. J Rheum 1991; 18:1199–1206.
63. Fauci AS, Katz P, Haynes BF, Wolff SM. Cyclophosphamide therapy of severe systemic necrotizing vasculitis. N Engl J Med 1979; 301:235–238.
64. Scott DGI, Bacon PA. Intravenous cyclophosphamide plus methylprednisolone in treatment of systemic rheumatoid vasculitis. Am J Med 1984; 76:377–384.
65. Turner AN, Whittaker S, Banks I, et al. Plasma exchange in refractory cutaneous vasculitis. Br J Dermat 1990; 122:41–45.
66. Sawada K, Segal AM, Malchesky PS, et al. Rapid improvement in a patient with leukocytoclastic vasculitis with secondary mixed cryoglobulinemia treated with cryofiltration. J Rheum 1991; 18:91–94.
67. Cupps TR, Springer RM, Fauci AS. Chronic, recurrent small-vessel cutaneous vasculitis. JAMA 1982; 247:1994–1998.
68. Saulsbury FT. Corticosteroid therapy does not prevent nephritis in Henoch-Schönlein purpura. Arthr Rheum 1992; 35:S189.
69. Lunardi C, Bambara LM, Biasi D, et al. Elimination diet in the treatment of selected patients with hypersensitivity vasculitis. Clin Exp Rheum 1992; 10:131–135.
70. Callen JP. Cutaneous leukocytoclastic vasculitis in a patient with an adenocarcinoma of the colon. J Rheum 1987; 14:386–389.
71. Kulp-Shorten CL, Rhodes RH, Peterson H, Callen JP. Cutaneous vasculitis associated with pheochromocytoma. Arthr Rheum 1990; 33:1852–1856.
72. Callen JP. Colchicine is effective in controlling chronic cutaneous leukocytoclastic vasculitis. J Am Acad Dermat 1985; 13:193–200.
73. Callen JP, Spencer LV, Burruss JB, Holtman J. Azathioprine: an effective, corticosteroid sparing therapy for patients with recalcitrant cutaneous lupus erythematosus or with recalcitrant cutaneous leukocytoclastic vasculitis. Arch Dermat 1991; 127:515–522.
74. Heurkens AHM, Westedt ML, Breedveld FC. Prednisone plus azathioprine treatment in patients with rheumatoid arthritis complicated by vasculitis. Arch Intern Med 1991; 151:2249–2254.
75. Jorizzo JL, White WL, Wise CM, et al. Low-dose weekly methotrexate for unusual neutrophilic vascular reactions: cutaenous polyarteritis and Behçet's disease. J Am Acad Dermat 1991; 24:973–978.
76. Geltner D, Kohn RW, Gorevic P, Franklin EC. The effect of combination therapy (steroids, immunosuppressives and plasmapheresis) on 5 mixed cryoglbulinemia

patients with renal, neurologic, and vascular involvement. Arthr Rheum 1981; 24:1121–1127.
77. Levey JM, Bjornsson B, Banner B, et al. Mixed cryoglobulinemia in chronic hepatitis C infection. Medicine 1994; 73:53–67.
78. Dupin N, Chosidow O, Lunel F, et al. Essential mixed cryoglobulinemia. Arch Dermat 1995; 131:1124–1127.
79. Misani R, Bellarita P, Fenili D, et al. Interferon alfa-2a therapy in cryoglobulinemia associated with hepatitis C virus. N Engl J Med 1994; 330:751–756.
80. Novack SN, Pearson CM. Cyclophosphamide therapy in Wegener's granulomatosis. N Engl J Med 1971; 284:938–942.
81. Fauci AS, Wolff SM, Johnson JS. Effect of cyclophosphamide upon the immune response in Wegener's granulomatosis. N Engl J Med 1971; 285:1493–1496.
82. Valeriano-Marcet J, Spiera H. Treatment of Wegener's granulomatosis with sulfamethoxazole-trimethoprim. Arch Intern Med 1991; 151:1649–1652.
83. Stegeman CA, Tervaert JWC, Sluiter WJ, et al. Association of chronic nasal carriage of *Staphylococcus aureus* and higher relapse rates in Wegener granulomatosis. Ann Intern Med 1994; 120:12–17.
84. Hoffman GS, Leavitt RY, Kerr GS, Fauci AS. The treatment of Wegener's granulomatosis with glucocorticoids and methotrexate. Arthr Rheum 1992; 35:1322–1329.
85. Gordon M, Luqmani RA, Adu D, et al. Relapse in patients with a systemic vasculitis. Q J Med 1993; 86:779–789.
86. Jayne DRW, Davies MJ, Fox CJV, et al. Treatment of systemic vasculitis with pooled intravenous immunoglobulin. Lancet 1991; 337:1137–1139.
87. Jayne DRW, Ensault VLM, Lockwood CM. ANCA anti-idiotype antibodies and the treatment of systemic vasculitis with intravenous immunoglobulin. J Autoimmun 1993; 6:207–219.

17
Hyperprolifterative Skin Diseases

Charles J. McDonald
Brown University, Providence, Rhode Island

I. PSORIASIS

Psoriasis is a very common chronic skin disease that is estimated to occur in 1–2% of most western European populations (1). In West African and African American populations the prevalence of psoriasis is estimated to be considerably less (2). Multiple factors influence the onset and course of the disease. Among these are heredity, environment, psyche, physical and emotional trauma, and abnormal inflammation. Based on inheritance or lack of inheritance, psoriasis patients are often divided into two groups. Type I psoriasis has an early onset associated with a strong family history of psoriasis and an associated *HLA-CW6* genotype. Type II psoriasis has its onset late in life and has little or no association with the *HLA-CW6* genotype. Type I tends toward a more severe outcome. These associations have been found most commonly in northern Europeans.

Psoriasis characteristically presents as isolated, or a cluster of red, scaling papules that ultimately coalesce to form plaques. The nature of the disease is such that it enters periods of extreme activity followed by periods of complete quiescence. Early lesions tend to occur on the scalp, elbows, and knees and they are often bilaterally symmetrical. Hidden lesions often occur within the umbilicus and between the gluteal folds just superior to the anal orifice. In males, lesions may also occur on the genitalia. Trauma to the skin is sometimes followed by the appearance of typical psoriatic papules and plaques (the Koebner isomorphic response). A wide variety of acute infectious diseases may be followed by the appearance of scattered "drop-like" or guttate lesions. This is particularly true of group A streptococcal infections.

Psoriasis may also occur in pustular forms and in the absence of any associated or causative bacteria. Localized pustular disease, principally found on the palms and soles or around inflamed joints of the digits, is most commonly observed. Generalized pustular disease may occur secondary to the withdrawal of systemic corticosteroids, after extensive topical corticosteroid use, or following generalized drug eruptions. Psoriasis involving the entire integument may also result in erythrodermic disease, often indistinguishable from erythroderma caused by other disease.

There is an arthritis that may be found in up to 25% of patients with psoriasis. Its onset may precede the appearance of psoriasis by many years, or it may begin many years after the onset of psoriasis. Psoriatic arthritis is characteristically seen involving distal interphalangeal joints of the hands and feet, as well as the sacroilium and larger joints at the waist. A negative rheumatoid factor is found in this disease. In any single patient arthritis may progress slowly or rapidly, occasionally ending in severe arthritis mutilans.

A. Etiology and Pathogenesis

Psoriasis is a disease in which multiple defects are found within the epidermis and dermis. The nature of the disease within the epidermis is characterized by increased cellular proliferation of epidermal keratinocytes and accelerated and incomplete epidermal cell differentiation (3). The ultimate outcome is marked scaling and shedding of the involved skin. Dermal disease is characterized by inflammation and the presence of abnormal cutaneous vasculature (4,5). Dermal disease is associated with extravasation of monocytes, lymphocytes, and neutrophils into the dermis and enhancement of infiltrates of neutrophils and activated T lymphocytes throughout the epidermis and dermis. Neutrophils within the epidermis often form microcollections or microscopic abscesses, particularly within the subcorneal layer of epidermis. Macrocollections may also occur, resulting in macroabscesses or the typical clinical lesions of pustular psoriasis. Directed leukocyte migration to epidermis appears to be due in part to altered leukocyte extracellular matrix interactions (6). In active psoriasis peripheral blood leukocytes show decreased adherence to extracellular dermal components, especially those of the basement membrane as collagen types I and IV, laminin, and fibronectin.

There is evidence that helper T lymphocytes play a very active role in the pathogenesis of psoriasis. Activation of T lymphocytes appears to precede epidermal proliferation. Lymphocytes within the epidermis and dermis are primarily of two types: $CD4^+$ (75%) and $CD8^+$ (25%) (7). Among infiltrating cells of the epidermis, $CD4^+$ cells appear to dominate in early disease, whereas $CD8^+$ cells appear to be dominant in chronic disease. In the dermis, particularly the papillary layer, $CD4^+$ cells are dominant in early and chronic disease (8). A markedly decreased $CD4^+/CD8^+$ ratio is seen in the epidermis in the chronic phase of the disease. Regulatory cytokines produced by activated T cells include

IL-2, IFN-γ, and tumor necrosis factor (TNF). CD1$^+$ Langerhans type cells (dendritic) appear to be most numerous in chronic stage disease. The expression of *HLA-DR* and *HLA-DQ* antigens on infiltrating cells appears to be similar in early and late stage disease. *HLA-DR* antigens and intracellular adhesion molecule 1 (ICAM-1) are more strongly expressed on epidermal keratinocytes in the chronic stage of the disease than in the acute stage. Integrin alpha 4 beta 1 positive cells (VLA-4) are expressed more abundantly in the epidermis in the early phase. The expression of ICAM-1 E-selectin and vascular cell adhesion molecule 1 (VCAM-1) on endothelial cells of subpapillary and papillary microvessels is augmented in psoriatic lesions. The number of helper-inducer/memory T cells that accumulate around subpapillary and papillary microvessels appears to be correlated with the degree of expression of E-selectin and VCAM-1 on papillary and subpapillary microvessels in the initial psoriasis lesion (9).

These observations suggest a number of possibilities relative to the pathogenesis of psoriasis, such as the chronic phase of psoriasis appears to be very active immunologically and is possibly more active than during early onset. CD4$^+$ cells, through the production of active cytokines, play an important role in the early onset of psoriasis and that role may be attenuated in late stage disease only to be assumed by active CD8$^+$ cells. Activated T cells produce a variety of regulatory cytokines such as IL-2, IFN-γ, and TNF. In addition to their active participation in the inflammatory process, some cytokines can stimulate proliferation of epidermal keratinocytes. It is also suggested that E-selectin and VCAM-1 expression on endothelial cells of the papillary microvessels may be critical for the initial trafficking of memory T cells and other cell types into psoriatic lesions. Lastly, there is some suggestion that the lymphocyte function-associated antigen-1α/ICAM-1 pathway may play an important role with regard to cell adhesion of infiltrating cells in psoriasis during disease exacerbation or prolongation.

Other investigations on the pathogenesis of psoriasis have demonstrated that activated keratinocytes of the epidermis have the ability to synthesize and release a variety of cytokines, as IL-1 and IL-6, and granulocyte-macrophage colony stimulating factor (GM-CSF), which can stimulate local T-cell activation (10,11). Locally activated T cells expressing markers as high levels of major histocompatibility complex (MCH) class IV molecules and CD25 IL-2 receptors are attracted to and recruit other inflammatory cells that ultimately infiltrate the epidermis, thus accounting for the presence of inflammatory infiltrates in great quantities within the epidermis. Local triggering of activated T cells within the skin may lead to additional proliferation and biochemical activation of epidermal keratinocytes through ordinary cytokine pathways in a process very much like that which occurs in an activated cellular immune reaction.

Type 1 psoriasis (genetically inherited), seen most often in some northern European groups, is strongly associated with the inheritance of certain specific

HLA class I alleles as *HLA-Cw6, -B13, -BW17, -BW16,* and *-BW37* (12,13). In this form of psoriasis, antigens presented on class I molecules may activate $CD8^+$ lymphocytes. Activated $CD8^+$ lymphocytes produce a variety of cytokines that may act on epidermal keratinocytes, thus psoriasis may also present as a primary autoimmune disease in which activated $CD8^+$ lymphocytes act directly or through elaborated cytokines on the skin, thereby initiating an injury repair system in altered keratinocytes. This repair system is characterized by epidermal hyperplasia, activation of the regenerative pathway of keratinocyte differentiation, and accumulation of acute and chronic inflammatory cells locally in the skin. During the process of wound healing a similar kind of injury repair mechanism takes place. A number of investigators have concluded that events that occur in an active plaque of psoriasis serve as evidence that psoriasis is primarily an epidermal disease in which keratinocyte activation precedes any other alterations, and that epidermal activation triggers local inflammation (14).

Excellent therapeutic responses have been induced in clinically active psoriasis by a variety of immune-modulating agents such as FK-506, cyclosporine, and DAB_{389} IL-2 (15–17). The responsiveness of active psoriasis to this group of immune-modulating drugs lends considerable support to the hypotheses that there is a large role played by T lymphocytes and other immunological cells in the pathogenesis of psoriasis. Cyclosporine has been shown to diminish activation of T cells within psoriatic lesions. It has also been observed that the number of T lymphocytes, especially $CD4^+$ and $CD8^+$ T cells, as well as those expressing the IL-2 receptor, are reduced in psoriasis lesions after cyclosporine administration. Cyclosporine also decreases antigen presentation by epidermal cells and inhibits keratinocyte proliferation, but only at dosage levels much higher than those required to inhibit T-cell activity. FK-506 is an agent that is under study for its effect on the immune response. It appears that FK-506 selectively decreases T-cell activation. DAB_{389} IL-2 toxin has been shown to reduce the intraepidermal population of $CD3^+$ and $CD8^+$ T cells in psoriasis. In addition to exerting an antiproliferative effect on epidermal keratinocytes it is possible that drugs such as methotrexate (MTX) and hydrea similarly affect T-cell function and production of lymphokines, cytokines, and other proteins that may induce T-cell expression and activation.

B. Pathology

The histopathological picture in early stage psoriasis is often not characteristic. Parakeratosis, lymphocytes and macrophages invading the epidermis, and a moderate infiltration of lymphocytes and macrophages in the papillary dermis may be all that is seen. There may also be dilatation of capillaries and edema within dermal papillae.

In a mature psoriasis plaque more characteristic pathology is seen. There is thickening of the epidermis due to overall elongation of the rete ridges and a compensatory elongation of the dermal papillae. Thinning of the supra-papillary portion of the epidermis, absence of a granular layer in the epidermis, parakeratosis, and the presence of microabscess within the epidermis are seen. The rete ridges are elongated and bulbous at the base. The number of mitoses per unit surface area is increased. Dermal capillaries are dilated and tortuous. There is a monomorphous inflammatory infiltrate surrounding dermal blood vessels. The number of inflammatory cells within the epidermis increases to the extent that microcollections of leukocytic cells will produce microscopic intraepidermal clusters, many containing neutrophils.

C. Indications for Use of Immunomodulatory and Cytotoxic Agents

The vast majority of patients with psoriasis can be effectively treated with the large number of topical agents that are available over the counter or by prescription. In the treatment of psoriasis it should be remembered that most patients will experience periodic episodes of clearing, alternating with periods of disease exacerbation. Treatment is primarily required to "carry" patients through periods of disease exacerbation. Based on extensive clinical experience it is estimated that only 5–10% of patients with psoriasis will require at some time treatment with immunomodulatory and cytotoxic drugs. Immunomodulatory and cytotoxic drugs should be reserved for patients who in the past have undergone appropriate intensive and extensive treatment with a variety of topical agents and regimens and have failed to show evidence of clinical response, have experienced some adverse event during such treatment, or have experienced rapidly recurring bouts of disease after successful treatment. In general these patients should have extensive and debilitating disease or have disease that impairs the performance of normal daily activities, that is, it affects the patient's economic, psychosocial, or physical

Table 1 Indications for Systemic Therapy in Psoriasis

Psoriasis of any type refractory to intensive topical treatment, including inpatient or outpatient Goeckerman regimen
Photosensitive psoriasis
Erythrodermic psoriasis
Pustular psoriasis, acute generalized
Pustular psoriasis, localized
Psoriatic arthritis
Psoriasis that jeopardizes economic, psychosocial, or physical well being

well being (Table 1). For example, the latter group may include a salesperson or a nurse with severe hand psoriasis who is expected to use or expose his/her hands while carrying out assigned tasks. In theses circumstances, severely affected psoriatic hands may be repulsive to customers of the salesperson, or may not permit the nurse to perform routine "scrubs" without adversely affecting the status of his/her psoriasis.

D. Method and Rationale for Treatment

Every physician should develop a plan or a series of plans that can be engaged when a patient presents with one of the myriad varieties of psoriasis. Localized plaque psoriasis requires a different regimen versus that used for extensive plaque disease, or pustular psoriasis of the localized or generalized type, or guttate psoriasis, or erythrodermic psoriasis. Agents that may be used in the topical treatment of psoriasis include crude coal tar (3–5%), anthralin (0.1–2%), ammoniated mercury (5%), and calcipotriene (0.005%). Emollients alone and as simple as petrolatum often work "miracles" in treating some patients with extensive disease. The simultaneous use of an emollient in any treatment regimen (topical or systemic) is almost a necessity. Either of the topical agents above may be used alone or in combination with ultraviolet light B (UVB) in suberythema dosages. This treatment regimen may be initiated in the outpatient setting. A more rapid and complete response can be arrived at using a day care program or inpatient treatment regimen. Topical corticosteroids of any strength are to be used sparingly and for very short periods, if at all, except in the treatment of lichenified psoriasis or psoriasis of the scalp. Rarely do topical corticosteroids clear or partially clear anything but the mildest of psoriasis. In most patients the number and type of potential adverse effects from constant to long-term use of topical corticosteriods far outweigh their effectiveness. *There are few, if any, indications for use of systemic corticosteroids in the treatment of psoriasis.*

The failure of a patient to respond to the agents and regimens above should lead one to a consideration of the use of systemic psoralen and ultraviolet light A (PUVA), or topical psoralen (solution or bath) and UVA. Based on experience, the efficacy of the PUVA regimen is often exceeded by the number and severity of short- and long-term adverse reactions experienced by some patients (18). Many knowledgeable therapists will bypass this regimen and proceed to the use of systemic immunomodulatory and cytotoxic agents for treatment of severe recalcitrant psoriasis.

There are several moderately effective to effective systemic agents available for general use in psoriasis. These include the cytotoxic agents methotrexate (MTX), hydroxy urea (hydrea), and the combination of methotrexate and 5-fluorouracil. The vitamin A derivative etretinate has been used extensively in severe psoriasis. It has been used as a single agent or in combination with

UVB or PUVA (REPUVA). Cyclosporine has been tested extensively in severe psoriasis. It was found to be highly effective and has been recommended for approval with psoriasis as an indication by an Advisory Committee to the Food and Drug Administration (FDA). However, in early 1995 the manufacturer of cyclosporine elected to withdraw its new drug application from consideration by the FDA. Cyclosporine remains available in the United States for its primary indication, prevention of transplantation rejection.

A rather large number of immunomodulatory agents remain under study in the United States and may, in time, be made available for use in psoriasis. Among the agents under study that show promise are DAB_{389} IL-2, a fusion protein composed of human IL-2 and fragments of diphtheria toxin. DAB_{389} IL-2 acts through a process in which IL-2 binds to cells having IL-2 receptors as activated T lymphocytes. Once bound to the target cell the fusion toxin penetrates and kills the affected cell or T lymphocytes, thus selectively blocking the growth of activated lymphocytes. SD2 IMM 125 is the hydroxyethyl derivative of d-serine-cyclosporin. In experimental studies, the immunosuppressive properties of this agent are at least equivalent to that of cyclosporine, and it appears the new agent is better tolerated, especially with regard to renal function. BCX-34 is a small-molecule drug that inhibits purine nucleoside phosphorylase, an enzyme necessary for T-cell proliferation. Topical and systemic formulations are now being tested in psoriasis and show promise of having a favorable efficacy/toxicity ratio.

1. Methotrexate

As of today MTX remains the "gold standard" for systemic treatment of severe recalcitrant psoriasis. It is quite effective in controlling most forms of severe psoriasis and is quite safe in the properly monitored patient. There are very few contraindications to use of MTX (Table 2). Among these are known liver disease, severely compromised renal function, severe hematological disease, severe systemic infections, and most importantly, an unreliable patient. Caution must be

Table 2 Methotrexate Contraindications for Use

An unreliable patient
Excessive alcohol consumption
Acute or chronic liver disease
Severe renal disease*
Severe folate deficiency*
Females who wish to conceive a child
Severe hematological abnormalities

* Only a relative contraindication.

exercised in administering this agent to the elderly, who are often folic acid deficient and have poor renal function, and to females of childbearing age.

The pretreatment evaluation of a patient who is being considered for MTX is as follows (Table 3). It begins with a good history and physical examination to assess the patient's competence, emotional stability, and general medical status. A good history will also identify medications that may potentiate or interfere with the metabolism of MTX, and vice versa. A complete laboratory examination should include a hemogram with platelets, liver chemistries, and studies of renal function. A creatinine clearance is necessary in the elderly or in patients with known or suspected renal disease. A measure of the serum folate level is especially needed in the elderly whose diets are often deficient in folate.

A liver biopsy is a requirement at or very near the beginning of treatment. It is needed as a baseline indicator for the presence or absence of antecedent liver disease. There should be very few exceptions to this policy. Treatment of psoriasis with MTX is a very serious undertaking and should be approached in a serious manner. The exception is patients over 75 years of age whose life expectancy is such that an accumulative MTX toxic liver effect will not likely be reached.

A substantial number of physicians forego pretreatment liver biopsies, electing to give several months of treatment while determining if the patient will be able to tolerate MTX. In these patients, it is often quite difficult to extract an agreement to do a liver biopsy and many will wish to continue on a program of long-term use. At our institution, it is a rule that only in the rarest of circumstances will one initiate treatment with MTX prior to the patient submitting to liver biopsy. There are several reasons for taking this position. At least 10–20% of patients who submit to liver biopsies will show some form of liver abnormality. Often these abnormalities are indistinguishable from that attributed to MTX. The therapist should be aware of these pretreatment defects so that he/she, if electing to initiate or continue MTX, will be able to devise a treatment regimen that will include plans for a repeat biopsy prior to the accumulation of the standard total dosage ordinarily recommended for posttreatment liver biopsy. The latent discovery of typical psoriasis-MTX liver disease in a patient who has not pervi-

Table 3 Methotrexate Pretreatment Evaluation

Complete history and physical examination
Complete blood count, including platelets
Test of renal function: BUN, creatinine*
Liver biopsy
Routine blood chemistry profile, including liver function studies

* In the elderly or patients with known renal disease these studies are supplemented with a creatinine clearance.

ously submitted to a pretreatment biopsy places the therapist at considerable risk in our present litigious society. The patient who submits to pretreatment liver biopsy is clearly being informed of the seriousness of the treatment regimen he/she is about to undertake. Lastly, experience has shown it is quite rare to find a patient with severe psoriasis who does not tolerate MTX.

It has been recommended that in the absence of abnormal liver function tests, which should be repeated quarterly, a repeat liver biopsy should be done after an accumulative MTX dosage of 1500 mg. At our institution, liver biopsy is repeated after a total dosage of 2500 mg. Our return on finding MTX-associated liver disease before reaching an accumulative drug dosage of 2500 mg is nil. Some therapists have continued MTX after finding overt liver disease on liver biopsy and report no progression of the disease. In some patients, liver changes occur for the better after discontinuing alcohol and while continuing to receive MTX.

A complete blood count with platelets is repeated each week prior to the patient receiving MTX. A low white cell or platelet count calls for a temporary cessation of treatment until the count(s) returns to a normal level. (In the normal patient the white cell count should exceed 4000/mm^3 and the platelet count should exceed 100,000/mm^3). Often oral ulcerations will precede or accompany a drop in the white cell count, thus patients are asked to test this phenomenon on the days just preceding the administration of MTX. This may be done by ingesting orange, grapefruit, or tomato juice. If mouth ulcerations are detected, the patient is told to withhold the weekly dosage of MTX. In some patients, a reasonable profile of the white cell and platelet count will be achieved after several months of observation. In patients whose blood counts remain at or above the minimum during a prolonged period of treatment, consideration may be given to repeating their counts on a biweekly basis, although drug may be continued weekly. Frequent monitoring of hematological studies will prevent the sudden development of severe bone marrow toxicity (Table 4).

Although there is no correlation between standard liver function tests and the development of MTX-associated disease, these tests should be repeated quarterly to twice yearly. If found to be abnormal, repeat liver studies are done monthly for a period of 2–3 months. In patients whose studies do not return to normal on repeated examination, a repeat liver biopsy is done. In most patients who experience repeated liver chemistry abnormalities, a reminder that alcohol consumption is not allowed during treatment with MTX is usually followed by a return of liver chemistries to normal values. Liver function studies should not be drawn on days the patient is scheduled to receive MTX. Preferably they are done just prior to the patient receiving his/her weekly drug.

a. Dosing of MTX. All patients except those with compromised renal function and the elderly are started on a total dosage of 7.5 mg/wk. This may be taken as a single dose or in three doses of 2.5 mg each given at 12 h intervals.

Table 4 Methotrexate Ongoing Evaluation

Complete blood count with platelets, weekly, just prior to the administration of drug (in the exceptional patient this schedule may be modified). A low platelet or white cell count necessitates withholding of drug until count returns to normal. Repeat folate and B12 are done if low WBC persists.*
Chemistry profile to include liver function studies is done every 3–4 mo, and at least 7 d after the last dose of MTX. Abnormal liver function studies should be repeated. If abnormal after 3 consecutive months of testing the liver biopsy is repeated.
Repeat liver biopsy is done after a cumulative dosage of 1.5 g has been reached. This timing may vary based on each centers experience.
If evidence of cirrhosis is found liver biopsy should be repeated in 1 y.
Increased severity of cirrhosis on repeat liver biopsy requires termination of MTX.

* Frequent patient monitoring will prevent severe hematological abnormalities and bone marrow suppression.

Table 5 Cyclosporine Contraindications for Use

An unreliable patient
Preexisting hypertension
Preexisting renal disease
History of cancer (exception: nonmelanoma skin cancer)
Previous vascular disease
History of liver disease
Elderly

The single oral dose, especially in amounts above 10–15 mg, is often associated with nausea. This problem occurs rarely with divided doses. In patients who do not respond to 7.5 mg, the daily dosage may be increased gradually until acceptable clearing is achieved or mild toxicity is experienced. In general, one should not exceed a total dosage of 25 mg in 24 h, once weekly.

It is important to remember that the goal of the therapist is to reduce the disease burden enough to make the patient comfortable. The goal is not complete clearing of the disease.

Patients who respond to the initial 7.5 mg dose may be continued indefinitely at this level. If complete disease clearing is achieved, drug dosages should be reduced appropriately. This may be done by reducing the amount given weekly or by giving drug on alternate weeks. MTX may also be given by the parenteral route. Based on the excretion pattern of oral versus parenteral drug treatment, this route will usually require higher total dosages. Patients who are unreliable or who experience gastrointestinal symptoms may be treated by the parenteral route. Finally, an attempt should be made to stop treatment whenever possible and after the desired disease response has been achieved.

2. Hydroxy Urea (Hydrea)

Hydrea is a cytotoxic drug that was introduced as a treatment for psoriasis almost 25 years ago (19). When used alone hydrea often achieves minimal effect in severe psoriasis. Hence, it has very few modern day proponents. Very good to excellent results may be achieved when using hydrea in combination with intensive topical treatment (Goeckerman regimen) or with the vitamin A derivative etretinate. When used in recommended dosages of 1.0–1.5 g daily, hydrea has very few adverse effects. Its principal toxic effects are on the bone marrow; white cell and platelet counts may be affected. Megaloblastosis almost always occurs. At the onset of treatment, a few patients will describe a flulike syndrome consisting of fever, chills, and malaise associated with changes in liver enzyme plasma levels. This response precludes the further use of hydrea. Chronic hepatic toxicity does not occur.

When used along with an intensive tar and UVB regimen, hydrea may shorten the period required to clearing and will often aid in sustaining clearing with minimal continuing light exposure. When used with etretinate, hydrea will aid in reducing the dosage of etretinate required for clearing. Thus, it may aid in reducing the number and kinds of adverse effects experienced using etretinate. Hydrea has been used in combination with methotrexate. However, I would caution against using in a single patient two potent bone marrow suppressants whose efficacy is probably not synergistic, but whose marrow effect can be additive.

Since there are few adverse effects experienced using hydrea, monitoring for drug effect is quite simple. All patients should have a complete blood count with platelets done before the drug is given and weekly thereafter. Studies of liver function should be done at the start of treatment and quarterly thereafter. Hepatic toxicity will rarely necessitate termination of treatment.

a. Dosing of Hydrea. The standard dosage of hydrea is 1.0–1.5 g each day. This is most often divided into three doses of 500 mg each.

3. Cyclosporine

Although the new drug application (NDA) for use of cyclosporine in psoriasis has been withdrawn in favor of a new derivative SD2 IMM 125, with an improved risk benefit ratio, cyclosporine remains available for prescription use in the United States as an immunosuppressant following organ transplantation.

Although considerable toxicity is associated with both short- and long-term use of cyclosporine, it remains one of the most effective agents for clearing severe recalcitrant psoriasis. Eighty percent of patients receiving 7.5 mg/kg/d achieved complete clearing (20). Because cyclosporine toxicity does not generally overlap that of other systemic agents used in psoriasis, cyclosporine can be used for short-term achievement of control in patients with severe disease who may have experienced an adverse reaction from one or more agents. Disease control achieved through the use of cyclosporine may be followed immediately by continuing control using another systemic agent or an intensive topical regimen. Toxicity is dose and duration dependent, as is efficacy. Contraindications for use of cyclosporine are summarized in Table 5.

The most severe adverse effects are hypertension and induction of renal disease. Both blood pressure and renal function require constant monitoring and correction during treatment. Hypertension is usually reversible after cyclosporine use is ended. In most patients hypertension during treatment can be controlled using calcium channel blockers. Nephrotoxicity is a direct reflection of decreased glomerular filtration. An increasing blood urea nitrogen and serum creatinine are evidence of restricted filtration and increasingly severe renal disease. However, direct measurement of the glomerular filtration rate (GFR) is the most reliable indicator of the true renal effect of cyclosporine. Blood pressure and renal function studies should be assessed every 2 wk throughout the course of treatment (Tables 6 and 7). Other troubling but less severe adverse effects include hypertrichosis, gum hyperplasia, tremor, paresthesias, headache, nausea, and reduced magnesium blood levels. All of these effects are usually reversible when cyclosporine is discontinued.

a. Dosing of Cyclosporine. It is generally agreed that a low starting dosage followed by incremental increases (0.5 mg/kg/d) every 2–3 wk until a therapeutic response or maximum dosage is achieved is the best approach to the treatment of most patients. The adequacy of a treatment regimen can be determined by measurement of cyclosporine trough levels in the blood. A trough level of cyclosporine around 100 ng/ml is ideal and can be achieved with the administration of 3–5 mg/kg/d. A starting dosage should not exceed 5 mg/kg/d. The maximum tolerable dosage approximates 7.5 mg/kg/d. It is recommended that this dosage be approached only under rare circumstances and that it not be exceeded in a patient during the treatment of psoriasis. If the serum creatinine

Table 6 Cyclosporine Pretreatment Evaluation

Blood pressure, baseline
Blood chemistry profile to include creatinine, BUN, liver function tests, serum lipids, uric acid, electrolytes, and magnesium
Glomerular filtration rate (GFR)
Complete blood count, including platelets

Table 7 Cyclosporine Ongoing Evaluation

Test	Abnormality	Intervention
Blood pressure	Increasing	Treat (calcium channel blockers)
BUN or creatinine	Increasing	Reduce drug dosage
Lipids	Increasing	Dietary manipulations, reduce drug dosage
Potassium	Increasing	Reduce drug dosage
Magnesium	Decreasing	Replace
Cyclosporine trough levels	Over 200 ng/ml	Reduce drug dosage

rises above baseline by 30% during treatment, drug dosage should be reduced, or if the creatinine continues to rise after a dosage reduction, cyclosporine should be discontinued (Table 7).

4. Etretinate (Tegison)

Good to excellent results have been achieved using etretinate in a variety of types of psoriasis. Erythrodermic and pustular psoriasis have been described as especially responsive to etretinate. Plaque type psoriasis has a more variable response, with good to excellent clearing experienced by about 75% of patients treated. The efficacy of etretinate may be improved by combining it with PUVA, MTX, or hydrea. Contraindications to the usage of etretinate may be found in Table 8.

Adverse reactions to etretinate, although not severe, are seen in most patients. Among these are cheilitis, dry mouth, dry nostrils associated with epistaxis, dry and exudative eyes, ectropion, dry fragile skin, especially of the palms and soles where constant peeling may be described, hair loss, change in skin texture, and change in texture of the nails. More severe toxicity includes hypercholesterolemia, hypertriglyceridemia, bone pain, vertebral osteophytes, bony bridging, and teratogenicity. Teratogenicity can be prevented by withholding the drug from women of childbearing age or women who wish to conceive within 2 y of

Table 8 Etretinate Contraindications

Women who wish to conceive a child
Patients with severe liver disease
Patients with severe lipid abnormalities

receiving therapeutic dosages of etretinate. Bony defects can be prevented or reduced by periodic monitoring of appropriate areas using bony x-rays; that is, the spine and Achilles tendon. When persistent bone pain is experienced or evidence of bony defects appear, etretinate should be discontinued. Hyperlipidemia can often be reversed with simple changes in dietary habits. In the absence of change etretinate should be discontinued.

Some of the minor adverse effects such as cheilitis and fragile skin may be reduced with improved lubrication of the skin using appropriate emollients, by reducing drug dosage, or by reducing drug dosage and combining etretinate with another agent or treatment regimen.

a. Dosing of Etretinate. The optimum dosage of etretinate is 0.6–0.7 mg/kg/d. Efficacy is reduced below this range and adverse effects are increased in number and severity above this range. If clearing is achieved using 0.6–0.7 mg/kg/d then a reduction in dosage is in order. It has been noted that the number and severity of adverse reactions may be reduced by giving patients rest periods of 2–3 mo out of each 12 mo treatment period.

Patient evaluation prior to treatment includes studies of liver function, complete blood count, urinalysis, fasting cholesterol and triglycerides, and x-rays of joints, particularly those in which pain is often described (Table 9). Routine monitoring includes complete blood count, liver function tests, fasting cholesterol and triglycerides, and x-rays as indicated by descriptions of pain and immobility (Table 10).

Table 9 Etretinate Pretreatment Evaluation

Complete blood count, including platelets
Complete chemistry profile, including liver studies
Lipid profile

Table 10 Etretinate Ongoing Evaluation

Complete blood count with platelets	Every 2 wks
Complete chemistry profile	for 6 wks
Lipid profile	then monthly
Skeletal or Achilles tendon x-rays yearly and whenever severe bone pain is experienced.	

5. Combination and Rotational Therapy

In an attempt to reduce the number and types of adverse reactions experienced by patients with severe disease, and who require continuous treatment with systemic agents, Weinstein and White introduced the concept of rotational therapy (21). Recently this concept was broadened to include a single agent regimen and combination drug regimens. In the approach to rotational treatment the therapist changes each patients treatment program once each 2–3 y, regardless of the patient's disease status or adverse drug experience. For example, a patient on MTX for 3 y would be switched to etretinate, and if control is maintained the patient would remain on this agent for 2–3 y, after which he/she would be switched to another agent or treatment regimen or combination of agents and regimens. Theoretically, with this approach one would reduce the patients total exposure to a single agent or regimen and thus to the toxic effects of any one agent or regimen. Ultimately one may be able to span a period of 10 y or more during which a patient may be exposed to a single toxic agent less than one-third of the time, causing adverse effects that may have occurred during exposure to heal or progress at a slower rate. This concept deserves further thought and possible execution.

REFERENCES

1. Rea JN, Newhouse ML, Halil T. Skin disease in Lambeth: a community study of prevalence and use of medical care. Br J Prev Soc Med, 1976; 30:107–114.
2. Lomholt G. Psoriasis in Uganda: a comparative study with other parts of Africa. In: Farber EM, Cox AJ, eds. Psoriasis: Proceedings of an International Symposium. Stanford: Stanford University Press, 41–48.
3. Weinstein GD, McCullough JL. Cell proliferation kinetics. In: Roenigk HH Jr, Maibach HI, eds. Psoriasis. 2nd ed. New York: Marcel Dekker, 1991:327–342.
4. Cooper KD. Psoriasis: leucocytes and cytokines. Dermat Clin 1990; 8:737–745.
5. Braverman IM. Microcirculation. In: Roenigk HH Jr, Maibach HI, eds. Psoriasis. New York: Marcel Dekker, 1985:287–298.
6. el-Sherif AI, Krupinski P, Majewski S, Jablonska S. Leucocyte-extracellular matrix interactions in psoriasis. Int J Dermat 1994; 33:371–373.
7. Schlaak JF, Buslau M, Jochum W, Hermann E, Girndt M. T-cells in psoriasis vulgaris belong to the TH 1 subset. J Invest Dermat 1994; 102:145–159.
8. Onuma S. Immunohistochemical studies of infiltrating cells in early and chronic lesions of psoriasis. J Dermat 1994; 21:301–307.
9. Wakita H, Takigawa M. E-selectin and vascular cell adhesion molecule-1 are critical for initial trafficking of helper-inducer/memory T cells in psoriatic plaques. Arch Dermat 1994; 130:457–463.
10. Nickoloff BJ. The cytokine network in psoriasis. Arch Dermat 1991; 127:871–884.

11. Krueger JG, Krane JF, Carter DM, Gottlieb AB. Role of growth factors, cytokines and their receptors in the pathogenesis of psoriasis. J Invest Dermat 1990; 94(suppl):135S–140S.
12. Hensler T, Christophers E. Psoriasis of early and late onset. Characterization of two types of psoriasis vulgaris. J Am Acad Dermat 1995; 13:450–456.
13. Baadsgaaed O, Fisher G, Voorhees JJ, Cooper KD. The role of the immune system in the pathogenesis of psoriasis. J Invest Dermat 1990; 95(5)(suppl):32S–34S.
14. Weinstein GD, Krueger JG. An overview of psoriasis. In: Weinstein GD, Gottlieb AB, eds. Therapy of moderate to severe psoriasis. Portland, Ore: National Psoriasis Foundation, 1993:1–23.
15. Ackerman C, Abu-Elagd K, Venkataramanan K, Fung J, Todo S, et al. Recalcitrant psoriasis and pyoderma gangrenosum treated with FK 506. J Invest Dermat 1991; 96:536.
16. Ellis CN, Fradin MS, Messana JM, et al. Cyclosporine for plaque-type psoriasis. Results of a multidose, double blind trial. N Engl J Med 1991; 324:277–284.
17. Gottlieb SL, Gilleaudecere P, Johnson R, et al. Response of psoriasis to a lymphocyte-selective toxin (DAB $_{389}$ IL-2) suggests a primary immune, but not keratinocyte, pathogenic basis. Nature Med 1995; 1:442–447.
18. Morison WL. PUVA therapy. In: Weinstein GD, Gottlieb AB, eds. Therapy of moderate to severe psoriasis. Portland, Ore: National Psoriasis Foundation, 1993:23–38.
19. Leavell UW, Yarbro JW. Arch Dermat 1970; 102:144.
20. Ellis CN, Fradin MS, Messana JM, et al. Cyclosporine for plaque-type psoriasis. Results of a multidose, double-blind trial. New Eng J Med 1991; 324:277–284.
21. Weinstein GD, White GM. An approach to the treatment of moderate to severe psoriasis with rotational therapy. J Am Acad Dermat 1993; 28:454–459.

18
Pityriasis Rubra Pilaris

Leslie Robinson-Bostom and Charles J. McDonald
Brown University, Providence, Rhode Island

Pityriasis rubra pilaris (PRP) is an uncommon heterogeneous papulosquamous disorder of unknown etiology. All races are affected, with a male/female ratio of 1:1. The point prevalence for sporadic PRP ranges from 1/3500 to 1/5000 among newly presenting dermatology patients (1,2). There is a bimodal age presentation with peaks in the first and fifth decades (2). Although no specific HLA patterns have been reported, genetic factors have been considered in the pathogenesis of some cases of PRP (3).

Some authors suggest that certain exposures may precipitate PRP in a genetically predisposed individual (2–4). Examples include viral or bacterial infection, sun exposure, electrical or chemical burns, parturition, and postsurgical complications (5). Affected relatives are not found in the classical acute onset varieties. An autosomal dominant inheritance pattern with variable expression and reduced penetrance has been documented in some patients with atypical juvenile onset disease (6). Isolated cases have been reported in association with numerous medical diseases including leukemia, hypothyroidism, celiac sprue, hydronephrosis, syringomyelia, and HIV infection (7–10).

Griffith has classified PRP into five types based on clinical appearance, behavior, and prognosis (2). These include type I—classical adult, type II—atypical adult, type III—classical juvenile, type IV—circumscribed juvenile, and type V—atypical juvenile (2). This discussion will focus on type I classical adult onset, which accounts for the largest number of reported cases. Typically in these patients one or several erythematous plaques on the upper half of the body spread caudally over weeks or months as large zones of follicular hyperkeratosis. Follicular acuminate papules evolve into flat-topped papules that coalesce into sheets of erythema and scale, often progressing to generalized erythroderma (2).

Characteristic 1 cm islands of normal appearing skin remain interspersed between the erythematous areas ("islands of sparing").

Follicular hyperkeratosis persists longest on the dorsal phalanges and has been regarded as pathognomonic for PRP, but is also seen in ichthyosiform erythroderma and follicular ichthyosis. Keratoderma of the palms and soles in usually present and may occur first (2,11,12). The erythema, which is distinctively orange or yellowish rather than pink, is best viewed on the palms and soles.

The scaling is fine, powdery, or branlike on the upper half of the body and course on the lower half. Plaques on the elbows and knees become psoriasiform as the disease progresses. Ectropion may be present with extensive facial disease. Nail dystrophy consists of subungual hyperkeratosis, splinter hemorrhage, and longitudinal riding (13). According to Griffiths, prognosis is excellent with approximately 80% of patients clearing in 3 y (2).

Type II, atypical adult onset PRP, affects only 5% of patients. Although follicular hyperkeratosis is prominent in some areas, eczematous changes and ichthyosiform scaling on the legs occur frequently. The prognosis is less favorable, lasting up to 20 y.

Type III, classical juvenile onset PRP, occurs in the first decade of life, affects 10% of cases, and shares the clinical features of type I. Rapid onset after acute infection has been reported (14). Although Griffith originally reported a poor prognosis for this subtype (6% remission within 3 y), others have reported rapid clearing in 1–2 y (15).

Type IV, circumscribed PRP, occurs in prepubertal children and affects approximately 25% of cases. Transient scaly erythematous plaques on the trunk and well-demarcated follicular hyperkeratotic plaques resembling follicular psoriasis are seen on the knees and elbows. Progression to erythroderma does not occur. The 3 y remission rate is approximately 32%.

Type V, atypical juvenile onset PRP, affects only 5% of patients. This disease runs a chronic course and presents at birth or infancy with follicular hyperkeratosis, erythema, and keratoderma. Sclerodermic-like changes of the digits have been reported in several patients (3). Most cases of familial PRP belong to this subtype. There is clinical overlap with ichthyotic disorders and the erythrokeratodermas (2,6).

I. ETIOLOGY AND PATHOGENESIS

Although the cause of pityriasis rubra pilaris is unknown, one fundamental abnormality is epidermal hyperproliferation. Enhanced epidermal proliferative activity as measured by the mitotic index (MI) and the flash labeling index (FLI) using tritiated thymidine is found in both PRP and psoriasis (16). Kinetic data reveal that the proliferative indices for PRP are lower than for psoriasis. This may explain the less dramatic response of PRP to antimetabolite therapy as compared to psoriasis.

Labeling indices reported for PRP in vivo range from 9.7 to 27.3 compared to normal controls of approximately 3. In one study enhanced FLIs have been demonstrated in the islands of apparently normal skin (16).

Vanderhooft et al. studied four patients in a family with PRP (1). Immunoblot analysis revealed expression of the hyperproliferative keratins, K6/K16, extreme broadening of the spinous keratins, K1 and K10, a doublet corresponding to keratin K14/16, and a 45 Kd acidic keratin felt to be K17. Keratin 17 is normally expressed in basal and myoepithelial cells of complex epithelia, but not in stratified squamous epithelia. This keratin has been detected in psoriasis (1), basal cell carcinoma, and other malignancies. Additional immunoblot studies of both familial and sporadic PRP are needed to help interpret these data.

The histological similarity between clinical vitamin A deficiency and PRP prompted several investigators to utilize vitamin A as a therapy (17,18). Beneficial effects observed in some patients treated with vitamin A in the 1970s and 1980s encouraged others to postulate that the pathogenesis of PRP was related to a deficiency of vitamin A (19). This has been refuted, as measured plasma levels of vitamin A and carotenoids are normal (20). Other authors have reported reduced levels of retinol binding protein and have speculated that defective synthesis or deficiency of this protein accounted for the lack of clinical response to oral vitamin A in a percentage of patients (21). Anabolic steroids, including stanazol, have been used in an effort to increase circulating levels of retinol binding protein, and thus increase tissue delivery of retinol to tissues (22). These attempts yielded mixed results (22,23). Evaluation of retinoic acid nuclear and cytoplasmic receptors, cytokine production, and expression of adhesion molecules has not been studied (24). It seems likely that high doses of vitamin A and retinoids improve PRP pharmacologically through nonspecific antikeratinizing effects.

Whether immunological factors play a role in the pathogenesis of PRP is yet to be elucidated. Several case studies have reported immunological abnormalities associated with PRP. For example, Shvili reported normal numbers of T helper and suppressor lymphocytes, decreased functional activity of helper inducer cells, and elevated spontaneous suppressor activity in a 6-year-old boy with PRP (25).

A unique form of PRP is seen in patients with HIV infection. Dramatic keratotic spines and severe nodulocystic inflammatory folliculitis or furunculosis similar to acne conglobata occur acutely and simultaneously (5,10,26–28).

Although two cases of furunculosis and PRP have been reported in the absence of HIV infection (26), these patients seem to demonstrate a single disorder of follicular keratinization. Additionally, while most papulosquamous disorders reported in HIV-positive patients occur with severe immunosuppression (T4 counts less than 100 or 150), PRP may occur as the initial manifestation of HIV infection or in patients with relatively high CD4 counts (less than 500). The interaction of PRP and HIV infection may provide insight to help clarify the pathogenesis of PRP.

II. PATHOLOGY

The histological features of classical adult pityriasis rubra pilaris are distinctive. As summarized by Soeprono (29), these characteristics include a) alternating orthokeratosis and parakeratosis, both vertically and horizontally; b) intact granular layer or hypergranulosis, even beneath parakeratotic scale; c) thick suprapapillary plates; d) broad rete ridges; e) narrow dermal papillae; and f) a sparse superficial perivascular lymphohistiocytic infiltrate. Follicular plugging with parakeratosis in the perifollicular shoulders has also been reported.

Although pityriasis rubra pilaris shares histological features with psoriasis, that is, psoriasiform hyperplasia and a superficial perivascular infiltrate, the characteristics listed above are usually sufficient to help differentiate these separate papulosquamous disorders. Mounds of parakeratotic scale with neutrophils, thin suprapapillary plates, broad dermal papillae, and tortuous capillaries are all features of psoriasis that are not seen in pityriasis rubra pilaris.

The histology of PRP varies in different stages of the disease, therefore, biopsies from multiple sites in the single patient may differ. In late lesions, acanthosis is less pronounced, while compact or laminated orthokeratosis predominates over alternating parakeratosis (29).

III. INDICATIONS FOR USE OF IMMUNOMODULATORY AND CYTOTOXIC AGENTS

The low prevalence and varying clinical severity and clinical course of pityriasis rubra pilaris make evaluation of therapy difficult. Although most patients clear within 3 y, there are reports of cases lasting up to 20 or 30 y. Immunomodulating and cytotoxic therapy should be reserved for patients with disabling erythroderma or incapacitating keratoderma.

The plethora of therapeutic suggestions for PRP attends to the lack of uniform response to any single agent. Currently retinoids and antimetabolites appear to be the most successful therapies.

High-dose oral vitamin A (150,000–300,000 IU/d) improves disease in approximately one-third of patients, however, data regarding long-term treatment and incidence of vitamin A toxicity have not been reported (30). Toxic doses of oral vitamin A (1 million IU/d for 5–14 d) has resulted in complete desquamation of the hyperkeratotic plaques in 10–14 d, followed by erythema which lasts for several months. Symptoms associated with this regimen include headaches, chills, and diarrhea. Transient elevated triglycerides, WBC, and SGOT are seen in some patients (31). Of note, vitamin A is teratogenic at doses as low as 10,000 IU, and unlike synthetic retinoids, is stored in the liver.

Interestingly, Kellun et al. describe a Tunisian patient who improved with emulsified agueous vitamin A and d-α-tocopherol acetate, but experienced rapid exacerbations while receiving the lipid soluble vitamin A formulions (32). Some investigators have found a synergistic effect of vitamins A and E. They claim that in patients with PRP unresponsive to oral vitamin A, prompt clearance is often achieved with the addition of 800–1600 IU of d-α-tocopherol acetate (32). However, the role of d-α-tocopherol acetate (vitamin E) as adjuvant treatment with vitamin A is unproven in controlled clinical trials.

As previously stated, Finzi et al. have reported reduced levels of retinol binding protein in patients with PRP (21), however, these results have been disputed. Stanozol and other anabolic steroids have been used effectively to treat patients with PRP while increasing levels of retinal binding protein, although several other authors have found no beneficial effect (33).

The oral retinoids, isotretinoin, and etretinate are less toxic than vitamin A, while retaining its pharmacological action. Both isotretinoin and etretinate have been reported as effective therapies for PRP. Most data are derived from case reports, small series, and rctrospective studies. Clinical improvement ranges from 60–95% of patients 4–6 mo after starting isotretinoin. The largest prospective trial of isotretinoin for PRP was a multicenter study reported by Goldsmith et al. in 1982 (34). The mean daily dose of isotretinoin was 2.13 mg/kg/d, significantly higher than the doses used today. Marked improvement in the degree of erythema, induration, and scaling was noted in more than half the patients (28 of 45) within 4 wk, however only 6 patients cleared completely. In this study response rate did not correlate with pretreatment duration of disease. Dickens reported the results of a large retrospective study of various therapies for PRP (30). Patients responding favorably to isotretinoin had a shorter duration of disease prior to initiating treatment, compared with those who were unresponsive (30).

As stated above, clinical improvement of PRP may be seen during the first month of therapy, although significant clinical improvement may require completing 4–6 mo of treatment (12).

Several authors report that etretinate may be superior to isotretinoin in the treatment of both adult and childhood onset PRP. Borok and Lowe (35) noted faster clearance at lower dosages (0.5%) in a study comparing etretinate to isotretinoin therapy for PRP. Marks et al. (36) and Kenerva et al. (37) report response rates of 67% and 80%, respectively, with etretinate. In juvenile PRP, response to etretinate is often dramatic; lesions may resolve in several weeks and do not relapse. Etretinate is stored in adipose tissue and has been detected in blood for more than 2 yr after discontinuation of therapy. Because of its prolonged half-life, women of childbearing age are at unknown risk of subsequent teratogenicity. Skeletal abnormalities such as premature epiphyseal closure, slender long bones, and osteoporosis have been reported in children. These side effects, in addition to the other well known adverse effects, should be considered carefully before initiating treatment.

Methotrexate has also been used to treat patients with PRP. The dose schedule and route of administration have varied. Historically, early reports describing methotrexate therapy have included dose schedules that would not be utilized today. For example, Knowles and Chernasky (38) supported the use of long-term daily oral administration of methotrexate, alternating 5 mg one day and 2.5 the next without a rest period for several months. Currently, dose schedules comparable to what are used in treatment of psoriasis are advocated. Clinical response rates of PRP to methotrexate therapy have not been as consistent as those reported for psoriasis. This may be related to the slower epidermal turnover rate of affected skin in PRP. Griffiths reported no response in 27 out of 44 patients treated with MTX (19). Others have reported more favorable response rates (38,39). Clinical improvement has been observed after 4–6 wk of therapy, with complete response after approximately 4 mo. Many patients relapse when treatment is discontinued. Clinical and laboratory monitoring is as required for psoriasis, including liver biopsy if necessary.

Pityriasis rubra pilaris has also been treated successfully with azathioprine. Hunter and Forbes treated five erythrodermic patients with azathioprine in doses ranging from 50 mg b.i.d. to 50 mg t.i.d. (40), Decreased erythema was noted within 1 wk of therapy. Complete clearance was reported within 3 mo. Prolonged remission was observed in half of these patients. Side effects in this series included acute gastric intolerance and transient neutropenia which responded to a reduced dose. Increased susceptibility to infections was not seen with these doses. The authors speculate that an immunosuppressive mechanism accounts for the observed beneficial effect (40). Griffiths has reported similar results.

In general, the use of cyclosporine A for PRP has shown minimal or no beneficial effects. Meyer et al. report lack of effect of cyclosporine after 18 wk of therapy in one patient (41). In a multicenter prospective trial, Gupta et al. reported minimal response to cyclosporine in all three patients with PRP (42). Side effects included dysesthesia, fatigue, hypertrichosis, nausea, and flushing. HTN and renal difficult all of which normalized within 1 mo of discontinuing therapy. Biopsies were obtained at pretherapy, when clinical improvement was first noted, and on completion of cyclosporine therapy. Specimens were stained with hematoxylin-eosin, and immunophenotyping was performed using the monoclonal antibodies ICAM-1, HLA-DR, and HLA-DQ. At pretreatment, biopsies demonstrated a superficial perivascular inflammatory infiltrate composed of T lymphocytes with a CD4/CD8 ratio of 5:1. Most of the dermal lymphocytes were HLA-DR$^+$. Two of the three patients demonstrated focal ICAM-1 expression. At the end of therapy there were no changes in the dermal infiltrate, however ICAM-

1 and HLA-DR expression by keratinocytes decreased. This is in contrast to psoriasis where the dermal infiltrate of T cells and HLA-DR expression of T cells is diminished after cyclosporine therapy. The authors suggest that the pathogenesis of PRP may not be T-cell mediated or is modulated by a noncylosporine-sensitive T-cell product.

Two positive case reports using cyclosporine for PRP have been reported. In both cases the patients had been previously treated with etretinate. Ghazi and Laso-Dosal do not specify the washout interval, but report dramatic response to cyclosporine within 1 wk followed by complete clearance after 4 wk (43). In the case report by Rosenbach and Lowe, cyclosporine was started 7 wk after cessation of etretinate (44). The half-life of etretinate is 80–160 d, therefore a 7 wk washout period is insufficient to attribute the patients improvement to the cyclosporine. The authors suggest limiting the use of cyclosporine to patients with debilitating PRP who have failed conventional therapy.

Many other systemic and topical agents have been used with variable success. Phototherapy, including both UVB and PUVA, is generally unsuccessful either as primary or adjuvant measures (19). PUVA has rarely been reported as beneficial (19).

Recently, topical calcipotriol, the vitamin D analog, has been effective in one patient with circumscribed juvenile PRP. Improvement was reported after 1 mo of therapy, with lesions resolving after 2 mo (45). This treatment is limited to those with localized disease, as the maximum topical dose is 100 g/wk. Calcipotriol in vitro has been shown to interfere with various aspects of cutaneous inflammation, epidermal proliferation, and keratinization. Specifically, inhibition of T-cell activation, inhibition of keratinocyte growth in culture, and enhancement of the cornified envelop formation occur. In one patient studied by Vanderkorhot, calcipotriol treatment did not result in a reduction of recruitment of cycling cells, but rather enhanced this process. It is unlikely that a direct effect on epidermal proliferation is relevant to the code of action of calcipotriol in PRP.

IV. METHOD AND RATIONALE FOR TREATMENT

Therapy for PRP can be logically guided toward individual patients. Localized disease can be controlled with emollients or topical calcipotriene. Topical steroids do not uniformly improve localized lesions. Tar and anthralins are of no benefit. Patients with debilitating disease (incapacitating keratoderma or erythroderma) can be managed with systemic retinoids or immunosuppressive medications.

Guidelines for the appropriate use of methotrexate, etretinate, and cyclosporine are described in detail in the previous section on psoriasis.

The monitoring guidelines for isotretinoin (Accutane) are similar to those followed for etretinate (37). However, isotretinoin is not lipophilic and has a shorter half-life (10–20 h) than etretinate. This drug can be used safely in women of childbearing potage if adequate contraception is used consistently for 1 mo prior to therapy, throughout treatment, and for 1 mo after stopping therapy. A serum pregnancy test should be negative within 2 wk of starting therapy, and should be repeated each month during therapy and 1 mo after completion. Treatment should be initiated on the third day of the menstrual cycle. A CBC with differential, SMA-12, fasting cholesterol, and triglycerides should be checked prior to therapy and repeated each 4–6 wk (34). Some authors suggest checking triglycerides every 2–3 wk until stable. Dosing of isotretinoin is similar to doses used in acne (1 mg/kg/d). Occasionally, higher doses (up to 2 mg/kg/d) are required. Although many patients improve within the first month of therapy, some require at least 4–6 mo of treatment before improvement occurs. Side effects were discussed in the previous section.

Azathioprine is a synthetic purine analog. Its main clinical application is in transplantation rejection. Azathioprine has been utilized in numerous dermatological disorders and has both immunosuppressive and anti-inflammatory properties. Adverse effects include dose-related bone marrow suppression, nausea, vomiting, diarrhea, and abdominal pain. Hepatotoxicity occurs in less than 1% of dermatology patients. Hypersensitivity reactions such as pancreatitis, urticaria, and morbilliform rash have been reported. Opportunistic infections are more common in transplant patients. Although oncogenic potential is well documented in transplant patients, this risk is only slightly increased in dermatology patients (40).

Azathioprine should not be used in pregnant and lactating patients unless the benefit outweighs the risk. Drug interactions include allopurinol, which inhibits its metabolism. The usual starting does is 1–2 mg/kg/d in two divided doses. If there is no beneficial effect in 6–8 wk, the dose may be increased by 0.5 mg/kg every 4 wk to a maximum of 3 mg/kg/d. If there is no beneficial effect after 12–16 wk at the maximum dose, the medication should be discontinued. Once the disease has stabilized, the doses may be decreased by 0.5 mg/kg every 2–4 wk.

Monitoring requires a baseline physical exam, CBC with differential, platelets, BUN, creatinine, electrolytes, LFTs, and urinalysis. The CBC and platelets should be repeated weekly for 8 wk and then every 2 wk, if stable. The white blood count nadir occurs at approximately 7–14 d after treatment. Liver function tests and renal tests should be repeated each month.

REFERENCES

1. Vanderhooft SL, Francis JS, Holbrook KA, Dale BA, Fleckman P. Familial pityriasis rubra pilaris. Arch Dermat 1995; 131:448–453.
2. Griffiths WAD. Pityriasis rubra pilaris. Clin Exp Dermat 1980; 5:105–112.

3. Goldsmith LA, Weinrich AE, Shupack J. Pityriasis rubra pilaris response to 13-cis-retinoic acid (isotretinoin). J Am Acad Dermat 1982; 6:710–715.
4. Stanoeva L, Konstantinov D, Ristov R. Clinical aspects of pityriasis rubra pilaris in childhood. Dermatologica 1971; 142:1–6.
5. Martin AG, Weaver CC, Cockerell CJ, Berger TG. Pityriasis rubra pilaris in the setting of HIV infection: clinical behavior and association with explosive cystic acne. Br J Dermat 1992; 126:617–620.
6. Griffiths WAD. Pityriasis rubra pilaris. An historical approach. Clin Exp Dermat 1976; 1:37–45.
7. Aguilar AR, Gomez F, Balsa FT, Framil JP, Oubina PN. Pityriasis rubra pilaris with muscle and joint involvement. Dermatologica 1973; 146:361–366.
8. Tunnessen WW Jr, Neburg PI, Voorhess ML. Hypothyroidism and pityriasis rubra pilaris. Response to thyroid hormone. J Pediatr 1976; 88:456–458.
9. Reinhardt LA, Rosen T. Pityriasis rubra pilaris and the initial manifestation of leukemia. Cutis 1983; 31:100–102.
10. Blauvelt A, Nahass GT, Pardo RJ, Kerdel FA. Pityriasis rubra pilaris and HIV infection. J Am Acad Dermat 1991; 24:703–705.
11. Dolezal JF. Pityriasis rubra pilaris, a case report and photo essay. Cutis 1980; 26:37–40.
12. Dickens C. Isotretinoin treatment of pityriasis rubra pilaris. J Am Acad Dermat 1987; 16:297–301.
13. Sonnex TS, Dawber RPR, Zachery CB, Millard PR, Griffiths WAD. The nails in adult type I pityriasis rubra pilaris. J Am Acad Dermat 1986; 3:446–451.
14. Griffiths WAD, Leigh IM, Marks R. In: Champion RH, Burton JL, Ebling FJG, eds. Textbook of dermatology, 5th ed. New York Blackwell Scientific 1992:1358–1362.
15. Gelmetti C, Schiuma AA, Cerri D. Pityriasis rubra pilaris in childhood—a long term study of 29 cases. Pediatr Dermat 1986; 3:446–451.
16. Griffiths WAD, Pilris S. Pityriasis rubra pilaris—an acute radiographic study. 1982; 107:665–667.
17. Griffiths WAD. Retinal binding protein and pityriasis rubra pilaris (letter). Br J Dermat 1982; 107:125–127.
18. Gross DA, Laundau JW, Newcomer VD. Pityriasis rubra pilaris. Arch Dermat 1969; 99:710–716.
19. Cohen PR, Prystowsky JH. Pityriasis rubra pilaris: a review at diagnosis and treatment. J Am Acad Dermat 1989; 20:801–807.
20. Niemi KM, Kowsa M, Storgards K. Pityriasis rubra pilaris. A clinical pathological study with a special reference to autoradiography and histocompatability antigens. Dermatologica 1976; 152:109–118.
21. Finzi AF, Altomere G, Bergamaschine L, Tucci A. Pityriasis rubra pilaris and retinal-binding protein. J Dermat 1981; 104:253–256.
22. Bergamaschini L, Tucci A, Colombo A, Agostoni A, Finzi AG. Effect of stanozolol in patients with pityriasis rubra pilaris and retinal-binding protein deficiency (letter). N Engl J Med 1992; 306:546–547.
23. Van Voorst Vades PC, Van Oostveen F, Houthaft HJ, Marrink J. Pityriasis rubra pilaris, vitamin A and retinol-binding protein: a case study. Acta Dermat Vener (Stockh) 1984; 64:430–432.

24. Griffiths WAD. Pityriasis rubra pilaris: the problem of its classification (letters, comment). J Am Acad Dermat 1992; 26:140–142.
25. Shvili D, David M, Mimouni M. Childhood onset pityriasis rubra pilaris with immunologic abnormalities. Pediatr Dermat 1987; 4:21–23.
26. Cerstgnet J, Lacour JPH, Perrin C, Brun P, Ortonne JP. Juvenile pityriasis rubra pilaris associated with hypogammaglobulinemia and furunculosis. Br J Dermat 1994; 131:717–719.
27. Auffret N, Quirt L, Domert P, Dubertret L, Lecam JY, Binet O. Pityriasis rubra pilaris in a patient with human immunodeficiency virus infection. J Am Acad Dermat 1992; 27:260–261.
28. Resnick SD, Murrel DF, Woosley JT. Pityriasis rubra pilaris, acne angiomata, and elongata follicular spines: an HIV associated follicular syndrome? (letter, comment). J Am Acad Dermat 1993; 29:283.
29. Seeprono FF. Histologic criteria for the diagnosis of pityriasis rubra pilaris. Am J Dermat Pathol 86; 8:277–283.
30. Dickens, CH. Treatment of classic pityriasis rubra pilaris. J Am Acad Dermat 1994; 31:997–999.
31. Randle HW, Diaz-Perez JL, Winkelmann RK. Toxic doses of vitamin A for pityriasis rubra pilaris. Arch Dermat 1980; 116:888–892.
32. Kewllum, RE. Possible significance of aqueous emulsified vitamin A in effective therapy for pityriasis rubra pilaris. J Am Acad Dermat 1989; 20:126–128.
33. Brice SL, Spencer SK. Stanozolol in the treatment of pityriasis rubra pilaris. Arch Dermat 1985; 21:1105–1106.
34. Goldsmith LA, Weinrich, AE, Shupack J. Pityriasis rubra pilaris response to 13-cis-retinoic acid (isotretinoin). J Am Acad Dermat 1992; 6:710–715.
35. Borok M, Lowe NJ. Pityriasis rubra pilaris. J Am Acad Dermat 1990; 22:792–795.
36. Marks
37. Kanerva L, Lautaranta J, Niemi KM, Lassus A. Ultrastructure of pityriasis rubra pilaris with observations during retinoid (etretinate) treatment. Br J Dermat 1983; 108:653–663.
38. Knowles WR, Chernasky ME. Pityriasis rubra pilaris, prolonged treatment with methotrexate. Arch Dermat 1970; 102:603–612.
39. Brown J, Perry HO. Pityriasis rubra pilaris. Treatment with folic acid antagonists. Arch Dermat 1966; 94:636–638.
40. Hunter GA, Forbes IJ. Treatment of pityriasis rubra pilaris with azathioprine. Br J Dermat 1972; 87:42–45.
41. Meyer P, VanVoorst Vader PC. Lack of effect of cyclosporin A in pityriasis rubra pilaris. Acta Dermat Vener (Stockh) 1989; 69:272–275.
42. Gupta AK, Ellis C, Nickoloff BJ, Goldfarb MT, Rocher LL, Griffith CEM, Cooper K, Voorhess J. Oral cyclosporine in the treatment of inflammatory and noninflammatory dermatoses. Arch Dermat 1990; 126:339–350.
43. Ghazi A, Laso-Dosal F. Cyclosporin A and pityriasis rubra pilaris. Acta Dermat Venerol (Stockh) 1990; 70:181–183.
44. Rosenbach A, Lowe NJ. Pityriasis rubra pilaris and cyclosporine. Arch Dermat 1993; 129:1346–48.
45. Van DeKerhof PCM, Steijlen PM. Topical treatment of pityriasis rubra pilaris with calcipotriol. Br J Dermat 1994; 130:675–678.

19
Ichthyosis

Leslie Robinson-Bostom and Charles J. McDonald
Brown University, Providence, Rhode Island

I. ICHTHYOSES

The ichthyoses are a group of inherited and acquired skin disorders characterized by persistent noninflammatory scaling. The term ichthyosis is derived from the Greek word for fish. This chapter will discuss two types of ichthyoses which result from epidermal hyperproliferation: lamellar ichthyosis and epidermolytic hyperkeratosis.

A. Lamellar Ichthyosis

Lamellar ichthyoses have been classified into several autosomal recessive, and more recently, autosomal dominant subtypes (1,2). Autosomal recessive lamellar ichthyosis affects approximately 1 in 300,000 people. The autosomal recessive types can be divided into nonerythrodermic and erythrodermic variants—classic lamellar ichthyosis (LI) and nonbullous congenital ichthyosiform erythroderma (CIE), respectively (2). Bergers et al. have subtyped recessive lamellar ichthyosis into nonerythrodermic autosomal recessive lamellar ichthyosis (NEARLY) and erythrodermic autosomal recessive lamellar ichthyosis (EARLI) (3). It is unclear whether the EARLI patients can be grouped as a subtype of nonbullous congenital ichthyosiform erythroderma.

Clinically both LI and CIE usually present at birth encased in a collodion membrane that subsequently desquamates over the next 2 wk. Infants with classic lamellar ichthyosis then develop generalized large parchment or shield-like scale with flexoral prominence. The palms and soles demonstrate hyperkeratosis with fissuring. Severe facial involvement results in ectropion and deformed "crumpled" ears. Scarring alopecia and sparse body hair may be seen. Hyperpyrexia may occur secondary to sweating abnormalities (2,4). There is no tendency for improvement throughout life.

Nonbullous congenital ichthyosiform erythroderma represents a heterogeneous disorder. As stated above, infants usually present at birth, but occasionally erythroderma is delayed until after the neonatal period. The characteristic findings include generalized erythroderma and fine white scale. Erythema tends to decrease after puberty and may clear in middle age, although scaling is persistent. The joints may demonstrate hyperkeratosis. Ectropion occurs only in severely affected cases (2,4).

1. Etiology and Pathogenesis

The original kinetic studies performed by Frost et al. demonstrated both germinative cell hyperplasia and decreased epidermal transit time in lamellar ichthyosis (5,6). However, no distinction was made between classic lamellar ichthyosis and nonbullous congenital ichthyosiform erythroderma (5,6). Williams and Elias demonstrated a small increase in the rate of keratinocyte production in classic lamellar ichthyosis as compared with CIE, that is, tritiated thymidine autoradiographic labeling indices of 9.36 and 19.70, respectively (4). Analysis of scale lipids has also produced differentiating results for LI and CIE. Elevated levels of sterol and free fatty acids were reported for classic lamellar ichthyosis, while scale from CIE demonstrates elevated increased n-alkanes (2), although these findings have been disputed. Recently, mutations of the gene encoding transglutaminase type I have been identified in lamellar ichthyosis (7).

2. Pathology

The histopathology of classic lamellar ichthyosis is not diagnostic but may simulate biopsies obtained from the normal palm or sole. Dramatic hyperkeratosis without parakeratosis or rare foci is consistently noted. On scanning magnification the stratum corneum appears thicker than the underlying epidermis. The epidermis may be of normal thickness or show psoriasiform hyperplasia. The granular layer is usually normal or increased, although hypogranularis has rarely been reported (4). A sparse superficial mononuclear cell infiltrate may be present. Biopsies from some patients demonstrate dilated and tortuous capillaries, indistinguishable from the pattern observed in psoriasis (4).

Nonbullous CIE demonstrates psoriasiform epidermal acanthosis with overlying parakeratotic scale. The epidermis appears thicker in CIE than in classic lamellar ichthyosis (4).

3. Indications for the Use of Immunomodulatory and Cytotoxic Agents

Treatment regimens for lamellar ichthyosis are guided by the disease severity. Topical therapy is important in all forms of lamellar ichthyosis. Some patients with mild cases of CIE may respond to various topical agents used as monotherapy. These include emollients, urea-containing creams, and various keratolytic agents (8). Unfortunately, in most patients with classic lamellar ichthyosis topical therapy is unsatisfactory.

Several studies have addressed the efficiency, tolerability, and safety of calcipotriol ointment in disorders of keratinization (9,10). Two randomized, double-blind, vehicle-controlled, right/left comparative studies demonstrated moderate improvement in patients with lamellar ichthyosis. Patients were studied for a period of 12 wk; no follow-up data was provided. Larger, long-term studies are needed to confirm these results. Calcipotriol ointment must be limited to a weekly dose below 100 g (9,10). Therefore, twice daily application is not practical in patients with generalized disease.

Azelaic acid, a dicarboxylic acid, has significant normalizing effects on the process of keratinization, including dose-dependent inhibition of DNA and protein synthesis (11). Other pharmacological properties include and antibacterial effects and anti-inflammatory effects via inhibition of hydroxy and superoxy radicals. Azelaic acid is available in the United States as a 20% cream. Oral forms have been administered to patients in dosages of up to 15 mg/d for 6 mo. Side effects have only included gastric irritation. Hematological variables including blood counts, liver function tests, blood chemistries, and urine analysis have not resulted in pathological changes (12,13). This drug may prove to be useful in the treatment of ichthyosis.

Although metothrexate is effective, the life-long duration of this disease precludes its continuous use. Intermittent courses may be used as in psoriasis. Rotational therapy, as described in the psoriasis chapter, may reduce single agent toxicity (14).

Numerous studies have demonstrated efficiency of the oral retinoids, isotretinoin, and etretinate at moderate to high dose(2 mg/kg/d) (15–17). Dramatic clinical improvement may occur, although optimal benefit seldom results in complete clearing. Systemic therapy should be reserved for patients with severe disease. Some authors recommend initation of therapy in the first few years of life to prevent the development of persistent ectropion (15). These children require chronic therapy and therefore are at risk to develop premature closure of the epiphyses. Skeletal changes resembling diffuse idiopathic skeletal hyperostosis have rarely been reported in children. Withdrawal of the retinoids results in rapid relapse, without rebound.

4. Method and Rationale for Treatment

Topical therapy is an integral component of treatment for all types of ichthyosis. For mild cases of CIE, tap water soaks followed by an ointment, such as petrolatum, provide minimal clinical improvement. Urea creams have been advocated by some authors as softening agents. Keratolytics, including alpha hydroxy acids, B hydroxy acids, and 40–60% propylene glycol in water provide some symptomatic improvement. These agents are more effective when treating the retention icythyosis, that is, linked ichthyosis and ichthyosis vulgaris (18).

Topical retinoic acid has been minimally effective in treating lamellar ichthyosis, but can cause significant irritation.

Calcipotriol can also be utilized as monotherapy or combined with systemic agents. Weekly topical doses should not exceed 100–120 g. If twice daily doses are utilized, approximately 15–20% of an adult's body can be treated. Daily applications have not been evaluated to date.

For patients with severe lamellar ichthyosis, the retinoids carry immeasurable physical, psychological, and social benefits. Early therapy can prevent persistant ectropion, and children under 1 y of age have been treated successfully. The pretreatment evaluation is described in the chapter on psoriasis. The subsequent risk of teratogenicity should be considered in the treatment of young girls. Therefore, isotretinoin therapy should be attempted before etretinate.

When isotretinoin is used, dosing begins at 0.5 mg/kg/d and is then increased as needed. Doses of 2 mg/kg/d are frequently required. Lower doses of etretinate are usually sufficient (0.5–1.0 mg/kg/d). Desquamation begins approximately 1 wk after beginning either drug. An optimal effect is usually reached after 2–3 wk (27).

Laboratory monitoring has already been described. There are no definitive monitoring guidelines for diffuse idiopathic skeletal hyperostosis or other skeletal changes. Paige et al. has advocated a baseline selective skeletal survey, excluding skull views, with follow-up radiology restricted to those with pretreatment radiological abnormalities or those who develop muscular skeletal symptoms (19). Most other authors recommend yearly x-rays of achilles tendons and the lateral thoracic spine. A child's growth should be monitored using a standarized growth curve.

B. Epidermolytic Hyperkeratosis

Epidermolytic hyperkeratosis (EH) or bullous congenital ichthyosiform erythroderma is a rare group of autosomal dominately inherited diseases occurring with a point prevalence of 1:200,000–300,000. However, up to 50% of new cases represent spontaneous mutations (20). At least three variants have been described: bullous ichthyotic erythroderma of Brocq, ichthyosis bullosa of Siemens, and ichthyosis hystrix of Curth-Macklin. DiGiovanna has categorized EH into six different subtypes showing varying amounts of palmoplantar hyperkeratosis, presence or absence of erythroderma, quality of scale, extent of involvement, and presence of digital contracture and posture/gait abnormalities (21).

General features of the diseases include erythema, blistering, and scale evident at birth. Bullae tend to form at sights of trauma. Hyperkeratotic, verrucous, malodorous plaques develop in flexoral areas. Normal appearing skin may be seen in the centers of the plaques. Severely affected individuals develop ectropion. Blistering usually resolves by age 8, however 20% of adults continue to develop recurrences. Bacterial overgrowth or infection may be responsible for the unpleasant odor and some blister formation. Palmoplantar hyperkeratosis may be disabling (21).

1. Etiology and Pathogenesis

Significant advances have been gained toward understanding the etiology of epidermolytic hyperkeratosis. Several different avenues of research have implicated epidermal differentiation in the pathogenesis of this heterogeneous disease. Frost et al. was the first to classify EH as a hyperproliferative disease based on histopathological and biometric observations (5, 6). Ultrastructural studies have revealed clumped keratin intermediate filaments in the malpighian layer of the epidermis. These have been identified as the differentiation-specific keratins, K1 and K10 (22). Mutations of these keratins produce a weakened cytoskeleton that results in cell fragility and lyses. Transgenic mice expressing mutant K1 and K10 genes develop abnormalities resembling human epidermolytic hyperkeratosis (23). More recently, genetic linkage to the type II keratin region on chromosome 12 has been reported (20). Several authors have identified point mutations in K1 and K10 genes. DiGiovanna has correlated some specific point mutations with clinical phenotypes of EH (20). In some cases, disease severity has also been correlated with the extent to which a mutation interferes with keratin network formation (24).

2. Pathology

The histopathological features of epidermolytic hyperkeratosis or bullous congenital ichthyosiform erythroderma are characteristic and diagnostic of this type of ichthyosis. Similar features are seen in bullous and nonbullous skin. The spinous and granular layers of the epidermis demonstrate various sized clear spaces surrounding keratinocyte nuclei. These cells show indistinct boundaries formed by amphophilic-staining cytoplasmic material or keratohyalin granules. The granular layer is greatly thickened and contains increased numbers of irregularly sized and shaped trichohyalin-like and keratohyalin-like granules. Compact hyperkeratosis without parakeratosis overlies the epidermis. Bullae arise intraepidermally through rupture of large clear-staining keratinocytes (20). These histological features may also be seen in a variety of processes including epidermal nevi, benign keratoses, palmoplantar keratoderma, or incidentally.

On electron microscopic examination large amounts of perinuclear endoplasmic reticulum with numerous canaliculi, ribosomal particles, and mitochondia are seen in the cells of the granular and spinous layers (25). As stated above, irregularly clumped tonofilaments are seen suprabasally. The keratin intermediate filaments 1 and 10 have been identified in these aggregates (22). In the granular layer, numerous keratohyalin granules are found embedded in shell-like formations of tonofilaments. Although the desmosomes appear normal, tonofilament attachments are disrupted. For example, a desmosome may be attached to only one keratinocyte.

3. Indications for the Use of Immunomodulatory and Cytotoxic Agents

Epidermolytic hyperkeratosis is the most recalcitrant ichthyosis to treatment. Topical regimens are minimally effective alone, but serve an integral role in all treatment plans. Pyogenic infection is common and may produce blistering. Topical antibacterial products and appropriate antibiotics should be adminstered liberally. In addition, fungal colonization can be treated with topical antifungal medications. The efficiency of calcipotriol ointment has not been adequately evaluated.

In the future, it may be possible to directly target the keratin mutations. At present, in severe cases of epidermolytic hyperkeratosis, retinoids may represent the only effective therapy. Unfortunately, dramatic clinical improvement as in lamellar ichthyosis may not occur. Additionally, there have been numerous reports of increased blistering while on retinoid therapy (15).

4. Method and Rationale for Treatment

Topical therapy, including emollients, urea creams, and keratolytics are utilized as in other ichthyoses. Antibacterial products, including soaps and washes, decrease bacterial overgrowth, help control odor, and decrease the incidence of infections.

Retinoids are administered to individuals with severe disease. As in other forms of ichthyosis, chronic therapy is required. Guidelines were discussed in the previous section. The increased blistering associated with retinoid use can occasionally be controlled with antibiotics. Relapse occurs rapidly when the medications are discontinued. Some children improve at puberty, therefore retinoid withdrawal may be attempted. Rotational therapy as described for psoriasis may also be attempted.

REFERENCES

1. Kolde G, Happle R, Traupe H. Autosomal-dominant lamellar icythyosis: ultrastructural characterics of a new type of congenital icythyosis. Arch Dermat Res 1985; 278:1–5.

2. Hazell M, Marks R. Clinical, histologic and cell kenetic discriminants between lamellar ichthyosis and nonbullous congenital ichthyosiform erythroderma. Arch Dermat 1985; 121:489–493.
3. Bergers M, Traupe H, Dunnwald SC, et al. Enzymatic distinction between two subgroups of autosomal recessive lamellar icythyosis. J Invest Dermat 1990; 94:407–412.
4. Williams ML, Elias PM. Heterogeneity in autosomal recessive ichthyosis: clinical and biochemical differentiation of lamellar ichthyosis and nonbullous congenital ichthyosiform erythroderma. Arch Dermat 1985; 121:477–488.
5. Frost P, Weinstein GD, Van Scott EJ. The ichthyosiform dermatoses: II. Autoradiographic studies of epidermal proliferation. J Invest Dermat 1966; 47:561–567.
6. Frost P, Van Scott EJ. Ichthyosiform dermatoses. Arch Dermat 1966; 94:113–126.
7. DiGiovanna JJ, Rogers GR, Steinert PM, et al. Mutations in the gene for transglutaminase I in autosomal recessive lamellar ichthyosis. Nat Genet 1995; 9:2279–2283.
8. Van Scott EJ, Uy RJ. Control of keratinization with alpha-hydroxy acids and related compounds. Arch Dermat 1974; 110:586–590.
9. Lucker GPH, VandeKerkhof PCM, et al. Effect of topical calcipatriol ointment on congenital ichthyosis. Br J Dermat 1994; 131:546–550.
10. Kragbelle K, Steiglen PM, et al. Efficacy tolerability and safety of calcipatriol ointment in disorders of keratinization. Arch Dermat 1995; 131:556–560.
11. Detmar PH, Muller R, Gasmuller H, et al. Effects of azelaic acid on protein synthesis and proliferation of cultered human keratinocytes. In: Orfanos CE, Stadler R, Gollnick H, eds. Dermatology in five continents. Proceedings of the XVII World Congress of Dermatology. Berlin; Springer Verlag, 1988:1169.
12. Greub HR. An open, non-controlled clinical multicenter study topical 20 percent azelaic acid cream in continous long-term treatment of acne vulgaris. Data on file. Schering AG, 1995.
13. Graupe K, Cunliffe WJ, et al. Efficacy and safety of topical azalaic acid (20 percent cream): an overview of results from European clinical trials and experimental reports. Cutis 1996; 57:20–35.
14. Weinstein GD, White GM. An approach to the treatment of moderate to severe psoriasis with rotational therapy. J Am Acad Dermat 1993; 28:454–459.
15. Tamayo L, Ruiz-Maldorado R. Oral retinoid (Ro10-9359) in children with lamellar ichthyosis, epidermolytic hyperkeratosis and symmetrical progressive erythrokertoderma. Dermatology 1980; 161:305–314.
16. Gilgor RS, Chiaramanti A, et al. Evaluation of 13-cis retinoic acid in lamellar ichthyosis, pityriasis rubra pilaris and Dariers disease. Cutis 1980; 25:380–385.
17. Baden HP, Burman MM, et al. Treatment of ichthyosis with isotretinoin. J Am Acad Dermat 1982; 6:716–720.
18. Baden HP, Goldsmith LA. Propylene glycol with occlusion for treatment of ichthyosis. JAMA 1972; 220:579–580.
19. Paige DG, Judge MR, et al. Bone changes and their significance in children with ichthyosis on long-term etretinate therapy. Br J Dermat 1992; 127:387–391.
20. DiGiovanna JJ, Bale SJ. Epidermolytic hyperkeratosis: applied moleculer genetics. J Invest Dermat 1994; 102:390–394.

21. DiGiovanna JJ, Bale SJ. Clinical heterogeneity in epidermolytic hyperkeratosis. Arch Dermat 1994; 103:1026–1035.
22. Ishida-Yamamoto A, Leigh IM, Lane EB, et al. Selective expression of the differentiation specific keratins K1 and K10 in the tonofilament clumps of bullous ichthyosis (epidermolytic hyperkeratosis). J Invest Dermat 1992; 99:10–25.
23. Vassar R, Coulombe PA, et al. Mutant keratin expression in transgenic mice causes marked abnormalities resembling human genetic skin disease. Cell 1991; 64:365–380.
24. Syder JA, Yu QC, et al. Genetic mutations in the K1 and K10 genes of patients with epidermolytic hyperkeratosis: correlation between location and disease severity. J Clin Invest 1994; 93:1533–1542.
25. Wilgram GF, Caulfield JB. An electron microscopic study of epidermolytic hyperkeratosis. Arch Dermat 1966; 94:127–143.

20
Kaposi's Sarcoma

Charles J. McDonald
Brown University, Providence, Rhode Island

Kaposi's sarcoma (Kaposi's hemorrhagic sarcoma, multiple idiopathic hemorrhagic sarcoma [Kaposi], and idiopathic multiple pigmented sarcoma) was formerly a rare neoplastic disorder that in the nonimmunocompromised host usually presents with quite typical cutaneous lesions. The cutaneous lesions are so typical that a definitive clinical diagnosis may be made on the basis of cutaneous findings alone. Kaposi's sarcoma and its classical cutaneous manifestations were first described by the Hungarian dermatologist Moricz Kaposi in 1872 p. (1). Until a decade ago, Kaposi's sarcoma was a medical oddity, largely unknown and of interest only to the dermatologist, the inquiring oncologist in equatorial Africa, and the occasional virologist with an interest in the role of viruses in the induction of human cancer.

Slightly more than 10 y ago an association with acquired immunodeficiency syndrome (AIDS) was identified and an intense medical interest in Kaposi's sarcoma began to develop. The intensive investigations now taking place, particularly on the association and relationship among viruses, immunodeficiency, and the development of cancers like Kaposi's sarcoma, have uncovered another substantial element in the puzzle of human neoplasia, its etiology and pathogenesis.

I. INCIDENCE AND EPIDEMIOLOGY

Until the outbreak of Kaposi's sarcoma in patients with AIDS was uncovered it was known to occur predominately in two forms. The most common is seen in populations of Europeans, principally North Americans, Central Europeans, and Italians, and is considered a benign indolent disease of men 50–60 y of age. In Europeans, 10–15 men will develop Kaposi's sarcoma for every woman affected.

In North America and Europe the reported incidence of Kaposi's sarcoma is 0.02–0.06 cases per 100,000 population (2,3). In North America, cases among Italian and Jewish men predominate, thus giving some credence to theories of racial and ethnic predispositions and the influence of genetics in the pathogenesis of this disease. Braverman offers a well-reasoned discussion of factors relative to racial predominance and ethnic background in European cases of Kaposi's sarcoma (4).

The second form is usually seen in African populations. Kaposi's sarcoma in Africa occurs principally south of the Sahara, in equatorial or tropical Africa. The highest incidence is found in populations of Uganda, Tanzania, Zaire, Kenya, and in the Bantu of South Africa, where Kaposi's sarcoma accounts for 6–10% of all malignant neoplasms in men (5–7). In females of the same region Kaposi's sarcoma makes up less than 0.6% of all cancers. Thus, in African populations Kaposi's sarcoma also affects men most often, but here the similarities between the African and European disease ends. In African men and women the disease tends to occur at an earlier age, occurring principally in the third and fourth decades, and it also appears to take a more aggressive and virulent course, much like the disease seen in patients with AIDS (3,7).

In the United States Kaposi's sarcoma has been reported in 34% of homosexual men with human immunodeficiency virus (HIV) infection and AIDS, and in only 6% of patients in all other HIV-infected groups (8). Kaposi's sarcoma is the most common neoplasm occurring in patients with AIDS. In these patients Kaposi's sarcoma is a fairly virulent disease and is often referred to as "epidemic" Kaposi's sarcoma. In spite of its increased virulence, patients with HIV-associated Kaposi's sarcoma appear to have an improved survival rate over those experiencing infectious complications of HIV disease. In San Francisco, Rutherford et al. (9) have reported a declining proportion of patients with AIDS-related Kaposi's sarcoma.

On numerous occasions it has been reported that black African children suffer a higher incidence of Kaposi's sarcoma than children of other races; Templeton (7) does not agree, stating that children account for approximately 4% of cases in both Caucasian (North American and European) and African groups. Dutz and Stout (10) report that children under 6 y of age account for approximately 3.3% of all described cases and most of these have come from the African continent. In children the disease shows much less male over female predominance, occurring in a ratio of 1–3:1 male to female.

Even in regions of Africa where the prevalence rate of Kaposi's sarcoma is high in native blacks, the disease incidence is low or nonexistent in whites. There is considerable speculation on the disparity between incidence rates in blacks in the Americas—North, Central, and Caribbean—and in black Africans. In black populations in the Americas, Kaposi's sarcoma occurs at a rate equal to or somewhat lower than in the white population. Often disparate incidence figures are used to refute genetic as well as racial factors that may be important in the pathogenesis of Kaposi's sarcoma. However, a closer look at these figures, keeping in mind earlier forced immigration patterns and the West African origin of most blacks in the Americas, lends support for both genetic and racial factors in the development of Kaposi's sarcoma. With few exceptions blacks in the Americas are descendants of blacks from western Africa. In the indigenous population of western Africa the incidence of Kaposi's sarcoma is about equal to that found in black Americans, and is much lower than that found in black's of equatorial Africa.

II. ETIOLOGY AND PATHOGENESIS

Despite more than a decade of intensive study the etiology of Kaposi's sarcoma remains obscure. The wealth of recent observations on the role of infection, immunosuppression, and the immune deficiency state, along with previously recorded observations, will possibly provide some important clues to the etiology of Kaposi's sarcoma. The acral parts and the lower extremities below the knees are the most commonly observed sites for lesions in typical non-HIV-related nodular type Kaposi's sarcoma, hence trauma and stasis associated with prolonged periods of standing in outdoor occupations have been proposed as prime etiological factors. To date there is no scientific evidence to support this hypothesis.

Substantial evidence has emerged to support a primary etiological role for bacterial and viral infection, immunosuppression, or an immunodeficient state in genetically predisposed hosts (11–17). A large number of immunological abnormalities have been described in HIV-infected persons. The major defect is a persistent profound quantitative and functional defect of a lymphocyte subset characterized by the expression of the $CD4^+$ antigen (helper-inducer T cells) (18). HIV has a selective tropism for helper-inducer T cells, infecting these as well as other peripheral blood cells such as the Langerhans cell and macrophages (19,20). Additionally, HIV appears to have a marked cytopathic effect on infected helper T cells. Thus, helper T-cell infection by HIV leads to severe and irreversible immunodeficiency. In a genetically predisposed host immune deficiency leads to unregulated growth of tumors like Kaposi's sarcoma.

Based on results from studies designed to assess immune function in a spectrum of patients with Kaposi's sarcoma, Martin et al. conclude the data suggests that immunosuppression is not required for the development of Kaposi's sarcoma (21). However, its presence predisposes an individual to an aggressive form of the disease.

Cytomegalovirus has been implicated as a primary etiological agent in the pathogenesis of Kaposi's sarcoma based on findings in serological studies (22), on the finding of cytomegalogenome in Kaposi's sarcoma tissue (16), and on the finding of virus particles in tissue culture of Kaposi's sarcoma material (23). In a group of 13 male homosexual patients with AIDS, disseminated cytomegalovirus infection was found in 12 and Kaposi's sarcoma in 12. In two patients Kaposi's sarcoma was found in internal organs but not in skin (24). When seen in the tissues of adults cytomegalovirus inclusions are found prominently in association with and within vascular endothelial cells, thus suggesting cytomegalovirus tropism for endothelial cells. There is strong evidence showing that Kaposi's sarcoma is a primary tumor of vascular endothelial cells. These findings strongly suggest that cytomegalovirus may be the causal pathogen in Kaposi's sarcoma, however, its presence in vascular endothelium of an infected person may also represent an opportunistic infection in an immunocompromised host.

While engaged in a laboratory search for a specific viral agent that might induce Kaposi's sarcoma, Gallo and Nerurkar (17) found that human retrovirus-infected $CD4^+$ lymphocytes produce a heretofore unrecognized growth factor which, when applied in vitro to a mixed population of cells from Kaposi's sarcoma tumor, stimulated growth of a group of cells that closely resemble the characteristic spindle cells of Kaposi's sarcoma. In addition to producing a vast array of biologically active substances in culture, when inoculated into nude mice these cells also induce early human sarcoma-like tumors. These and other observations have led Gallo and Nerurkar (17) to the following hypothesis: HIV and other retrovirus infection of $CD4^+$ lymphocytes and macrophages cause release of several cytokines, including a growth factor that promotes activation and growth of cells of possible endothelial origin. Endothelial cells are induced to undergo changes that result in formation of cells with Kaposi's sarcoma spindle cell morphology. These cells in turn produce and release self-perpetuating growth factors and cytokines. Ultimately a characteristic tumor is produced.

Friedman-Kien and Harte have described cases of six homosexual men who have Kaposi's sarcoma but show no evidence of infection with HIV (25). Some investigators cite these cases as evidence that the AIDS virus cannot be considered the primary pathological agent for Kaposi's sarcoma. Others suggest that a sexually transmitted pathogen yet to be identified is the causative agent. The sarcoma is more common in people infected with the AIDS virus through sexual contact than by contaminated needles or blood.

There exists a highly significant association between the development of Kaposi's sarcoma and other neoplasms in non-HIV-infected persons, principally neoplasms of the lymphoreticular system such as lymphomas (particularly Hodgkin's disease), leukemias, and multiple myeloma (26–28). This association is relevant in the white (North American) or non-African populations among whom second neoplasms have been estimated to be the most common cause of death (28). Most second neoplasms are derived from lymphoreticular tissues and Kaposi's sarcoma develops either simultaneously or subsequently in these patients. This mutual occurrence, therefore, may be associated with known immunodeficiencies in patients with lymphomas, leukemias, and myeloma.

Finally, there is a vast array of literature describing the initial onset of Kaposi's sarcoma in patients who are being treated actively with cytotoxic or immunosuppressive agents. Many of these "acquired" tumors recede spontaneously upon dosage reduction or complete withdrawal of cytotoxic or immunosuppressive therapy.

III. PATHOLOGY AND NATURAL HISTORY

Kaposi's sarcoma presents with a diversity of clinical features, the nature of presentation depending primarily on the racial group affected, the age and gender of the patient, and the status of the host's immune system (Table 1). In elderly males of European extraction the disease classically presents with solitary or multiple red, brown, blue, or purple macules, papules, nodules, and plaques. Nodules and plaques vary in size and degree of firmness. Early lesions most often appear on acral parts, especially the fingers and toes. Some are occasionally found on the face, scalp, or genitalia. Acute lesions most commonly occur on the lower extremities where they tend to be distributed bilaterally. As the lesions age, macules develop into plaques and papules into nodules. Large plaques frequently lose their characteristic color and become covered with a thick pale hyperkeratotic (scaly) surface. Occasionally, plaque-like lesions resolve spontaneously, leaving large atrophic telangiectatic and hyperpigmented patches. On the surface of some lesions the epidermis becomes atrophic and ulcerates, particularly on large nodular lesions or clusters of nodular lesions. Eventually a large fungating, necrotic tissue mass will become prominent at the site of ulceration. In spite of diversity of appearance, most individual lesions are quite characteristic and are not difficult for the dermatologist to diagnose. The differential diagnosis of Kaposi's cutaneous lesions include hemangioma, lymphangioma, granuloma pyogenicum, glomus tumor, and melanoma.

A brawny type of edema is often associated with upper and lower extremity lesions, particularly as the lesions enlarge. Edema may result from microscopic as well as macroscopic dermal lymphatic obstruction by tumor.

In patients of European extraction visceral organ disease, though infrequent, may involve the gastrointestinal tract. This involvement may be so extensive that occult gastrointestinal bleeding may be the presenting sign. In cases with gastrointestinal disease, typical blue to purple blebs and nodules may be found on the tongue, buccal mucosa, and throughout the gastrointestinal tract. Other organ involvement is rare and generally asymptomatic. Involvement of the central nervous system has not been reported.

Table 1 Characteristics of Various Clinical Forms of Kaposi's Sarcoma

Type of Disease	Histologic Pattern	Age Distribution	Gender Predominance	Race Predominantly Affected	Response to Therapy*
1. Indolent					
A. Papules Plaques Nodules	Mixed cellularity	>50 y	Male	C	Good
B. Nodules	Mixed cellularity	>50 y	Male	B	Good
2. Aggressive					
A. Florid (exophytic ulcerative)	Mixed cellularity; monocellular; anaplastic	>50 y	Male	B	Excellent
B. Infiltrative	Monocellular	>50 y	Male	B	Poor
C. Lymphadenopathic	Mixed cellularity	0–10	Male, female	C,B	Excellent
D. Cutaneous; lymphadenopathic; systemic	Mixed cellularity	20–40 y	Male, female	B†	Poor

* Response to radiotherapy or chemotherapy.
† Now found to be the dominant disease type in patients with the acquired immune deficiency syndrome (AIDS), nearly all of whom are young Caucasian males.
C = Caucasian; B = blacks.
Source: McDonald CJ. Malignant neoplasms of the skin. In: Calabresi P, Schein PS, eds. Medical oncology, 2nd ed. New York: McGraw-Hill, 1993:536.

In children, Kaposi's sarcoma rarely occurs on the skin, but most often involves the lymphoreticular system. Most children present with strikingly diffuse, discrete, nontender lymphadenopathy and hepatosplenomegaly. Occasionally the eyelids, lacrimal glands, and parotid glands may be involved (6). In young African and Haitian adults widespread cutaneous and systemic involvement is characteristic and is associated with a rapidly fatal course (7). This pattern of disease is also seen in HIV-associated disease and in immunosuppressed patients (3).

Although most patients with Kaposi's sarcoma present with clusters of lesions that develop at various times, the origin of distant disease is thought to be multicentric rather than metastatic. Regional lymph node metastases are rare, but aggressive lesions often diffusely infiltrate surrounding subcutaneous tissues and bone (7).

Due to the variability of clinical expression in the African-type Kaposi's sarcoma, Taylor et al. (14) developed a morphological classification that identifies disease according to clinical presentation, histopathological pattern, clinical course, and response to therapy (see Table 1). Four types are identified and include nodular, florid (exophytic or ulcerative), infiltrative, and lymphadenopathic. The nodular type is most commonly encountered and is quite indolent. Florid disease occurs principally as rapidly growing exophytic ulcerating tumors. This type of tumor is often deeply invasive and frequently involves bone. Infiltrative disease, seen more often in European populations, results from widespread tumor infiltration of skin and subcutaneous tissues. It is usually confined to one or more extremities and is often associated with firm nonpitting edema in the affected part. The lymphadenopathic type is seen most commonly in children. Tumor infiltrates are confined to lymphoreticular tissues. Cutaneous and other organ involvement are rare. To these four can be added an additional type best described as cutaneous lymphadenopathic Kaposi's sarcoma. This disease occurs almost exclusively in young adult males and females (10,12,14). The prognosis is poor; the disease is very difficult to treat, and death occurs rapidly in a very high percentage of cases.

In patients infected with HIV the clinical picture may differ. Atypical lesions may be solitary or disseminated. Color can vary from light tan to deep purple, and macules may be more common than nodules. Lesion distribution varies; 29% are found on the lower extremities, 19% on the upper extremities, 9% on the trunk and lymph nodes, and 7% on oral mucous membranes (29). Surprisingly, survival of patients with lymph node involvement has been better than that of patients with skin disease only. Follicular, zosteriform, or liner patterned lesions may be seen.

Histopathologically lesions of Kaposi's sarcoma show one of three basic cellular patterns: mixed cellularity, monocellular or spindle cell, or anaplastic disease (30). The mixed cellular pattern is the most common and most typical pattern. Mixed tumors are composed of interlacing bundles of spindle-shaped cells, many having the appearance of endothelial cells, especially when lining well-defined vascular channels. Other cells lie in aggregates. Sometimes the tumor is composed predominantly of endothelial-lined vascular spaces. Early lesions show an intense perivascular as well as diffuse cellular infiltrate composed of lymphocytes, plasma cells, and histiocytes. Clusters of extravasated red blood cells and hemosiderin may be scattered throughout the lesion. As the tumor grows, spindle cells and vascular channels proliferate and the inflammatory component lessens. Lesions of mixed cellularity are seen in most patients with "nodular disease," in all patients with "lymphadenopathic disease," and in patients with "florid disease."

Monocellular or spindle cell tumors are characterized by a predominance of spindle cells and the virtual absence of endothelial cell and vascular channel proliferation. In most of these lesions typical mixed cellularity Kaposi's tissue may be seen at the periphery (7). Histopathologically this lesion is very difficult to distinguish from a number of other mesenchymal tumors. It may resemble fibrosarcoma or leiomyosarcoma, as well as spindle cell variants of squamous cell carcinoma and spindle cell amelanotic melanoma (31). The pleomorphic or anaplastic variant contains numerous anaplastic cells showing nuclear pleomorphism and multiple mitoses. Although the anaplastic pattern is associated almost exclusively with florid-type lesions, it is an unusual presentation in Kaposi's sarcoma tissue.

The histopathological features of Kaposi's sarcoma in AIDS patients are very similar to those seen in all forms of Kaposi's sarcoma (32).

Since Kaposi's original description of this disease in which he proposes a vascular origin, numerous discussions have arisen over the exact origins of tumor cells. Both a lymphoreticular origin (33–35) and a direct origin from Schwann cells have many proponents (36,37). The current more widely supported view is that Kaposi's sarcoma originates from an angioformative or pluripotential endothelial cell (24,38–40). A large body of evidence, including electron microscopic observations of tumor cell type, tends to support a vascular origin, at least in part. Spindle cells and vascular channel lining cells of Kaposi's sarcoma tissue show reactivity to monoclonal antibodies that recognize endothelial cell surface antigens (40). Factor VIII-related antigen has been demonstrated in neoplastic cells in Kaposi's sarcoma (24). Endothelial cells were shown to synthesize factor VIII (41). Finally, cytomegalovirus inclusions when found in human tissues are nearly always located in vascular endothelial cells. Cytomegalovirus tropism for endothelial cells has been suggested, further adding to the evidence supporting the viral (cytomegalovirus) etiology of Kaposi's sarcoma.

IV. DIAGNOSIS

The clinical diagnosis of Kaposi's sarcoma is not difficult in either the European or African variety. In 90% of cases the characteristic clinical features described earlier are present. In the other 10% of cases diagnosis can be made on the basis of characteristic histopathological findings. In most cases the typical mixed cellular type of histological pattern is seen, even in the clinically recognizable florid form of the disease. The pleomorphic or anaplastic type of Kaposi's sarcoma is very rare and histological diagnosis may be difficult.

Patients with HIV-associated Kaposi's sarcoma often present with a wide variety of atypical cutaneous lesions that may be scattered over the entire integument. Any new cutaneous eruption in individuals at risk for the development of HIV infection should arouse suspicion and the eruption should be biopsied. Histological examination is usually confirmatory.

In any diagnostic evaluation of patients with cutaneous lesions, the gastrointestinal tract and the respiratory tract must be examined, because extracutaneous involvement is most common in these systems. This is particularly true in the European or non-African variety of Kaposi's sarcoma. In children all elements of the reticuloendothelial system may be involved, therefore a thorough examination of the lymph nodes, liver, spleen, and parotid glands is in order. Rarely are other systems involved in this population. In young adults disseminated disease is most common, therefore all organ systems must be examined.

Thallium-201 scintigraphy is a potentially useful procedure for detecting extracutaneous Kaposi's sarcoma in AIDS patients. Thallium appears to show an avidity for Kaposi's sarcoma tissue in lymph nodes, lung, mucosa, and the vagina (42).

V. STAGING

It has become widely recognized that a system for staging AIDS-associated Kaposi's sarcoma is definitely required to uniformly evaluate pretreatment patient characteristics, clinical status, and subsequent clinical responses. Classifying patients into limited or extensive disease categories allows a clinician to properly select appropriate local or systemic therapy. Krigel et al. proposed a practical system for staging Kaposi's sarcoma using estimates of tumor extent and observed rate of progression (43). Four primary staging groups were described. This system was found appropriate for staging traditionally encountered disease. However, as the number of HIV-associated Kaposi's sarcoma patients increased, its inadequacies soon became apparent. For example, clinical symptoms were initially omitted and the presence or absence of immunological and virological influences on disease state were not considered. Recognizing these deficiencies Chachova et al. have proposed a new system of staging with many modifications of the original system (44).

Meanwhile Krown and members of the National Institute of Allergy and Infectious Diseases (NIAID)-sponsored AIDS Clinical Trials Group (ACTG) have suggested a new and more comprehensive system (45). Members of ACTG have proposed standardized criteria for the evaluation of HIV-associated disease response in ACTG therapeutic trials. Limitations in this system are readily acknowledged, but it is unlikely that any system will be comprehensive enough to satisfy all criteria in such a multifaceted disease.

VI. TREATMENT

Kaposi's sarcoma of the indolent type, principally confined to limited areas of the skin, is radiosensitive to both gamma rays and electrons (46,47). A correlation appears to exist between the treatment given and the likelihood of long-term response.

Patients with either form of indolent cutaneous disease who do not respond to radiation therapy may be responsive to a single chemotherapeutic agent, as may patients with indolent disease involving other organ systems (48–51). Of the single agents reported to date, vinblastine appears to be the most widely used. Weekly intravenous vinblastine is effective in controlling both localized and generalized forms of the disease in elderly patients without inducing serious systemic toxicity. The major disadvantage of vinblastine therapy is the necessity for protracted use of the drug.

Various combinations of chemotherapeutic drugs have been used for control of the more aggressive forms of the disease as well as for control of widespread indolent disease in patients with nonepidemic Kaposi's sarcoma. The most impressive results using combination chemotherapy has been reported by Olweny (50). Of 32 patients receiving a three-drug combination of actinomycin-D, vincristine, and DTIC, 30 achieved complete remission, 1 a partial remission, and 1 did not respond to therapy. Similar results were reported in children. Two patients with very aggressive disease were treated with a three-drug combination consisting of vincristine, actinomycin-D, and bleomycin. Both achieved complete disease remission.

Patients with Kaposi's sarcoma and AIDS also respond to cytotoxic chemotherapy. Single-agent regimens using either vinblastine, vincristine, or etoposide have shown substantial efficacy, with response rates of nearly 90% in some trials (52). Excellent response rates, however, are often accompanied by moderate to severe adverse reactions, including an increased incidence of opportunistic infections and further immune suppression, problems that are not encountered in non-AIDS-associated Kaposi's sarcoma.

In an attempt to reduce adverse effects, combinations of chemotherapeutic agents have been studied. An alternating regimen of vinblastine and vincristine shows considerable promise (52). A combination using adriamycin, bleomycin, and vincristine has produced complete or partial responses in a majority of advanced cases of epidemic Kaposi's sarcoma while causing relatively mild and tolerable toxicity (53). Gompels et al. report on the treatment of 46 severely ill patients using vincristine and bleomycin (54). They conclude that the regimen is effective and has low toxicity in AIDS patients.

As reports of successful treatment of epidemic Kaposi's sarcoma continue to appear, it is important to recall that Kaposi's sarcoma is rarely the cause of death in HIV-infected patients. Treatment is rarely curative, hence drug treatment should not negatively influence survival. There is at least one study which concludes that appropriately given chemotherapy, even in severely affected patients, does not increase survival (55).

The initial report of the successful use of purified human interferon in epidemic Kaposi's sarcoma has led to a proliferation of studies using this agent in a single-drug regimen, as well as in a variety of combinations with cytotoxic drugs (56). Interferon-α, at first glance, appears to be an ideal drug for use in patients who have developed tumors subsequent to immunosuppression. However, in studies using IFN-α alone, therapeutic results to date can at best be considered modest (57,58). Krown has described a subset of epidemic Kaposi's sarcoma patients who appear most likely to benefit from IFN-α treatment alone (59). They lack such systemic symptoms as fever, weight loss, and night sweats, have not experienced opportunistic infections, and have relatively good preservation of immune function (total CD4 lymphocyte count greater than 200/mm and T4/T8 cell ratios greater than 0.5).

The efficacy of high-dose versus low-dose IFN-α continues to be debated. So does the use of IFN-α combined with a cytotoxic agent. There are proponents of combination therapy who feel that there is data to suggest that IFN-α plus one or more standard chemotherapeutic drugs allows maximization of the therapeutic potential of each individual agent (58). Others suggest that there is no convincing evidence to support the concept that a combination of IFN-α and any cytotoxic drug improves clinical response, nor does it reduce drug toxicity (57,59). Other investigations have described an improved outcome with the addition of zidovudine to the treatment regimen using IFN-α in combination or as a single agent (60).

Radiation therapy using photons or orthovoltage has been reported as successful in palliating disease in patients with extensive cutaneous lesions (61). Likewise intralesional injections of vinblastine, IFN-α, and IL-2 may offer some palliative effect (62,63).

Surgery has been of limited use in localized disease. It may be well to conclude this section on treatment of Kaposi's sarcoma with a referral to a recent publication of Miles et al. (64) in which improved survival of patients with AIDS-related Kaposi's sarcoma appears to be occurring irrespective of the treatment used.

REFERENCES

1. Kaposi M. Idiopathisches multiples pigmentsarkom der haut. Arch Dermat Syph 1872; 4:265–273.
2. Oettle AG. Skin cancer in Africa. Natl Cancer Inst Monogr 1963; 10:197–214.
3. Friedman-Kein AE. Disseminated Kaposi's sarcoma syndrome in young homosexual men. J Am Acad Dermat 1981; 5:468–471.
4. Braverman IM. Kaposi's hemorrhagic sarcoma. In: Braverman IM, ed. Skin signs of systemic disease. Philadelphia: W.B. Saunders 1981.
5. Taylor JF, Smith PG, Bull D, Pike MC. Kaposi's sarcoma in Uganda: geographic and ethnic distribution. Br J Cancer 1972; 26:483–497.
6. Olweny CLM, Toya T, Katongole-Mbidde E, Lwanga SK, Owor R, Kyalwazi S, Vogel CB. Treatment of Kaposi's sarcoma by combination of actinomycin-D, vincristine and imidazole carboxamide (NSC-45388): results of a randomized clinical trial. Int J Cancer 1974; 14:649–656.
7. Templeton AC. Kaposi's sarcoma. Pathol Annu 1981; 16:315–336.
8. Curran JW, Morgan WM, Hardy AM, Jaffe HW, Darrow WW, Dowtle WR. The epidemiology of AIDS: current status and future prospects. Science 1985; 229:1352–1357.
9. Rutheford GW, Schwarcz SK, Lemp GF, Barnhart JL, Rauch KJ, Warner WL, Piland TH, Werdegar SD. The epidemiology of AIDS-related Kaposi's sarcoma in San Francisco. J Infect Dis 1989; 159:569–572.
10. Dutz W, Stout AP. Kaposi's sarcoma in infants and children. Cancer 1960; 13:684–694.
11. Masters SP, Taylor JF, Kyalwazi SK, Ziegler JL. Immunological studies in Kaposi's sarcoma in Uganda. Br Med J 1970; 1:600–602.
12. Haim S, Friedman-Birnbaum R, Better OS, Tuma S. Skin complications in immunosuppressed patients: follow up of kidney recipients. Br J Dermat 1973; 89:169–173.
13. Taylor JF. Lymphocyte transformation in Kaposi's sarcoma. Lancet 1973; 1:883–884.
14. Taylor JF, Templeton AC, Vogel CL, Ziegler JL, Kycelwazi SK. Kaposi's sarcoma in Uganda: a clinicopathological study. Int J Cancer 1971; 8:122–135.
15. Giraldo G, Beth E, Kyalwazi SK. Etiological implications of Kaposi's sarcoma. Antibiot Chemother 1981; 29:12–31.
16. Boldogh I, Beth E, Huang ES, Kyalwazi SK, Giraldo G. Kaposi's sarcoma. IV. Detections of CMV DNA, CMV RNA and CMNA in tumor biopsies. Int J Cancer 1981; 28:469–474.
17. Gallo RC, Nerurkar LS. Human retroviruses: their role in neoplasia and immunodeficiency. Ann NY Acad Sci 1989; 567:82–94.
18. Cavaille-Coll M, Messiah A, Klatzmann D, Rosenbaum W, Lachiver D, Kernbaum S, Brisson B, Chapuis F, Blanc C, Debra P, Glucksman JD. Critical analysis of T-cell subset and function evaluation in patients with persistent generalized lymphadenopathy in groups at risk for AIDS. Clin Exp Immunol 1984; 57:511–19.
19. Tenner-Racz K, Racz P, Dietrich M, Kern P. Altered follicular dendritic cells and virus-like particles in AIDS and AIDS-related lymphadenopathy. Lancet 1985; 1:105–106.

20. Gyorkey F, Melnick JL, Sinkovics JG, Gyorkey P. Retrovirus resembling HTLV in macrophages of patients with AIDS. Lancet 1985; 1:106.
21. Martin ME, Solodnik T, Rosenthal CJ. Role of immune disregulation in Kaposi's sarcoma. Proc Annu Meet Am Soc Clin Oncol 1988; 7:A23.
22. Giraldo G, Beth E, Kourilsky FM, Henle G, Mike V, Hurauy JM, Andersen HK, Gharbi MR, Kyalwazi SK, Puissant A. Antibody patterns to herpes virus in Kaposi's sarcoma: serological association of European Kaposi's sarcoma with cytomegalovirus. Int J Cancer 1975; 15:839–848.
23. Giraldo G, Beth E, Haguenau F. Herpes-type virus particles in tissue culture of Kaposi's sarcoma from different geographic regions. J Natl Cancer Inst 1972; 49:1509–1526.
24. Guarda LG, Silva EG, Ordones NG, Smith JL. Factor VIII in Kaposi's sarcoma. Am J Clin Pathol 1981; 76:197–200.
25. Friedman-Kien AE, Harte JS. Meeting report: American Academy of Dermatology symposium on AIDS, 1990. J Am Acad Dermat 1991; 25:1086–1091.
26. Reynolds WA, Winkelman RK, Soule EH. Kaposi's sarcoma: a clinicopathologic study with particular reference to its relationship to the reticuloendothelial system. Medicine 1965; 44:419–443.
27. Safai B, Mike V, Giraldo G, Betu E, Good RA. Association of Kaposi's sarcoma with secondary primary malignancies: possible etiopathogenic implications. Cancer 1980; 45:1472–1479.
28. Ulbright TM, Santa Cruz DJ. Kaposi's sarcoma: relationship with hematologic, lymphoid, and thymic neoplasia. Cancer 1981; 47:963–973.
29. Myskowski PL, Niedzwiecki D, Shurgot BA, Kaufman D, Krown SE, Nisce L, Safai B. AIDS-associated Kaposi's sarcoma: variables associated with survival. J Am Acad Dermat 1988; 18:1299–1306.
30. Lever WF, Schaumberg-Lever G. Histopathology of the skin, 6th ed. Philadelphia: JB Lippincott, 1983.
31. Hutt MSR. Pathology of Kaposi's sarcoma. Antibiot Chemother 1981; 29:32–37.
32. Egbert B. Histologic features of AIDS-related Kaposi's sarcoma and its clinical and histopathologic mimics. Semin Dermat 1986; 5:308–315.
33. Dorffel J. Histogenesis of multiple idiopathic hemorrhagic sarcoma of Kaposi. Arch Dermat Syph 1932; 26:608–634.
34. Tedeschi CG. Some consideration concerning the nature of the so-called sarcoma of Kaposi. Arch Pathol 1958; 66:656–684.
35. Dayan A, Lewis PD. Origin of Kaposi's sarcoma from the reticuloendothelial system. Nature 1967; 213:889–890.
36. Mackee GM, Cipollaro AC. Idiopathic multiple hemorrhagic sarcoma (Kaposi). Am J Cancer 1936; 26:1.
37. Becker BJP. The histogenesis of Kaposi's sarcoma. Acta Un Int Cancer 1962; 18:477–486.
38. Hashimoto K, Lever WF. Kaposi's sarcoma: histochemical and electron microscope studies. J Invest Dermat 1964; 43:539–549.
39. Nadji M, Morales AR, Ziegles-Weissman J, Pennys NS. Kaposi's sarcoma: immunohistologic evidence for an endothelial origin. Arch Pathol Lab Med 1981; 105:274–275.

40. Scully PA, Steinman HK, Kennedy C, Trueblood K, Frisman DM, Voland JR. AIDS-related Kaposi's sarcoma displays differential expression of endothelial surface antigens. Am J Pathol 1988; 130:244–251.
41. Jaffee EA. Endothelial cells and the biology of factor VIII. N Engl J Med 1977; 296:377–383.
42. Lee VW, Rosen MP, Baum A, Cohen SE, Cooley TP, Liebman HA. AIDS-related Kaposi's sarcoma: findings on thallium-201 scintigraphy. Am J Radiol 1988; 151:1233–1235.
43. Krigel RL, Laubenstein LJ, Muggia FM. Kaposi's sarcoma: a new staging classification. Cancer Treat Rep 1983; 67:531–534.
44. Chachova A, Krigel RL, Lafleur F, Ostreicher R, Speer M, Laubenstein L, Wernz J, Rubenstein P, Zang E, Friedman-Kien A. Prognostic factors and staging classification of patients with epidemic Kaposi's sarcoma. J Clin Oncol 1989; 7(6):774–780.
45. Krown SE, Metroka C, Neruz JC, and AIDS Clinical Trials Group Oncology Committee. Kaposi's sarcoma in the acquired immunodeficiency syndrome: a proposal for uniform evaluation, response, and staging criteria. J Clin Oncol 1989; 7:1201–1207.
46. Nisce LZ, Safai B, Poussin-Rosillo H. Once weekly total and subtotal skin electron beam therapy for Kaposi's sarcoma. Cancer 1981; 47:640–644.
47. Cooper JS. The influence of dose on the long-term control of classic (new-aids associated) Kaposi's sarcoma by radiotherapy. Int J Radiat Oncol Bial Phys 1988; 15:114–116.
48. Vogel CL, Primack A, Dhru D. Treatment of Kaposi's sarcoma with actinomycin D and cyclosphosphamide: results of a randomized clinical trial. Int J Cancer 1971; 8:136–143.
49. Vogel CL, Primack A, Owor R, Kyalwazi SK. Effective treatment of Kaposi's sarcoma with 5-(3,3-dimethyl-1-triazeno) imidazole-4carboxamide (NSC-45388). Cancer Chemother Rep (part I) 1973; 57:65–71.
50. Olweny CLM. Management of Kaposi's sarcoma: chemotherapy II. Antibiot Chemother 1981; 29:88–95.
51. Solan AJ, Greenwald ES, Silvay O. Longterm complete remissions of Kaposi's sarcoma with vinblastine therapy. Cancer 1981; 47:637–639.
52. Volberding PA. The role of chemotherapy for epidemic Kaposi's sarcoma. Semin Oncol 1987; 14:23–26.
53. Gill P, Deyton L, Rarick M, Larelo C, Ray J, Levine AM. Results of a prospective trial of adriamycin, bleomycin and vincristine in the treatment of epidemic Kaposi's sarcoma. Proc Am Soc Clin Oncol 1987; 6:A18.
54. Gompels MM, Hill A, Jenkins P, et al. Kaposi's sarcoma in HIV infection treated with vincristine and bleomycin. AIDS 1992; 6:1175–1180.
55. Volberding F, Kusick P, Fevgal DW. Effect of chemotherapy for HIV-associated Kaposi's sarcoma on longterm survival. Proc Am So Clin Oncol 1989; 8:A11.
56. Krown SE, Real FK, Cunningham-Rundles S, et al. Prelim observations on the effect of recombinant leucocyte A interferon in homosexual men with Kaposi's sarcoma. N Engl J Med 1983; 308:1071–1076.
57. Abrams DI, Volberding PA. Alpha interferon therapy of AIDS-associated Kaposi's sarcoma. Semin Oncol 1987; 14:43–47.

58. Kern P, Meigel W, Racz P, Gotteslbeu A, Dettke T, Dietrich M. Interferon alpha in the treatment of AIDS-associated Kaposi's sarcoma. Onkologie 1987; 10:50–52.
59. Krown SE. The role of interferon in the therapy of epidemic Kaposi's sarcoma. Semin Oncol 1987; 14:27–33.
60. Paredis J, Krown SE. Interferon alpha therapy in patients with Kaposi's sarcoma and the acquired immunodeficiency syndrome. Int J Immunopharmacol 13 (suppl) 1991; 1:77–81.
61. Chak LY, Hill CK, Gill PS, Meyer PR, Levine AM, Petrovich Z. Radiation therapy for Kaposi's sarcoma in patients with acquired immune deficiency syndrome. Proc Am Soc Clin Oncol 1987; 6:A9.
62. Newman SB. Treatment of epidemic Kaposi's sarcoma with intralesional vinblastine injections. Proc Am Soc Clin Oncol 1988; 7:A19.
63. Gayka G, Alecy M, Halalau F, Comau G. Intralesional human leucocyte interferon treatment alone or associated with IL-2 in non-AIDS-related Kaposi's sarcoma. J Dermat 1992; 19:35–39.
64. Miles SA, Wang H, Elashoff R, Mitsuyasu RI. Improved survival for patients with AIDS-related Kaposi's sarcoma. J Clin Oncol 1994; 12:1910–1916.

21
Malignant Melanoma

Ruth Oratz and Jean-Claude Bystryn
New York University Medical Center, New York, New York

I. INTRODUCTION

The rate of increase in the incidence of malignant melanoma is greater than that of any other cancer in the United States, except for lung cancer in women. By the end of this decade the lifetime risk for an American of developing melanoma will reach about 1 in 90 (1). Currently, effective curative therapy is limited to complete surgical excision of early stage melanoma. Once melanoma metastasizes to sites beyond the primary and regional draining lymph nodes, treatment is less effective, prognosis is guarded, and average survival is measured in months. Efforts to define active therapy for systemic metastases have been directed toward cytotoxic chemotherapy regimens and immunotherapy with biological response modifiers.

Melanoma can metastasize to almost any soft tissue site or organ. Common locations include lung, liver, and brain, but bowel, adrenal, breast, and kidney metastases are not infrequently seen (2–4). Prognosis is related to the site of the first distant metastases and the number of metastases. For those with skin and soft tissue disease only, and one site of involvement, survival averages at about 7 mo; for those with two or more sites and visceral involvement median survival is often less than 6 months (5,6).

Given the poor prognosis of patients with systemic metastases, research efforts have been directed toward developing new therapeutic approaches. Currently cure is still not a realistic aim, with median survival of 6–8 mo. Furthermore, the median age of patients with melanoma is 45 years—relatively young adults who are often fully employed and are primary providers for their families. Treatment decisions must follow careful evaluations of the patient's extent of disease, other medical conditions and requirements for relief of pain or other symptoms, and improvement in the qualify of life. Careful consideration must be given to the impact of treatment and its toxicity on this group of patients.

II. CHEMOTHERAPY

Chemotherapy remains the mainstay of systemic treatment for metastatic malignant melanoma. It is at best palliative and often toxic, but no other treatment has yet been shown to produce longer disease-free or overall survival for a greater number of patients.

Several cytotoxic agents have shown activity in metastatic melanoma. Single agent activity has been shown with dacarbazine (DTIC), the nitrosoureas, platinum compounds, and the tubular toxins. In general response rates range from 10–25% (7), with complete responses being rare. Patients who respond to treatment generally have longer survivals than nonresponders (8,9). Responses are seen more often in patients with skin, subcutaneous tissue, lymph node, and lung metastases, and these patients generally have a better prognosis from the time of presentation.

A. Single-Agent Chemotherapy

1. Dacarbazine

The single most active agent for treating disseminated melanoma is dacarbazine (DTIC). DTIC is 5-(3,3-dimethyl-1-triazeno)-imidazole-4-carboxamide and is an analog of 5-amino-imidazole-4-carboxamide, which is an intermediate in purine biosynthesis. DTIC functions as an alkylating agent. The drug is metabolized by hepatic microsomal-mediated demethylation, which leads to active metabolites that interfere with purine synthesis. It may also inhibit purine nucleoside incorporation into DNA (10,11). The specific mechanism of activity of DTIC on the malignant cell is uncertain, but it appears to kill cells in all phases of the cell cycle and shows little or no cell cycle dependency. In addition to cytotoxic effects, DTIC and other triazine compounds, in sublethal doses, may induce differentiation of malignant cells (12). The drug is given by intravenous infusion. DTIC is generally well tolerated. The most common toxicity is nausea and vomiting, which now may be more readily controlled with new antiemetic regimens including odansetron. Myelosuppression is generally moderate and not dose limiting. Other side effects including local pain at the infusion site and a mild flu-like syndrome. Rarely hepatic veno-occlusive disease with acute hepatic necrosis has been reported (13).

The activity of single agent DTIC has been well defined in malignant melanoma. In a number of series, response rates range from 15–25% (8,9,14–17).

Patients with involvement of skin, subcutaneous tissue, and lymph nodes respond most frequently, although lung metastases also may be responsive to DTIC. Only about 5% of patients achieve complete response and median duration of response is less than 6 mo to this single-agent therapy.

A new imidazole, teniozolamide, is currently undergoing clinical investigation in single-agent drug trials (18). It may show promise as another antimelanoma alkylating agent.

2. Platinum Analogs

cis-Platin and the platinum analogs have shown significant activity in the treatment of melanoma. *cis*-Diamminedichloroplatinum (II) is a cytotoxic agent that exerts its effect through interactions with DNA. It is the only heavy metal compound used in cancer therapeutics. Three types of *cis*-platin DNA lesions have been defined: DNA-protein cross-links, DNA interstand cross-links, and DNA intrastrand cross-links. In vitro data indicates that these lesions may cause cytotoxicity by blocking DNA replication (19).

A number of single-agent studies show response rates of *cis*-platin ranging from 10–20% (20–22). Although no absolute dose response relationship has been shown, response rates to high single-agent platinum, with doses reaching 200 mg/m^2, seem to be higher. This may suggest a schedule dependency rather than a dose dependency (23).

Single-agent platinum in high doses given in combination with WR 2721, a thiol derivative that is protective of normal host tissues, has been reported to give high objective response rates of 53%. However, the median duration of these response was short at 4 mo (24). Based on this preliminary report, the Eastern Cooperative Oncology Group (ECOG) conducted a phase II randomized trial of *cis*-platin 120 mg/m^2 or *cis*-platin 150 mg/m^2 with WR2721. Although both regimens were active, both were associated with significant toxicity (Glover D, unpublished data). The optimum *cis*-platin regimen is yet to be defined.

cis-Platin is given by intravenous infusion. Its major side effect is nephrotoxicity which may be acute, is dose related, and is also cumulative. *cis*-Platin is excreted in the urine following glomerular filtration. Renal toxicity may be minimized by aggressive hydration regimens including mannitol and furosemide, or by administering smaller divided doses of *cis*-platin. Nephrotoxicity has been reported in up to 30% of patients treated with 50–75 mg/m^2 per course of *cis*-platin without adequate hydration (25).

Nausea and vomiting are also frequently seen with *cis*-platin administration. Although acute toxicity may be alleviated with concomitant administration of antiemetics, prolonged nausea and anorexia for up to 1 wk following drug administration is a common and difficult to manage problem.

Other toxicities include distal sensory neuropathy, which develops following several courses of treatment and is dose related and cumulative. Acute hypersensitivity reactions characterized by urticaria, wheezing, and hypotension may be seen.

cis-Platin analogs have been studied to a lesser extent in malignant melanoma. Carboplatin produced a response rate of 19% in one phase II trial (26). Thrombocytopenia was the dose-limiting toxicity. Early reports using iproplatin (CHIP) (27) and oxalato-platinum (L-OHP) (28) have been less promising.

3. Nitrosoureas

Another group of chemotherapeutic agents with antimelanoma activity is the nitrosoureas. These include carmustine (BCNU), lomustine (CCNU), and semustine (methyl CCNU). The nitrosoureas are highly lipid soluble and chemically reactive compounds. Their metabolic intermediates from single-strand adducts with DNA as well as DNA cross-links. In this regard they resemble classic alkylating agents. However, nitrosoureas also act by yielding isocyanates following their decomposition, and these isocyanates in turn react with amine groups, depleting glutathione and thus inhibiting DNA repair and RNA maturation (29–31).

Nitrosoureas, because of their extreme chemical reactivity, are rapidly excreted following intravenous administration. Their high lipid solubility allows for CNS penetration and activity against primary intracranial tumors. Although this advantage has not been proven for melanoma metastases to the brain. Objective response rates of single-agent nitrosoureas range from 13%–18% (32–39). Sites of response and duration are similar to that for DTIC. The predominate toxicity is hematological with more profound and long-lasting suppression of all cell lines than DTIC.

One new nitrosourea, fotemustine (S10036, Servier Laboratories, France) has been intensively studied in Europe. Clinical trials have begun in the United States. Phase II studies show promising response rates of 20–30% (40). Median duration of response is reported at 22 wk and myelosuppression is more modest than that seen with other nitrosoureas (41,42).

4. Tubular Toxins

Another important class of compounds that has been shown to be active against melanoma are those that interfere with microtubular function and cell mitosis: the vinca alkaloids and taxol. The vinca alkaloids, including vinblastine and vincristine have shown modest response rates as single agents in melanoma ranging from 12–15%, and they have been widely used in combination therapies. Vindesine, a newer analog of vinblastine, has been studied by the Southwest Oncology Group with a 20% response rate (43). As single agents these drugs have very limited if any use in treating disseminated melanoma.

Taxol, a recently introduced agent also active at the level of microtubule assembly, has undergone preliminary testing in melanoma. In a limited phase II study the objective response rate was 14% and the duration of responses ranged from 6–38 mo. Two patients achieved complete response for 25 and 38 mo, respectively (44). Taxol is given by long intravenous infusion. Like the other tubular toxins there is associated peripheral neuropathy, but the toxicity of taxol is predominantly hematological. Anaphylaxis may occur with administration of taxol, and patients should be premedicated with steroids, diphenhydramine, and H_2 blockers (cimetidine). More data from controlled clinical trials will be needed to establish a role for this agent in the treatment of metastatic melanoma.

B. Combination Chemotherapy

Single-agent chemotherapy has been minimally effective in the treatment of metastatic disease, leading to the use of a number of combination regimens with the hope of increasing the response. In phase II clinical trials many of these regimens have shown higher response rates and improved overall survival. These results must be evaluated in the context of prospective controlled phase III trials in order to convincingly demonstrate a therapeutic advantage, given the higher response rates but increased toxicity of the combinations compared to the single-agent results. Examples of these clinical results are summarized.

The first group of combination chemotherapy trials are those that include active single agents based largely around DTIC with the addition of one or two other active agents including either a vinca alkaloid or *cis*-platin. In general, the response rates of these trials ranged from 12–32% (45–47) and were not significantly different from those of any single-agent DTIC trial. There is no clear advantage or synergistic antitumor effect demonstrated in these trials.

A second group of combination regimens have been developed using four drugs. Initially published by De Prete et al., and often referred to as the Dartmouth regimen, this four-drug treatment includes DTIC, *cis*-platinum, BCNU, and tamoxifen (48). In 1984 an initial trial reported 55% of patients with objective responses, including four complete responses and seven partial responses (48). These results were impressive, and subsequently were confirmed in follow-up studies (49). However, a significant toxicity (perhaps related to the tamoxifen) was seen in this group of patients: deep vein thrombosis and pulmonary embolism.

The tamoxifen was eliminated from the combination in a subsequent study and the response rate dropped back 10% (50). This observation has led to an interesting question as to the role of tamoxifen in this and other chemotherapeutic regimens for melanoma. It is clear that tamoxifen is not effective as a single agent in the treatment of melanoma, but it has been shown to enhance the antineoplastic effects of *cis*-platin in vitro and perhaps also to modulate the pharmacokinetics of BCNU. The mechanism of action of the former may be related to inhibition of protein kinase C and of the latter through modulation of calmodulin.

In addition, tamoxifen has been shown to add to the activity of single-agent DTIC. In a randomized study comparing DTIC alone to DTIC in combination with tamoxifen, Cocconi et al. demonstrated a significant advantage from the addition of tamoxifen to DTIC (51). There were relatively low response rates in both arms of this trial; however, the tamoxifen arm fared significantly better with a survival and response rate advantage (51). The role of tamoxifen in combination with chemotherapy is being analyzed in a number of cooperative group trials at this time. ECOG is studying the effect of tamoxifen when added to DTIC in a prospective randomization which also will test IFN-α. The North Central Cancer Treatment Group is testing the combination of DTIC, *cis*-platinum, and BCNU, with or without tamoxifen, in conjunction with chemotherapy.

The consensus among most is that DTIC as a single agent is still a reasonable standard to practice, but that there is increasing evidence that DTIC-based combinations with *cis*-platin, BCNU, and tamoxifen are probably more effective. The results of the ongoing clinical trials will be reassuring to those who have made the clinical judgment that the combinations are a standard of practice based on controlled, often single institution, results. On the other hand, those who await the results of the prospective, often multi-institution, clinical trials must be supported in their judgment that the standard of chemotherapy practice is DTIC as a single agent.

C. High-Dose Autologous Bone Marrow Transplantation

As an alternative approach, very high-dose intense chemotherapy has been explored in a number of other solid tumors, and dose intensity certainly has been shown to be an important factor in achieving response rates. However, in malignant melanoma very intensive regimens have not been shown to produce survival benefits, and autologous transplant programs have shown response rates at the rate of 40–50% with complete responses of about 15%. Toxicity, however, is substantial, and response duration is quite brief with no significant impact on patient survival (52–56). Therefore, high-dose chemotherapy with autologous bone marrow support is not recommended as a standard treatment for metastatic melanoma. Combinations with new agents remain to be tested.

III. IMMUNOTHERAPY

A. Interferon

Interferons are a group of lymphokines produced by activated cells that possess a broad spectrum of biological activity including immunomodulatory, antiviral, and antiproliferative properties. There are three major classes of interferons. Interferon-α is produced by macrophages and non-B, non-T lymphocytes; IFN-β is produced by fibroblasts and epithelial cells; and IFN-γ is produced by T lymphocytes and natural killer cells. Interferons were the first group of lymphokines to be tested as potential antitumor agents. The rationale for their use is their ability to inhibit the growth of cells, to interfere with the expression of oncogenes, and to modulate immune responses to tumors. The later includes stimulation of tumor cell-surface antigen expression, augmentation of antibody production, and regulation of cytotoxic effector cells.

IFN-α is the product that has been the most extensively studied in patients with malignant melanoma. Initial clinical trials were conducted with human leukocyte interferon. Since the advent of recombinant technology, commercially prepared recombinant IFN-α has been available in large quantities. After phase I toxicity and feasibility studies were completed, investigators conducted a series of phase II trials in order to define the most effective dose and schedule. A wide range of IFN-α dosage schedules have been tested, ranging from 3×10^6 units/m^2 to 100×10^6 units/m^2 given intravenously or subcutaneously, either as an intermittent 5 d course at 3 wk intervals, daily, or thrice weekly (59–63). The thrice weekly schedule has been shown to be more effective than the intermittent 5 d courses, and in general interferon seems to have more antitumor activity against melanoma when given in intermediate-dose levels two or three times a week. Creagan et al. reported a 22% response rate in 96 patients with advanced melanoma treated at a single institution using two different doses of IFN-α on a thrice-weekly schedule (57). Median time to disease progression and survival was short at 1.5 and 5 mo, respectively. Responses were most often seen with soft tissue metastases. The dosage of interferon did not influence treatment outcome. These observations are representative of those reported in other trials (53,59,60,62). Almost all patients treated with interferons experience "flu-like" symptoms: fever, chills, fatigue, malaise, muscle aches, and anorexia. The effects, which are dose related, tend to improve with continued treatment (tachyphylaxis) can be controlled with acetaminophen, are generally tolerated, and are rapidly reversible upon discontinuation or modification of therapy. Other toxicities include transient decreased blood counts, asymptomatic elevation of liver enzymes, confusion, somnolence (more prevalent among the elderly), mild low blood pressure, and occasional nonmalignant arrhythmias.

Immunotherapy of metastatic melanoma with interferons has been of limited efficacy. There has been no overall prolongation in survival and the response rate is no greater than what can be achieved by conventional chemotherapy, although with perhaps less toxicity. Because complete remissions have been induced in a small proportion of patients with disseminated disease, efforts to improve this approach are being continued. This involves evaluation of different doses and schedules, administration to patients with smaller tumor loads, and use in combinations with different interferons or with other immunotherapeutic agents. At New York University, we conducted a phase I trial of IFN-α-2a in combination with low weekly doses of *cis*-platinum. We found the maximally tolerated dose in patients with all types of cancer to be 5×10^6 units/m^2 of interferon given subcutaneously three times a week and *cis*-platinum at 25 mg/m^2 given intravenously once a week. One partial response and two mixed responses were seen in patents with metastatic melanoma (64). A phase II trial of this combination in patients with malignant melanoma was conducted. Patients received treatment as above on 5 wk cycles: 3 wk on treatment followed by a 2 wk rest. All patients experienced the expected interferon-associated constitutional symptoms; many have declined in performance status. Both complete and partial responses have been documented (65) and have similar patterns of toxicity and response.

Promising results have been seen from the addition of IFN-α to DTIC. Initial trials published by McLeod et al. and Kirkwood et al. (66,67) have failed to demonstrate any significant advantage for the combination of these agents. More recently, however, Falkson et al. (68) have shown induction IFN followed by a combination of IFN-α-2 and DTIC produced a significant response advantage when compared to DTIC alone. The combination arm of the 64 patients studied achieved 16 total responses with 12 complete responses, compared to the single-agent DTIC arm which only achieved 6 total responses and 2 complete responses. Because both response rate and survival for the combination were significantly improved, this study has led to several large randomized trials in order to confirm these findings. The dose of IFN-α was quite high in this study and toxicity was formidable. Currently ECOG is testing the combination of DTIC with and without IFN-α and with or without tamoxifen in order to definitively establish the presence of a possible synergistic action of these two agents when combined with DTIC.

The combination of IFN-α and 13-*cis*-retinoic acid has shown significant activity against a number of human tumors including squamous cell carcinomas. The differentiating agent retinoids have shown considerable activity in premalignant and malignant skin disorders (69–71). In vitro and preclinical animal studies of 13-*cis*-retinoic and all *trans*-retinoic acids have shown toxicity against melanoma cell liver and animal tumor models (72,73). Topical application of retinoids caused some clinical response in dysplatic nevi and malignant melanoma lesions as well as oral lesions (74–76). In view of these findings and the previously reported synergistic effect of *cis*-retinoic acid and IFN-α in other malignancies, a phase II trial of this combination was conducted in patients with metastatic melanoma (77). Only 11 patients were treated and no responses were seen. Further testing of the retinoids alone and in combination with interferon is ongoing. A trial is currently being conducted at NYU Medical Center.

IFN-β has also been tested in metastatic melanoma. It has a spectrum of toxicity similar to IFN-α, but may not be as clinically effective (78). IFN-γ, which is also an immune interferon and binds to different receptors than IFN-α and IFN-β, has shown little activity in melanoma in preliminary trials (79). Schiller et al. (unpublished data) completed a randomized phase II study to investigate an optimum biological dose correlated with in vitro measures of immune response. This study confirmed the low level of clinical activity.

B. Interleukin-2

Interleukin-2 (IL-2) is a soluble polypeptide cytokine, produced by lymphocytes, which functions to help regulate normal growth and differentiation of immune system cells. IL-2 binds specifically to a high-affinity cell surface receptor expressed on activated T cells and certain malignant lymphocytes. It has a broad range of immunological effects including activation of cytotoxic lymphoid populations, inducing proliferation of activated T cells, and inducing IFN-γ, tumor necrosis factor, and a number of other secondary cytokines (80,81). Both natural killer (NK) and cytotoxic T lymphocytes are activated by IL-2 and these compromise part of the population of cytotoxic cells which mediated "lymphokine-activated killing" (LAK). Hence, these IL-2 induced/activated cells are referred to as LAK cells. LAK cells are cytotoxic to fresh, noncultured tumors and also to autologous, allogeneic, and syngeneic primary and metastatic tumors (81). Preclinical in vitro and in vivo studies have demonstrated the ability of LAK cells plus IL-2 to kill tumor cells. Another cytotoxic population of immune cells that are augmented and activated by IL-2 is the tumor-infiltrating lymphocyte (TIL) cell population. These are lymphocytes that infiltrate primary or metastatic tumors; they can be isolated from these tumors and grown ex vivo in the presence of IL-2. TIL cells are 50–100 times more effective than LAK cells in animal models (82).

In preclinical animal models, single-agent IL-2 is active against a variety of tumors including melanoma. IL-2 antitumor activity is related to tumor burden, immunogenicity of the tumor cell, and the status of the host immune system. IL-2 has greatest activity against low tumor burden, and sustained low doses seem more effective than high-dose bolus dose schedules (83–85).

Tumor cells (such as melanoma) expressing high levels of class I major histocompatibility complex (MHC) antigens are more responsive than non-class I bearing tumors (86). Moreover, in animals with impaired immune system function, IL-2 antitumor activity is decreased (86). It appears in animals that IL-2 activity is enhanced by addition of LAK cells (87).

In humans, IL-2 has shown activity in malignant melanoma and renal cell carcinoma. Initial clinical trials tested IL-2 in high doses administered in conjunction with LAK cells. At the National Cancer Institute (NCI) Rosenberg et al. treated 48 patients with malignant melanoma with high dose IL-2 LAK (88). They observed an 8% complete response and 13% partial response rate.

The duration of complete response ranged from 18–52 mo in three patients and the median duration of partial response was 6 mo. The sites most responsive to therapy were skin, soft tissue, and lung.

In order to corroborate these findings the NCI IL-2 Extramural Working Group (ILWG) performed a subsequent phase II study in 36 patients with melanoma. Only one patient (3%) achieved a complete response and five patients (14%) had partial responses (89). Again the median duration of responses was relatively long—6 mo—and three patients maintained partial response for 21–24+ mo. Alterations in the schedule of IL-2 administration did not significantly effect response rates (90).

Toxicity on these treatment regimens was significant, with dose-limiting toxicity being hypotension requiring vasopressors, oliguria, fluid overload with associated capillary leak syndrome, and renal and hepatic dysfunction. These toxicities were generally reversible and less than 5% of patients died from treatment-related toxicity.

The next set of clinical trials studied continuous intravenous infusion of IL-2, rather than bolus administration, in an effort to induce greater in vivo LAK cell activation and proliferation. The ILWG again performed these studies in a phase I trial, but only 1 of 30 patients (3%) achieved a partial response and no complete response was seen (91). In a phase II study in melanoma the response rate was again disappointingly low at 3% (1 of 33 patients). Although the continuous infusion led to increased numbers of measurable LAK cells, clinical efficacy was not improved, and indeed seemed inferior (92).

Studies with single-agent IL-2, excluding LAK cells, yielded comparable clinical results. Rosenberg et al. reported no complete responses and 10 of 42 (24%) partial responses in a study of IV bolus IL-2 (88). In the extramural ILWG the response rates were 4% complete response and 17% partial response among 47 patients treated with IL-2 alone. It became evident that the addition of LAK cells in humans did not enhance the therapeutic antitumor activity of IL-2 (93). Randomized studies confirmed these findings (91,94,95).

Low-dose IL-2 treatment schedules have also been explored, offering the potential advantage of outpatient administration, less toxicity, and lower cost. In 27 patients treated with low-dose IV IL-2 and cyclophosphamide, 1 (4%) complete response and 5 (19%) partial response were achieved (96). Other studies at comparable doses reported response rates ranging from 6–11% (97–99).

Since TILs are many-fold more effective in LAK cells as tumor killing cells, clinical trials were then initiated combining TIL cells with IL-2. Rosenberg et al. at the NCI reported a 61% objective response rate (19 of 31 patients) (82). However, it was possible to isolate, culture, and grow TIL cells from only 50% of the patients who were entered on study and had tumors excised (100). Further studies with TIL cells, including genetic engineering studies, are ongoing. The hypothesis is that by inserting the gene for TNF into the TIL cell, high levels of TNF (or other cytokines) will be delivered to local tumor sites when the TIL cells traffic to the tumor. No clinical data has yet been published from these studies.

IL-2 has been combined with other cytokines and with monoclonal antibodies for treatment of metastatic malignant melanoma. In a combination of IL-2 and IFN-α Rosenberg et al. reported a 33% response rate (101). The extramural working group saw no differences in response rates or survival between patients randomly treated with high-dose IV bolus IL-2 alone or in combination with IFN-α (102).

A number of investigators have added IL-2 to chemotherapy. Patients treated with high-dose *cis*-platin combined with high-dose IV IL-2 achieved an overall response rate of 37%, with 11% (3/27) complete responses and 26% (7/27) partial responses. The complete responses were durable for 9, 16, and 30+ mo. Toxicity was significant (103). Other combinations of IL-2 plus *cis*-platin and dacarbazine regimens have yielded response rates ranging from 22–37% (104–108).

Overall, it appears that IL-2 produces objective responses in 10–20% of patients with metastatic malignant melanoma. This is comparable to the results of treatment with other cytotoxic or biological agents used singly or in combination. There is no clear advantage to the addition of LAK or TIL cells. Toxicity is significant. Of interest, responding patients may have long disease-free intervals. Further investigation should be directed toward better defining the immunobiology of response to the agent in an effort to identify which patients might benefit from IL-2-based treatment.

C. Monoclonal Antibodies

Monoclonal antibodies are directed against a single antigenic determinant. Their value is that they can be extremely specific in their action and thus recognize subtle differences between malignant and normal cells. They have the potential of being highly specific diagnostic and therapeutic agents that could detect small metastases or selectively kill tumor cells without damaging adjacent normal cells. Hybridoma technology can now generate monoclonal antibodies in large quantities, permitting their clinical potential to be examined. There are several possible mechanisms of antitumor activity for monoclonal antibodies: they can coat tumor cells and facilitate antibody or complement-dependent cellular cytotoxicity (109,110); they may interact with host effector immune cells, such as T cells and NK/LAK cells, and stimulate them to recognize and kill tumor cells (111); and they can serve as carrier molecules for chemotherapeutic drugs, toxins, or radiopharmaceuticals and selectively deliver these toxic agents to tumor cells.

The therapeutic activity of several murine monoclonal antibodies has been examined in patients with melanoma (112–117). The results indicate that they can bind preferentially to melanoma tumors in vivo, that they can be repeatedly administered to patients with acceptable toxicity, and that their use is in some cases associated with partial and rarely complete regression of metastatic lesions. A number of problems have emerged from studies with monoclonal antibodies. No monoclonal antibody is completely specific for melanoma. After intravenous infusion, monoclonal antibodies accumulate in melanoma nodules but also bind nonspecifically to the reticuloendothelial system, particularly in the liver and kidney. Some time is needed in order to clear the antibodies from these sites. In addition, most patients treated with murine monoclonal antibodies develop an immune response to the antibody that sharply reduces its half-life in the circulation and perhaps the duration of its effects. Patients are at risk for developing immune complex disease or serum sickness if the antibody is given again. Efforts are being made to circumvent these problems by using the Fab fragments of antibody molecules, inducing tolerance by frequent administration, generating human monoclonal antibodies or chimera antibodies, and/or administering immunosuppressive drugs along with the monoclonal antibodies.

The most extensive clinical trials of monoclonal antibody immunotherapy of human melanoma have been conducted by Houghton et al. using R-24, a mouse monoclonal IgG3 antibody (112,114). R-24 reacts with the disialoganglioside G_{D3}, which is strongly expressed by most melanomas and to a lesser extent by melanocytes, astrocytomas, and some sarcomas. In vitro, R-24 can inhibit the growth of melanoma cells and can kill these through complement-mediated cytotoxicity or antibody-dependent cell-mediated cytotoxicity. In humans, Houghton et al. (114) reported partial responses (50% reduction in all metastatic nodules) in 19% of 21 patients with disseminated disease and mixed responses (50% reduction of some but not all metastases) in two additional patients. The treatment appeared to induce an inflammatory response in melanoma metastasis, as suggested by the frequent development of pruritus and urticaria over cutaneous tumors in patients treated at the highest dosage of monoclonal antibodies and by the presence of an inflammatory cell infiltrate in tumor nodules removed during or after therapy. Side effects of this monoclonal antibody therapy are dose related and include nausea, diarrhea, abdominal pain, flu-like symptoms, and fever. Most patients develop antibodies to mouse immunoglobulin; in most cases this reaction seems well tolerated and does not preclude further treatment. Other investigators working with monoclonal antibodies to the p97 glycoprotein (116) and to the 250 kDR glycoprotein (118) have found little if any clinical efficacy. Clinical trials employing R-24 and IL-2 have not shown enhanced clinical activity (119).

Monoclonal antibodies are also being used to selectively target highly toxic agents to tumor cells. The theoretical advantages of this approach are that it should permit more selective delivery of toxic agents to tumor cells, and thus should decrease systemic toxicity, and that it does not rely on the ability of the monoclonal antibody to kill tumor cells. Various cytotoxic agents (vincristine, methotrexate, daunorubicin, and doxorubicin), protein toxins and cytotoxins (diphtheria toxin, ricin toxin), and radioisotopes (iodine 131) have been conjugated to monoclonal antibodies. Most of these investigations are still in preliminary phases of clinical testing.

Spitler et al. have conducted clinical trials of a murine antimelanoma monoclonal antibody conjugated to the A chain of ricin (115). Ricin is a protein toxin that consists of two polypeptides, the A and B chains. The A chain causes inhibition of protein synthesis and cell death. It is an extremely potent toxin; only one molecule is required to enter the cell to cause cell death. The B chain functions to facilitate entry of the A chain into virtually all types of eukaryotic cells. Without the B chain the A chain is poorly internalized and at least 1500 times less toxic than the whole ricin complex. The ricin A chain is attractive as a conjugate to monoclonal antibodies, because in the absence of the B chain it will not enter normal eukaryotic cells, while it will be internalized into those cells (i.e., tumor cells) that bind the monoclonal antibody. The ricin A chain was conjugated to a murine IgG2 monoclonal antibody that recognizes a cell surface glycoprotein of 240,000 kD present on most melanomas. By radioimaging studies this monoclonal antibody localized in melanoma and was safe to use (113).

Spitler et al. treated 22 patients with metastatic melanoma with this immunotoxin in a phase I study (115). There was one complete response with disappearance of pulmonary metastasis for at least 13 mo and four mixed responses. It is of interst to note that lesions regressed for prolonged intervals following a single course of immunotoxin without any additional therapy. Histological specimens examined within 24 h of immunotoxin infusion demonstrated intense antiricin A chain reactivity and murine immunoglobulin at the tumor site. Dose-limiting toxicity was a transient fall in serum albumin, with an associated fall in serum protein and weight gain and fluid shifts resulting in edema, which responded to conservative management. Most patients experienced mild to moderate malaise, fatigue, decrease in appetite, and fevers. Most patients also developed an immune response to both the murine immunoglobulin and to the ricin A chain. Further studies are ongoing to examine whether cyclophosphamide, azathioprine, or corticosteroids can abrogate host immune responses to the components of the immunotoxin monoclonal antibody conjugate and improve the efficacy of this type of immunotherapy. Oratz et al. completed a phase II study of this immunotoxin administered with cyclophosphamide (117). Twenty patients were treated with 0.4 μg/kg of the monoclonal antibody ricin—a chain immunotoxin followed by 1000 $\mu g/m^2$ of cyclophosphamide toxicity was similar to that seen in the phase I trial. There was a 20% overall response rate consisting of four partial responses lasting from 6–53 wk in patients with pulmonary and soft tissue metastases. Two other patients had mixed responses, one had a minor response, and three had stable disease. Ten patients had progressive disease. All patients mounted immune responses to both the murine immunoglobulin and the ricin A chain components of the immunotoxin. The combination of immunotoxin and cyclophosphamide appears safe and may be more effective than immunotoxin alone. At this time monoclonal antibody therapy remains limited to investigational use in clinical trials.

IV. MELANOMA VACCINES

A. Rationale for Melanoma Vaccines

Melanoma vaccines are intended to stimulate tumor protective immune responses and hence increase a patient's resistance to his own cancer. As the stimulation is specific, it is hoped it will be more effective than nonspecific immunotherapy with immunomodulators such as cytokines or interferon. The rationale for believing vaccines may be effective in the treatment of melanoma is that melanoma cells differ from normal adult pigment cells. These differences can be recognized by immunocompetent cells and stimulate antimelanoma immune responses, and the resulting immune responses can destroy melanoma cells in vitro. The most compelling evidence to support this hypothesis is that melanoma vaccines prevent this cancer in animals. Fifty to 100% of melanoma vaccine-treated mice survive challenge with otherwise lethal doses of melanoma cells (120,121). The protection is specific, indicating it is mediated by immune mechanisms.

B. Design of Melanoma Vaccines

A number of variables influence the effectiveness of melanoma vaccines. The most critical is the presence in the vaccine of melanoma tumor antigen(s) that can induce clinically effective tumor protective immune responses and that are expressed by the tumor to be treated. Unfortunately, the identity of the melanoma antigen(s) that stimulates protective immunity in man is unknown, and because of the antigenic heterogeneity of melanoma, the actual tumor antigen(s) expressed by the tumor to be treated is also usually not known. Another important consideration is the adjuvant selected to boost vaccine potency, as tumor antigens are usually poorly immunogenic. Several different types of vaccines are currently in clinical trials. These can be distinguished by the purity of the final preparation into nonpurified, semipurified, and purified vaccines.

The most common vaccines now in use are nonpurified or traditional vaccines consisting of whole melanoma cells or nonpurified extract of these cells (122–126). The major advantage of nonpurified vaccines is that they contain a broad representation of different tumor antigens, including presumably the as yet unidentified antigen(s) that stimulates tumor protective immunity. In addition, the broad range of tumor antigens in the vaccine may circumvent the antigenic heterogeneity of melanoma. Vaccines prepared from whole cells may also be inherently more immunogenic, as vaccines lose potency as they are purified. However, most of the material in nonpurified vaccines is irrelevant cellular material. This creates difficulties in reproducible manufacture and characterization of the vaccine, may decrease effectiveness due to the presence of suppressive factors or competitive inhibition of antitumor immune responses, and may increase side effects and the overall toxicity of the treatment.

A scientifically more elegant approach to formulate melanoma vaccines is to prepare them from purified tumor-associated antigens. Purified vaccines in clinical trials include preparations made from gangliosides (127), recombinant proteins, immunogenic peptides such as MAGE (128), or anti-idiotype monoclonal antibodies (129). The major advantage of this approach is that purified vaccines are easier to characterize and to manufacture in a reproducible manner, and they may be safer to use. Unfortunately, as the melanoma antigen(s) responsible for induction of protective immunity remains to be identified, the precise antigen(s) that should be selected and purified to formulate such vaccines is still unknown.

The third approach attempts to balance the advantages and disadvantages of nonpurified and purified vaccines. The concept is to prepare the vaccine from material enriched in cellular elements most likely to contain antigens relevant for vaccine effectiveness and depleted of those likely to be irrelevant. A polyvalent vaccine prepared from the material shed by viable melanoma cells, which is highly enriched in cell-surface antigens and depleted of cytoplasmic and nuclear material, is an example of this strategy (130). The major advantage of this approach is that it hopefully retains the most critical elements of vaccine effectiveness—the need to include a "cocktail" of antigens that can stimulate protective immunity and circumvent tumor antigenic heterogeneity—while being much purer than vaccines prepared from whole tumor cells.

None of these approaches is completely satisfactory as none fully satisfies the multiple requirements of cancer vaccines. In fact, these strategies often result in vaccine formulations with mutually exclusive desirable properties (see Table 1).

C. Clinical Trials with Melanoma Vaccines

Melanoma vaccines have now become accepted as an experimental treatment for surgically resected melanoma at high risk of recurrence. They are also being used in some patients with more advanced disease. The results of current clinical trials are encouraging, but not conclusive. Randomized phase III clinical trials to conclusively establish effectiveness have been initiated, but the results are still pending.

Melanoma vaccines can boost both antibody and/or cellular immune responses to melanoma. The type of immune response that is boosted and the frequency with which this occurs depends on the vaccine and adjuvant used.

Table 1 Relative Merits of Different Melanoma Vaccine Design Strategies

Desirable vaccine attribute	Crude vaccines	Semi-vaccines	Pure vaccine
Effectiveness			
Presence relevant antigens	+++	++	+
Presence multiple antigens	+++	++	+
Immunogenic potency of antigens	+++	++	+
Elegance of preparation			
Purity	+	++	+++
Reproducible manufacture	+	++	+++
Quality control	+	++	+++
Safety	++	++	++

Some vaccine formulations stimulate antibody but no cellular responses (123), while others stimulate cellular responses (127). In our own studies, a polyvalent vaccine prepared from shed antigens stimulated both antibody and cellular immune responses with similar frequencies (131). Vaccines can augment host responses to a patient's own tumor, as evidenced by the appearance of (TILs) in tumor nodules removed from vaccine-treated patients (132) or by the development of visible inflammation over cutaneous metastases (123).

There appears to be a correlation between the ability of melanoma vaccines to stimulate antimelanoma cellular and/or humoral immune responses and improved clinical outcome. This is reasonable, as vaccines are unlikely to be clinically effective unless they can induce strong immune responses to melanoma. Unfortunately, the immunogenicity of current vaccines is weak. They fail to boost immunity to melanoma in many patients. Thus there is an ongoing effort to discover safe but potent methods of increasing vaccine immunogenicity. Approaches currently being followed include the use of novel adjuvants such as QS-21, Detox, and DAF-M; encapsulating the vaccine into liposomes; modifying the biochemical properties of the vaccine; and administering it with immunomodulators such as IL-2.

D. Use of Vaccines for the Adjuvant Treatment of Localized or Regional Melanoma

Vaccines are particularly attractive for the adjuvant treatment of surgically resected high-risk primary melanoma or regional metastases because such patients usually do well for a variable length of time following their surgery. It is important that treatment of such patients be minimally toxic, a requirement which vaccines fulfill. In addition, immunotherapy is most likely to be effective in patients with minimal tumor load.

All melanoma vaccines currently in clinical trials appear to be relatively safe. No untoward effects from the vaccines themselves have been reported in hundreds of patients treated to date. The side effects that have occurred include ulceration at the site of immunization due to the use of potent adjuvants, such as BCG or Freund's complete adjuvant and infections due to bacterial or viral contamination of the vaccine. These side effects can be avoided by careful screening of vaccine preparation for pathogens and selection of adjuvants that cause less local or systemic inflammation. However, toxicity may increase in the future as novel and more potent adjuvants are being tried to increase vaccine effectiveness.

The clinical effectiveness of melanoma vaccines in delaying or preventing the recurrence of surgically resected melanoma is not known. However, the results of initial clinical trials are promising (122–127,131). Morton et al. prepared a nonpurified vaccine from three allogeneic melanoma cell lines selected for their high expression of protein and ganglioside antigens immunogenic in melanoma patients (122), administered with BCG as an adjuvant. Median survival of 61 vaccine-treated patients with surgically resected stage IIIA melanoma was 43.9 mo versus 28.7 mo for 126 historical control patients. Overall, 5 y survival was increased from 10% to 28% in patients with stage IIIA and from 7.5% to 23% in patients with stage IV melanoma in comparison to historical controls. Hersey prepared a nonpurified vaccine from the oncolysate of a single melanoma cell line infected with vaccinia (125). The 5 y overall survival of 80 patients with surgically resected AJCC stage III melanoma was 60% and 50% for 151 patients treated with vaccine plus cyclophosphamide in comparison to 34% for 151 historical controls and 34% for 55 concurrent but nonrandomized controls. Wallack and Sivanandham prepared another nonpurified vaccine from the oncolysate of four melanoma cell lines infected with vaccinia (126). The disease-free survival of 39 vaccine-treated patients with surgically resected AJCC stage II and III melanoma was significantly ($p = .04$) better than that of historical controls. Berd et al. prepared a nonpurified vaccine by conjugating dinitrophenol (DNP) to irradiated whole, autologous, melanoma cells (123). To increase immunogenicity, the vaccine was given with BCG as an adjuvant and with cyclophosphamide pretreatment to inactivate suppressor cells. The 2 y disease-free and overall survival of 41 patients with surgically resected melanoma was 59% and 85%, respectively; which was significantly better than that of 22 historical controls. Bystryn et al. prepared a semipurified vaccine from shed melanoma antigens, admixed with alum as an adjuvant (130). The median disease-free and overall survival of 94 vaccine-treated patients with surgically resected AJCC stage III melanoma was 30 mo and the 5 y overall survival was 50%, which were both approximately 50% longer than that of historical controls (131). Livingston conducted a series of trials using purified gangliosides administered either alone or combined with different adjuvants (127). A double-blind randomized study has been conducted in AJCC stage III melanoma patients pretreated with cyclophosphamide and given either a GM2 vaccine plus BCG, or BCG alone. There was no significant difference in either disease-free or overall survival between the two groups, but an encouraging trend in favor of the vaccine-treated patients was present. Outcome was significantly better in those patients who developed an antibody response to the vaccine.

The effect of vaccines on disease progression may be related to their ability to potentiate immunity to melanoma. We have found that survival of patients with surgically resected AJCC stage III melanoma is particularly prolonged among those who develop either a strong DTH or antibody response to vaccine treatment. Their median disease-free survival was more than 89 mo and 62 mo, respectively, which is 4.7 y and 2.5 y longer than that of nonresponders (131). These relations were independent of disease severity or of the immunological competence of the patients, suggesting the clinical benefits resulted from vaccine treatment.

E. Uses of Vaccines for the Treatment of Disseminated Disease

Though it is believed that vaccines will be most effective in patients with limited tumor load, they have been reported to induce regression or slow the progression of established metastatic lesions in some patients. Morton et al. reported clinical responses in 22% of 40 patients with AJCC stage IV disease, and a threefold increase in median survival in comparison to historical controls (122). Mitchell et al., using a nonpurified vaccine prepared from the lysates of two allogeneic melanoma cell lines, reported partial or complete responses in 19% of 106 evaluable patients with disseminated melanoma (124). While the overall survival of patients in the study was not increased, that of responding patients was prolonged. Berd et al. Mastrangelo used their irradiated autologous melanoma cell conjugated to DNP vaccine to treat 46 patients with metastatic AJCC stage IV melanoma (123). Twenty developed clinically apparent inflammation in superficial metastasis, suggesting that the treatment induced antimelanoma immune responses, and partial tumor regression occurred in five of the patients. Ferrone has constructed a purified melanoma vaccine from three anti-idiotype mouse monoclonal antibodies that harbor the internal image of several distinct determinants of the high molecular weight melanoma-associated antigen (129). Anti-idiotype antibodies recognize the antigen-combining region of another antibody and can act as surrogate antigens.

V. SUMMARY

While these results are promising, they are difficult to evaluate. The progression of melanoma is erratic, only a small number of patients have been studied, and no randomized, concurrently controlled study has been completed. Nonetheless, immunotherapy with tumor vaccines seems reasonable for melanoma patients with minimal disease but high risk of recurrence since the treatment is safe, there is no other effective alternative for such patients, and the current clinical data is promising.

REFERENCES

1. Rigel DS, Kopf AW, Friedman RJ. The rate of malignant melanoma in the U.S.: are we making an impact? J Am Acad Dermat 1987; 17:1050.
2. Lee YT. Malignant melanoma: patterns of metastasis. CA. 1980; 30:137.
3. Patel JK, Didolkar MS, Pickren JW, et al. Metastatic pattern of malignant melanoma: a study of 216 autopsy cases. Am J Surg 1978; 135:807.
4. Sacre R, Lejeune FJ. Patterns of metastases distribution in 173 stage I and II melanoma patients. Anticancer Res 1982; 2:47.
5. Balch CM, Soonj SJ, Shaw HM, et al. An analysis of prognostic factors in 4000 patients with cutaneous melanoma. In: Balch CM, Mi Hon GW, eds. Cutaneous melanoma: clinical management and treatment results worldwide. Philadelphia: JB Lippincott, p 1985:321.
6. Balch CM, Soong SJ, Murad TM, et al. A multifactorial analysis of melanoma: IV. Prognostic factors in 200 melanoma patients with distant metastases. J Clin Oncol 1983; 1:126.
7. Marsoni S, Hoth D, Simon R. Clinical drug development. An analysis of phase II trials, 1970–1985. Cancer Treat Rep 1987; 71:71.
8. Luce JK. Chemotherapy of malignant melanoma. Cancer 1972; 30:1604.
9. Costanza ME, Nathanson L, Schoenfeld D, et al. Results with methyl CCNU and DTIC in metastatic melanoma. Cancer 1977; 40:1010.
10. Montgomery JA. Experimental studies at Southern Research Institute with DTIC (NSC-45388). Cancer Treat Rep 1976; 60:125–134.
11. Hayward IP, Parson PG. Epigenetic effects of the methylating agent 5-(3-methyl-1-triazeno) imidazole-4-carboxamide in human melanoma cells. Austr J Exp Biol Med Sci 1984; 62:597–606.
12. Tisdale MJ. Induction of haemoglobin synthesis in the human leukemia cell line K562 by monomethyltriazenes and imidazotetrazinones. Biochem Pharmacol 1985; 34:2077–2082.
13. Feauz de Lacroix W, Runne U, Hauk H, et al. Acute liver dystrophy with thrombosis of hepatic veins: a fatal complication of dacarbazine treatment. Cancer Treat Rep 1983; 67:779–784.
14. Comis RL. DTIC (NSC-45388) in malignant melanoma: a perspective. Cancer Treat Rep 1976; 64:1123.

15. Wagner DE, Ramirez G, Weiss AJ. Combination phase I–II study of imidazole carboxamide (NSC-45388). Oncology 1971; 26:310.
16. Nathanson L, Wolter K, Horton J. Characteristics of prognosis and response to an imidazole carboxamide in malignant melanoma. Clin Pharmacol Ther 1971; 12:955.
17. van der Merwe AM, Falkson G, van Eden EB. Metastatic malignant melanoma: imidazole carboxamide in its treatment. Med Proc 1971; 17:399.
18. O'Reilly SM, Newlands ES, Slevers MF, et al. Teniozolomadene (CCRG81045; M and B39831; NSC 362856): a new oral cytotoxic agent with activity against melanoma, mycosis fungoides and high-grade glioma. Proc Am Assoc Cancer Res 1992; 33:1267.
19. Hansson J, Lewensohn R, Ringborg U. Cis-diamminedichloroplatinum (II) toxicity in human melanoma cells and lymphocytes as related to cellular platinum accumulation, DNA cross-linking and inhibition of DNA synthesis. Acta Oncol 1988; 27:383–392.
20. Goodnight JE Jr, Moseley HS, Eilber FR, et al. Cis-dichlorodiammine platinum (II) alone and combined with DTIC for treatment of disseminated malignant melanoma. Cancer Treat Rep 1979; 63:2005–2007.
21. Mortimer JE, Chestnut J, Higono CS, Goodman G. High dose cisplatin in metastatic melanoma: comparison of two schedules. Proc Am Soc Clin Oncol 1988; 7:254.
22. Murren JR, De Rosa W, Durivage HJ, et al. High dose cisplatin plus dacarbazine in the treatment of metastatic melanoma. Cancer 1991; 67:1514–1517.
23. Al-Sarraf M, Fletcher W, Oishi N, et al. Cisplatin hydration with and without mannitol diuresis in refractory disseminated malignant melanoma: a Southwest Oncology Group study. Cancer Treat Rep 1982; 66:31.
24. Glover D, Glick JH, Weiser C, et al. WR2721 and high dose cisplatin: an active combination in the treatment of metastatic melanoma. J Clin Oncol 1987; 5:574.
25. Madias NE, Harrington JT. Platinum nephrotoxicity. Am J Med 1978; 65:307–314.
26. Evans LM, Casper ES, Rosenbluth R. Phase II trial of carboplatin in advanced malignant melanoma. Cancer Treat Rep 1987; 71:171–172.
27. Abrams M, Eisenberger R, Kaplan R, Alsner J. A phase I study of iproplatin (CHIP) in advanced malignant melanoma. Proc Am Soc Clin Oncol 1988; 7:254.
28. Mathe G, Kidani Y, Triana K, et al. A phase I trial of trans-1-diaminocyclohexane oxalato-platinum (L-OHP). Biomed Pharmacother 1986; 40:372–376.
29. Ewig RAG, Kohn KW. DNA damage and repair in mouse leukemia L1210 cells treated with mitogen mustard, 1,3-bis (2 chloroethyl)-1-nitrosourea, and other nitrosoureas. Cancer 1977; 37:2114–2122.
30. Kahn HE Jr. Comparison of biochemical and biological effects of four nitrosoureas with differing carbomylating activities. Cancer Res 1978; 38:2363–2366.
31. Tew KD, Sudhakar S, Schein PS, Sonulson ME. Binding of chlorozotocin and 1-(2-chloroethyl)-3-cyclohexyl-1-nitrosourea to chromatin and nucleosomal fractions of hela cells. Cancer Res 1978; 38:3371–3378.
32. Ramirez G, Wilson W, Grage T, et al. Phase II evaluation of 1,3-bis(2-chloroethyl-nitrosourea) (BCNU); NSC-409962) in patients with solid tumors. Cancer Chemother Rep 1972; 56:787.
33. Ahmann DL, Hahn RG, Bisel HF. A comparative study of 1-(2-chloroethyl)-3-cyclo-hyxyl-1-nitrosourea (NSC-79037) and imidaxole carboxamide (NSC-45388)

with vincristine (NSC-67574) in the palliation of disseminated malignant melanoma. Cancer Res 1972; 32:2432.
34. DeVita VT, Carbone PP, Ownes AH Jr, et al. Clinical trials with 1,3-bis(2-chloroethyl)-1-nitrosourea, NSC-409962. Cancer Res 1965; 25:1875.
35. Hoogstraten B, Gottlieb JA, Caroli E, et al. CCNU (1-(2,chloroethyl)-3-cyclohexyl-1-nitrosourea, NSC-79037) in the treatment of cancer. Cancer 1973; 32:38.
36. Ahmann DL, Hahn RG, Bisel HF. Evaluation of 1-(2-chloroethyl-3-4-methyl-cyclohexyl)-1-nitrosourea (methyl-CCNU, NSC-95441) versus combined imidazole carboxamide (NSC-45388) and vincristine (NSC-67574) in palliation of disseminated melanoma. Cancer 1974; 33:615.
37. Wasserman TH, Slavik M, Carter SK. Review of CCNU in clinical cancer therapy. Cancer Treat Rev 1974; 1:131.
38. Young RC, Canellos GP, Chabner BA, et al. Treatment of malignant melanoma with methyl-CCNU. Cancer Pharmacol Ther 1974; 15:617.
39. Wasserman TH, Slavik M, Carter SK. Methyl-CCNU in clinical cancer therapy. Cancer Treat Rev 1974; 1:251.
40. Jacquillat C, Khayat D, Banzet P, et al. Final report of the French multicenter phase II study of the nitrosourea fotemustine in 153 evaluable patients with disseminated malignant melanoma including patients with cerebral metastases. Cancer 1990; 66:1873–1878.
41. Calabresi F, Aspro M, Becquart D, et al. Multicenter phase II trial of the single agent fotemustine in patients with advanced malignant melanoma. Ann Oncol 1991; 2:378.
42. Schallecuter KU, Wenzel E, Bressow FW, et al. Positive phase II study in the treatment of advanced malignant melanoma with fotemustine. Cancer Chemother Pharmacol 1991; 29:85.
43. Quagilana JM, Stephens M, Baker LH, Constanzi JJ. Vindesine in patients with metastatic malignant melanoma: a Southwest Oncology Group study. J Clin Oncol 1984; 4:316.
44. Binzig AJ, Hochster H, Wiernik PH, et al. A phase II study of taxol in patients with malignant melanoma. Invest New Drugs 1991; 9:59.
45. Fletcher WS, Daniels DS, Sandak VK, et al. Evaluation of cisplatin and DTIC in inoperable stage III and IV melanoma. A SWOG study. Am J Clin Oncol 1993; 16:359–362.
46. Luikart SD, Kennealey GT, Kirkwood JM. Randomized phase III trial of vinblastine, bleomycin, and cisdichlorodiammine-platinum versus dacarbazine in malignant melanoma. J Clin Oncol 1984; 2:164.
47. Oratz R, Speyer JL, Wernz SC, Hochster H, Meyers M, Mischak R, Spitler LE. Antimelanoma monoclonal antibody-ricin A chain immunoconjugate (XMMME-001-RTA) plus cyclophosphamide in the treatment of metastatic malignant melanoma: results of a phase II trial. Journal Biol Resp Mod 1990; 9:345–354.
48. De Prete SA, Maurer LH, O'Donnell J. Combination chemotherapy with cisplatin, carmustine, dacarbazine, and tamoxifen in metastatic melanoma. Cancer Treat Rep 1984; 68:1403.
49. McClay EF, Mastrangelo MJ, Bellet RE. Combination chemotherapy and hormonal therapy in the treatment of malignant melanoma. Cancer Treat Rep 1987; 71:1465.

50. McClay EF, Mastrangelo MJ, Berd D, Bellet RE. Effective combination chemo/hormonal therapy for malignant melanoma: experience with three clinical trials. Int J Cancer 1992; 50:553.
51. Cocconi G, Bella M, Calabresi F, et al. Treatment of metastatic malignant melanoma with dacarbazine plus tamoxifen. N Engl J Med 1992; 327:516.
52. Phillips GL, Fay JW, Herzig GP, et al. Intensive 1,3-bis(2-chloroethyl)-1-nitrosourea (BNCU), NSC-409962 and cryopreserve autologous marrow transplantation for refractory cancer. A phase I–II study. Cancer 1983; 52:1792.
53. Antman K, Eder JP, Elias A, et al. High dose combination alkylating agent preparative regimen with autologous bone marrow support: the Dana-Farber Cancer Institute/Beth Isral Hospital experience. Cancer Treat Rep 1987; 71:119.
54. Koeppler H, Pfleuger KH, Seitz R, et al. High dose chemotherapy with autologous bone marrow support in advanced malignant melanoma. Onkologie 1989; 12:277–279.
55. Peters WP, Stuart A, Klotman M, et al. High dose combination cyclophosphamide, cisplatin and melphalan with autologous bone marrow support. A clinical and pharmacologic study. Cancer Chemother Pharmacol 1989; 23:377–383.
56. Thatcher D, Lind M, Morgenstern G, et al. High-dose, double alkylating agent chemotherapy with DTIC, melphalan or ifosfamide and marrow rescue for metastatic malignant melanoma. Cancer 1989; 63:1296–1302.
57. Creagan ET, Ahmann DL, Frytak S, et al. Phase II trials of recombinant leukocyte A interferon in disseminated malignant melanoma: results in 96 patients. Cancer Treat Rep 1986; 70:619.
58. Dorval T, Palangie T, Jouve M, et al. Clinical phase II trial of recombinant DNA interferon (interferon alpha 2b) in patients with metastatic malignant melanoma. Cancer 1986; 58:215.
59. Hersey P, MacDonald M, Hall C, et al. Immunological effects of recombinant interferon alfa-2a in patients with disseminated melanoma. Cancer 1986; 57:1666.
60. Kirkwood JM, Ernstoff MS, Davis CA, et al. Comparison of intramuscular and intravenous recombinant alpha-2 interferon in melanoma and other cancers. Ann Intern Med 1985; 103:32.
61. Legha SS. Interferons in the treatment of malignant melanoma: a review of recent trials. Cancer 1986; 57:1675.
62. Robinson WA, Mughal T, Johnson TJ, et al. Treatment of advanced malignant melanoma with subcutaneous recombinant interferon. Proc Am Soc Clin Oncol 1986; 3:132.
63. Von Wussow B, Hartmann F, Deicher H. Intralesional interferon-alpha therapy in advanced malignant melanoma. Cancer 1988; 61:1071.
64. Walsh CM, Speyer JL, Wernz J, et al. Phase I study of the combination of alpha 2 interferon and cis-platinum. J Biol Resp Mod 1989; 8:11–15.
65. Oratz R, Dugan M, Walsh C, et al. Phase II trial of recombinant alpha-2a interferon and cis-platin in metastatic malignant melanoma. Proc Am Soc Clin Oncol 1989; 8:288.
66. McLeod GRC, Thomson DB, Hersey P. Recombinant interferon alfa-2a in advanced malignant melanoma: a phase I–II study in combination with DTIC. Int J Cancer 1987; 31(suppl).

67. Kirkwood JM, Ernstoff MS, Guiliano A, et al. Interferon alpha 2 and dacarbazine (DTIC) in melanoma. J Natl Cancer Inst 1990; 80:1062.
68. Falkson CI, Flakson G, Flakson HC. Improved results with the addition of interferon alfa-2b to dacarbazine in the treatment of patient with metastatic malignant melanoma. J Clin Oncol 1991; 9:1403.
69. Meyskens FL Jr, Gilmartin E, Alberts DS, Levine NS, Brooks S, Salmon SE, Surwit EA. Activity of isotretinoin against squamous cell cancers and preneoplastic lesions. Cancer Treat Rep 1982; 66:1315–1319.
70. Lippman SM, Kessler JF, Meyskens FL. Retinoids as preventive and therapeutic anticancer agents. Part I. Cancer Treat Rep 1987; 71:391–405.
71. Lippman SM, Kessler JF, Meyskens FL. Retinoids as preventive and therapeutic anticancer agents. Part II. Cancer Treat Rep 1987; 71:493–515.
72. Lotan R, Hendrix MJC, Lippman SM. Retinoids in the management of melanoma. In: Marks R, ed. Retinoids and cell differentiation. Oxford: Blackwell Scientific, 1990; 133–149.
73. Meyskens FL Jr, Salmon SE. Inhibition of human melanoma colony formation by retinoids. Cancer Res 1979; 39:4055–4057.
74. Edwards L, Jaffe P. The effect of topical tretinoin on dysplastic nevi. Arch Dermat 1990; 126:494–499.
75. Levine N, Meyskens FL Jr. Topical vitamin-A-acid therapy for cutaneous metastatic melanoma. Lancet 1980; 2:224–226.
76. Lippman SM, Shimm DS, Meyskens FL Jr. Nonsurgical treatment for skin cancer. J Dermat Surg Oncol 1988; 14:862–869.
77. Dhingra K, Papadopoulos N, Lippman S, et al. Phase II study of alpha interferon and 13-cis-retinoic acid in metastatic melanoma. Invest New Drugs 1993; 11:39–43.
78. Sarna GP, Figlin RA, Pertcheck M. Phase II study of betaseron (βser^{17}-interferon) as treatment of advanced malignant melanoma. J Biol Resp Mod 1987; 6:375.
79. Ernstoff MS, Trautman T, Davis CA, et al. A randomized phase I/II study of continuous versus intermittent intravenous interferon gamma in patients with metastatic melanoma. J Clin Oncol 1987; 5:1804.
79a. Lotze MT, Line BRM, Mathisen DJ, et al. The in vivo distribution of autologous human and murine lymphoid cells growth in T cell growth factor (TCGF): implications for the adoptive immunotherapy of tumors. J Immunol 1980; 125:238–245.
79b. Sondel PM, Kohler PC, Hank JA, et al. Clinical and immunological effects of recombinant interleukin-2 given by repetitive weekly cycles of patients with cancer. Cancer Res 1988; 48:2561–2567.
80. Shih Y, Konrad M, Warren K, Meyers FJ, Paradise C, Groves E. Serum lymphokine profiles in cancer patients before and after administration of pegylated interleukin-2. Proc Am Soc Clin Oncol 1990; 9:184.
81. Rosenstein M, Yvon I, Kaufman Y, Rosenberg SA. Lymphokine-activated killer cells: lysis of fresh syngeneic natural killer-resistant murine tumor cells by lymphocytes cultured in interleukin-2. Cancer Res 1984; 44:1946–1953.
82. Rosenberg SA, Spiess P, Lafreniere R. A new approach to adoptive immunotherapy of cancer with tumor infiltrating lymphocytes. Science 1986; 233:1318–1321.

83. Ettinghausen SE, Rosenberg SA. Immunotherapy of murine sarcomas using lymphokine activated killer cells: optimization of the schedule and route of administration of recombinant interleukin-2. Cancer Res 1986; 46:2784–2792.
84. Cheever MA, Thompson JA, Kern DE, et al. Interleukin-2 (IL-2) administered in vivo: Influence of IL-2 route and timing on T cell growth. J Immunol 1985; 134:3895–3900.
85. Nishimura T, Uchiyama Y, Yagi H, et al. Administration of slowly released recombinant interleukin-2: augmentation of the efficacy of adoptive immunotherapy with lymphokine-activated killer (LAK) cells. J Immunol Meth 1986; 91:21–27.
86. Papa MF, Vetto JT, Ettinghasen SE, et al. Effects of corticosteroid on the antitumor activity of lymphokine-activated killer cells and interleukin-2 in mice. Cancer Res 1986; 46:5618–5623.
87. Lafreniere R, Rosenberg SA. Successful immunotherapy of murine experimental hepatic metastases with lymphokine-activated killer cells and recombinant interleukin-2. Cancer Res 1985; 45:3736–3741.
88. Rosenberg SA, Lotze MT, Yang J, et al. Experience with the use of high-dose interleukin-2 in the teatment of 652 cancer patients. Ann Surg 1989; 210:474–485.
89. Dutcher JP, Creekmore S, Weiss GR, et al. Phase II study of high dose interleukin-2 and lymphokine activated killer cells in patients with metastatic malignant melanoma. J Clin Oncol 1989; 7:477–485.
90. Bar MH, Sznol M, Atkins MB, et al. Metastatic malignant melanoma treated with combined bolus and continuous infusion interleukin-2 and lymphokine-activeated killer cells. J Clin Oncol 1990; 8:1138–1147.
91. McCabe MS, Stablein D, Hawkins MJ. The modified group C experience—phase III randomized trials of IL-2 vs IL-2/LAK in advanced renal cell carcinoma and advanced melanoma. Proc Am Soc Clin Oncol 1991; 10:213.
92. Gaynor ER, Weiss GR, Margolin KA, et al. Phase I study of high-dose continuous-infusion recombinant interleukin-2 and autologous lymphokine-activated killer cells in patients with metastatic or unresectable malignant melanoma and renal cell carcinoma. J Natl Cancer Inst 1990; 82:1397–1402.
92a. Dutcher JP, Gaynor ER, Boldt DH, et al. A phase II study of high dose continuous infusion interleukin-2 with lymphokine activated killer cells. J Clin Oncol 1991; 9:641–648.
93. Parkinson DR, Abrams JS, Wiernik PH, et al. Interleukin-2 therapy in patients with metastatic malignant melanoma: a phase II study. J Clin Oncol 1990; 8:1650–1656.
94. Rosenberg SA, Lotze MT, Yang JC, et al. Prospective, randomized trial of high-dose interleukin-2 alone or in conjunction with lymphokine-activated killer cells for the treatment of patients with advanced cancer. J Natl Cancer Inst 1993; 85:622–631.
95. Richards JM, Bajorin DF, Vogelzang NJ, et al. Treatment of metastatic melanoma with continuous intravenous IL-2 $\pm$ LAK cells: a randomized trial. Proc Am Soc Clin Oncol 1990; 9:279.
96. Mitchell MS, Kempf FA, Harel W, et al. Effectiveness and tolerability of low-dose cyclophosphamide and low-dose intravenous interleukin-2 in disseminated melanoma. J Clin Oncol 1988; 6:409–424.

97. Lindemann A, Hoffken K, Schmidt RE, et al. A phase II study of low dose cyclophosphamide and recombinant interleukin-2 in metastatic renal cell carcinoma and malignant melanoma. Cancer Immunol Immunother 1989; 28:275–281.
98. Whitehead RP, Kopecky KJ, Samson MK, et al. A phase II study of IV bolus recombinant interleukin 2 in metastatic malignant melanoma: a Southwest Oncology Group study. Proc Am Soc Clin Oncol 1989; 8:284.
99. Perez EA, Scudder SA, Meyers FA, Tanaka MS, Paradise C, Gandara DR. Weekly 24-hour continuous infusion interleukin-2 for metastatic melanoma and renal cell carcinoma: a phase I study. J Immunother 1991; 10:57–62.
100. Rosenberg SA. The immunotherapy and gene therapy of cancer. J Clin Oncol 1992; 10:180–199.
101. Rosenberg SA, Lotze MT, Yang JC, et al. Combination therapy with interleukin-2 and alpha-interferon for the treatment of patients with advanced cancer. J Clin Oncol 1989; 7:1863–1874.
102. Sparano JA, Fisher RI, Sunderland, et al. Randomized phase III trial of treatment with high-dose interleukin-2 either alone or in combination with interferon alfa-2a in patients with advanced melanoma. J Clin Oncol 1993; 11:1969–1977.
103. Demchak PA, Mier JW, Robert NJ, O'Brien K, Gould JA, Atkins MB. Interleukin-2 and high-dose cisplatin in patients with metastatic melanoma: a pilot study. J Clin Oncol 1991; 9:1821–1830.
104. Shiloni E, Pouillart P, Janssen J, et al. Sequential dacarbazine chemotherapy followed by recombinant interleukin-2 in metastatic melanoma. A pilot multicentre phase I–II study. Eur J Cancer Clin Oncol 1989; 25(suppl 3):45–49.
105. Stoter G, Shiloni E, Aamdal S, et al. Sequential administration of recombinant human interleukin-2 and dacarbazine in metastatic melanoma. A multicentre phase II study. Eur J Cancer Clin Oncol 1989; 25(suppl 3):41–43.
106. Dillman RO, Oldham RK, Barth NM, et al. Recombinant interleukin-2 and adoptive immunotherapy alternated with dacarbazine therapy in melanoma: a National Biotherapy Study Group trial. J Natl Cancer Inst 1990; 82:1345–1349.
107. Papadopoulos NEJ, Howard JG, Murray JL, et al. Phase II DTIC and interleukin 2 (IL-2) trial for metastatic malignant melanoma. Proc Am Soc Clin Oncol 1990; 9:1072A.
108. Flaherty LE, Robinson W, Redman BG, et al. A phase II study of dacarbazine and cisplatin in combination with outpatient administered interleukin-2 in metastatic malignant melanoma. Cancer 1993; 71:3520–3525.
109. Hellstrom I, Braukorau V, Hellstrom E. Strong anti-tumor activation of IgG3 antibodies to human melanoma associated ganglioside. Proc Natl Acad Sci USA 1985; 82:1499.
110. Lowder JN, Meeher TC, Campbell M, et al. Studies in B-lymphoid tumors with monoclonal anti-idiotype antibodies: correlation with clinical responses. Blood 1987; 69:199.
111. Herlyn D, Koprowski H. IgG2a monoclonal antibodies exhibit human tumor growth through interaction with effector cells. Proc Natl Acad Sci USA 1982; 79:4761.

112. Bajorin D, Chapman P, Kunicka J, et al. Phase I trial of a combination of R24 mouse monoclonal antibody and recombinant interleukin-2 in patients with melanoma. Proc Am Soc Clin Oncol 1987; 6:210.
113. Engelstad B, Khentigan A, Rosendorf L, et al. Initial clinical experience with intravenous and subcutaneous indium-111 antimelanoma monoclonal radioimmunoimaging. Radiology 1985; 157:98.
114. Houghton AN, Mintzer D, Cordon-Cardo C, et al. Mouse monoclonal IgG3 antibody detecting GD_3 ganglioside. A phase I trial in patients with malignant melanoma. Proc Natl Acad Sci USA 1985; 82:1242.
115. Spitler LE, del Rio M, Khentyan A, et al. Therapy of patients with malignant melanoma using a monoclonal antimelanoma antibody-ricin A chain immunotoxin. Cancer Res 1987; 47:1717.
116. Goodman GE, Beaumier P, Hellstrom I, et al. Pilot trial of murine monoclonal antibodies in patients with advanced melanoma. J Clin Oncol 1985; 3:340.
117. Oratz R, Speyer JL, Wernz J, et al. Activity of an antimelanoma monoclonal antibody-ricin. A chain immunotoxin and cyclophosphamide in metastatic malignant melanoma. Berkeley, Calif.: Society of Biological Therapy, 1988.
118. Oldham RK, Foon KA, Morgan AC, et al. Monoclonal antibody therapy of malignant melanoma: In vivo localization in cutaneous metastatic after intravenous administration. J Clin Oncol 1984; 2:1235.
119. Bajorin D, Chapman P, Wong G, et al. Phase I evaluation of a combination of monoclonal antibody R24 and interleukin 2 in patients with metastatic melanoma. Cancer Res 1990; 50:7490–7495.
120. Bystryn J-C. Tumor vaccines. Cancer Met Rev 1990; 9:81–91.
121. Bystryn J-C. Antibody response and tumor growth in syngeneic mice immunized to partially purified B16 melanoma associated antigens. J Immunol 1978; 120:96–101.
122. Morton D, Hoon D, Nizze J, Foshag L, et al. Polyvalent vaccine improves survival of patients with metastatic melanoma. Ann Surg 1992; 216(4):463–482.
123. Berd D, Maguire H, Mastrangelo M. Treatment of human melanoma with a hapten modified autologous vaccine. Ann NY Acad Sci 1993; 690:147–150.
124. Mitchell M, Harel W, Kan-Mitchell J, Lemay L, et al. Active specific immunotherapy of melanoma with allogenic cell lysates. Ann NY Acad Sci 1993; 690:153–165.
125. Hersey P. Evaluation of vaccinia viral lysates as therapeutic vaccines in the treatment of melanoma. Ann NY Acad Sci 1993; 690:167–177.
126. Wallack M, Sivanandham M. Clinical trials VMO for melanoma. Ann NY Acad Sci 1993; 690:178–189.
127. Livingston P. Approaches to augmenting the IgG antibody response to melanoma ganglioside vaccines. Ann NY Acad Sci 1993; 690:204–213.
128. Coulie P, Weynets P, Muller C, Lehmann F, Herman J, Bauran JF, Boon T. Genes encoding for antigen recognition on human tumors by autologous cytolytic T lymphocytes. Ann NY Acad Sci 1993; 690:113–119.
129. Ferrone S. Human tumor associated antigen mimicry by anti-idiotypic antibodies. Ann NY Acad Sci 1993; 690:214–221.
130. Bystryn J-C, Jacobsen S, Harris MN, Roses DF, Speyer JL, Levin M. Preparation and characterization of a polyvalent human melanoma antigen vaccine. J Biol Resp Mod 1986; 5:221–224.

131. Bystryn J-C. Immunogenicity and clinical activity of a polyvalent melanoma antigen vaccine prepared from shed antigens. In: Specific immunotherapy of cancer with vaccines. Bystryn J-C, Ferrone S, Livingston P, ed. Ann NY Acad Sci 690:190–203.
132. Oratz R, Cockerell C, Speyer J, et al. Induction of lymphocytic cell infiltrate in human melanoma nodules by active immunization of melanoma antigen vaccine. Proc Am Assoc Cancer Res 1987; 28:374.

22
Treatment of Cutaneous Viral Infections

Omeed M. Memar and Stephen K. Tyring
University of Texas Medical Branch, Galveston, Texas

Monica L. McCrary
Medical College of Georgia, Augusta, Georgia

Skin lesions are a common presentation in viral infections. The most common viruses with cutaneous manifestations include the herpesviruses, papillomaviruses, pox viruses, parvovirus B19, enteroviruses, rubeola, rubella, and the human retroviruses, including HIV. In the past, no specific drugs were available for the treatment of viral infections, but in recent times, a wide selection of antiviral agents have become available. Most antivirals are effective against herpesviruses and retroviruses. Therefore, the correct diagnosis of viral infections is even more important than it used to be, due to the implications in therapy and prognosis. In this chapter, we will review the etiology, pathology, and treatment of lesions caused by the above mentioned viruses.

I. HERPES SIMPLEX VIRUSES

Acyclovir is indicated for the treatment of primary and recurrent genital and nongenital herpes simplex virus (HSV) infections in certain clinical situations.

Initial genital HSV infections, even in nonimmunocompromised hosts, can often be severe. The signs and symptoms may include pain, itching, fever, headache, stiff neck, mild photophobia, malaise, dysuria, urethral and vaginal discharge, inguinal adenopathy, myalgia, pharyngitis, prostration, central nervous system involvement, and urinary retention. Oral acyclovir at 200 mg five times daily for 10 d has been shown to be highly effective in reducing both the duration of viral shedding and lesion healing, and in some studies new lesion formation and pain duration (1–3). Patients with more severe signs and symptoms of initial genital HSV may be more appropriately managed with the more potent intravenous preparation at 5 mg/kg every 8 h for 7 d (4–6). Topical acyclovir therapy decreases viral shedding and time to lesion crusting, but does so less effectively than the alternate preparations (7,8). The efficacy of acyclovir administration may be increased by the early initiation of treatment. Acyclovir therapy of initial genital HSV does not alter the frequency of subsequent recurrences (9,10).

Recurrent HSV tends to be less severe than the primary episode and varies among patients in the frequency, intensity, and duration of episodes. The extent of the medical and psychosocial morbidity must be appreciated in the individual patient to best guide therapeutic management. Topical acyclovir ointment, while shortening the duration of viral shedding, is not an effective modality in the amelioration of the signs and symptoms of recurrent HSV (11,12). Since recurrent HSV tends to be milder and briefer than its primary counterpart, even when oral acyclovir treatment is instituted within 24 h of disease onset, the clinical benefits are minimal. Viral shedding and time to healing are slightly decreased, but the duration of symptoms is unaffected (3,13). Therefore, intermittent oral acyclovir at 200 mg five times daily for 5 d may be most appropriately offered to those individuals with frequent and moderately severe episodes that are preceded by discernible prodromes allowing for the early institution of therapy. For those patients with frequent (more than 6 per year) and/or particularly disconcerting episodes, continuous suppressive treatment of 400 mg of oral acyclovir twice daily is most appropriate and has been reported to effectively limit the frequency and severity of recurrences. Rarely, patients may require a higher dose of acyclovir to control symptoms. Effective suppression without serious side effects or cumulative toxicity for a period of up to 5 y has been shown (14). Asymptomatic viral shedding may occur during clinically successful suppressive treatment periods, and patients thus should be informed that even at those times infectious transmission may occur (15,16). The frequency and severity of HSV outbreaks tend to decrease with time. Every 12 mo patients should interrupt continuous suppressive therapy to determine whether the severity and frequency of the outbreaks necessitate continued treatment (17,18).

Chronic suppressive therapy with acyclovir has raised a number of issues. Acyclovir exhibits genetic toxicity by the induction of chromosome breaks in vitro and when administered in highly toxic doses to rodents (19). Chronic suppressive acyclovir therapy has not been shown to result in any such cytogenetic effects (20). The rebound effect after withdrawal of suppressive therapy described by Douglas et al. (21) has not been observed in other studies (22,23). After 1 y of chronic acyclovir treatment, the antibodies against the major proteins of HSV-2 (gB, gG, gD, gC/gE, VPIG) usually decrease. This decrease does not result in earlier and more severe recurrences after therapy termination (24). Those individuals with relatively high antibody levels to gB after therapy had relatively more severe first recurrences with treatment cessation (24). Chronic suppressive acyclovir treatment does not appear to have a clinically significant effect on sperm count, motility, or morphology (25). It is presently unanswered whether there is any mutagenicity or impairment of fertility with acyclovir administration in humans. Consequently, it is imperative to discuss these issues with the patient with reproductive potential.

The concerns that prolonged treatment might lead to acyclovir resistance moved from the laboratory to the clinic with the report of drug-resistant isolates identified during outbreaks from individuals on a suppressive acyclovir regimen (26). Subsequent studies that evaluated the sensitivity of HSV isolate before and after chronic acyclovir treatment in nonimmunocompromised patients found no change (27–29). This does not preclude the finding of an occasional patient who exhibits diminished sensitivity to acyclovir in the form of outbreaks during suppressive treatment, but at least in immunocompetent patients it is usually not the chronic treatment that predisposes them to their relative resistance. However, patients with AIDS and other severe immunodeficiencies are exhibiting acyclovir resistant HSV-2 infections with prolonged treatment of acyclovir. This resistance often can be clinically overcome with higher doses of acyclovir (18). On subsequent recurrences, after temporary discontinuation of a suppressive acyclovir regimen, resistant strains often revert and exhibit sensitivity to acyclovir (30,31). The nature of the resistance is usually a deficiency or absence of thymidine kinase. These viruses tend to be less virulent than the wild type, with a diminished ability to establish latency in the sensory ganglia (32). Other mechanisms of resistance include altered thymidine kinase (33) or DNA polymerase substrate specificity.

In addition to HSV genital infections, acyclovir is effective in other HSV-associated disease processes. Herpes simplex labialis (cold sore) can often prove to be both recurrent and vexing. It is often triggered by UV radiation or trigeminal surgery. Acyclovir has been shown to adequately treat (34) recurrent herpes simplex labialis and also to prophylaxis against its reactivation (35–37). Recurrent erythema multiforme is often a reaction to clinical or subclinical HSV infection. Oral acyclovir does prevent postherpetic-associated erythema multiforme (38–41).

Oral and intravenous acyclovir has been effective in treating herpetic tracheobronchitis (42,43). Eczema herpeticum, a potentially fatal disseminated HSV infection of compromised skin, can be treated with either intravenous or oral acyclovir (44–46).

Patients at risk for dermabrasion-induced HSV infections are frequently prophylaxed with acyclovir (47).

II. HERPES ZOSTER VIRUS

Herpes zoster (HZ) is caused by the reactivation of the varicella zoster virus (VZV) after latency in the dorsal root ganglia. Although HZ can be seen at any age, both its frequency and morbidity increase with age and degree of immunosuppression. The most serious complications of HZ often seen in the immunocompetent and immunocompromised patient are postherpetic neuralgia and hematogenous dissemination, respectively. Intravenous acyclovir in the immunocompromised host shortens the course of HZ and reduces the frequency of dissemination (48,49). Oral acyclovir (800 mg five times a day) has been shown in the immunocompetent patient to decrease both rash and acute pain duration (50). Postherpetic neuralgia has also been shown to be diminished with oral acyclovir (51). As with HSV infections, the maximal efficacy of acyclovir treatment is achieved when dosing is initiated soon after the start of the HZ outbreak.

Recurrent aphthous ulceration (RAU) of the oral mucous membrane may be caused by a local reactivation of VZV (52). While a double-blind study of oral acyclovir at 400 mg twice daily did not show efficacy in preventing RAU recurrence (53) an open trial of acyclovir at 800 mg twice daily did show benefit (54).

Varicella is a common, highly communicable viral disease for which no vaccine is commercially available. In the pediatric immunocompetent population varicella tends to be a self-limiting, low morbidity process, however there is a mortality rate of 2 per 100,000 childhood cases and 8 per 100,000 infant cases. Approximately 4000–6000 otherwise healthy individuals are admitted to hospitals each year with complications of primary varicella infection (55). The morbidity and mortality from this process increases dramatically with age and with degree of immunosuppression (56–58). Intravenous acyclovir has been shown to be efficacious for the treatment of varicella immunocompromised children and adults (50,51,59–63).

In a double-blind, placebo controlled study in immunocompetent varicella patients between 5 and 16 y of age who began oral acyclovir within 24 h of onset of their cutaneous eruption, the active group as compared with the placebo group experienced fewer and more rapidly healing cutaneous lesions and also less fever (64). The modest therapeutic efficacy of oral acyclovir in reducing the severity and symptoms of childhood varicella, including pruritus and constitutional illness, has also been shown in subsequent studies (65,66). The rate of complications or transmission of varicella did not differ among the treatment groups. This therapeutic intervention did not alter VZ-specific humoral or cellular immune responses measured a month and a year posttreatment (64).

The American Academy of Pediatrics committee on Infectious Diseases concluded in a recent position paper that because of the minimal efficacy of a rather expensive drug, which must be started within 24 h of disease onset, oral acyclovir is not recommended routinely for the treatment of uncomplicated varicella in otherwise healthy children (67). However, the report continues, those individuals who are more susceptible to experiencing an extreme course of varicella or its complications may warrant instituting, within 24 h of disease onset, oral acyclovir at a dose of 20 mg/kg (up to 800 mg) four times a day for 5 d. These individuals include otherwise healthy adolescents 13 y or older, children older than 12 mo with chronic cutaneous or pulmonary disorders, those receiving chronic salicylate therapy, and children receiving corticosteroid therapy, but specifically excludes those who are immunocompromised or are experiencing varicella virus-mediated complications for which intravenous acyclovir would be most appropriate.

In the treatment of infectious mononucleosis, a double-blind, placebo controlled study showed that acyclovir reversibly inhibited the oropharyngeal shedding of the Epstien-Barr virus and globally but not individually ameliorated symptoms (68).

Oral hairy leukoplakia (OHL) is an Epstien-Barri–induced asymptomatic benign white plaque with a verrucose surface seen on the inferiorlateral surface of the tongues of patients with HIV-induced immunodeficiency. Acyclovir induces regression of OHL, but recurrences are commonplace with treatment cessation (69,75).

The frequency and severity of herpetic infections varies directly with the degree of immunosuppression. Manifestations of severe herpetic involvement in the immunocompromised can include widespread cutaneous involvement, esophogitis, gastritis, tracheobronchitis, pneumonia, DIC, and encephalitis. Management approaches include early diagnosis with aggressive treatment and also prophylaxis. Transplant patients often experience severe episodes of herpes infections. Acyclovir prophylaxis has been shown to significantly decrease the frequency and severity of CMV infections in liver transplant patients (70–72) and herpes zoster infections in allogeneic bone marrow transplant patients (73–75).

The Acyclovir in Pregnancy Registry is maintained by the Burroughs Wellcome Company to track prospectively exposed pregnancies to evaluate exposure and outcomes and also to accumulate data on retrospective exposures. Through June 30, 1990, the Registry logged 312 prospective and 145 retrospective cases. No increase in the number of birth defects were seen in the prospective group over what was expected in the general population and no consistent pattern of abnormalities was recognized in the retrospective group (76). While these findings are reassuring, the number of cases was not large enough to draw definite conclusions regarding the safety of acyclovir during pregnancy. Consequently, it is still recommended to follow the CDC Sexually Transmitted Disease Treatment Guidelines from September 1989 (77) which limit the use of acyclovir in pregnancy to life-threatening maternal HSV infections (e.g., disseminated infections that include encephalitis, pneumonitis, and/or hepatitis).

A. Adverse Reactions

Topical acyclovir is well tolerated. The reports of mild pain and pruritus with acyclovir application to genital ulcers was not increased compared to placebo (78). Contact sensitization has rarely been reported (79,80).

Oral acyclovir is uncommonly associated with untoward effects. Clinical trial data from short-term oral acyclovir administration for genital HSV revealed nausea and vomiting (2.7%), headache (0.6%), diarrhea, dizziness, anorexia, fatigue, edema, skin rash, leg pain, inguinal adenopathy, medication taste, and sore throat (each 0.3%) (81). Long-term acyclovir (400 mg two times a day) administered for suppressive HSV therapy displayed adverse effects of nausea (4.8%), diarrhea (2.4%), headache (1.9%), and rash (1.7%) (81). When treating herpes zoster with 800 mg five times daily for 7–10 d the adverse effects were malaise (11.5%), nausea (8.5%), headache (5.5%), vomiting (2.5%), diarrhea (1.5%), and constipation (0.9%). Oral acyclovir has also been reported in the treatment of herpes zoster to cause bilateral pitting pedal edema (82) and acute renal failure (83,84).

Intravenous acyclovir is well tolerated. The most frequent adverse reaction is phlebitis (9%) (85). If the concentration of the acyclovir infusion is too high, a local vesicular eruption can be precipitated. Transient elevations of serum BUN and creatinine are seen (5–10%) (86). The renal insufficiency develops as the result of obstructive crystal nephropathy in the collecting ducts (87). Acyclovir crystalluria might be an early sign of acyclovir crystal nephropathy (88). The nephropathy is dose related and is often reversible by instituting hydration and/or by stopping further acyclovir administration. To prevent such adverse events, dosage modification is mandated in the setting of decreased creatinine clearance and patients must be adequately hydrated. Pruritus (2%), rash or hives (2%), and elevated transaminase (1–2%) also occur (85).

Neurotoxicity is a rare but potentially serious adverse effect. Lethargy, obtundation, tremors, confusion, hallucinations, agitation, seizures, or coma are seen (85). This neurotoxicity, which is reversible upon treatment cessation, has also been reported with oral acyclovir therapy (89,90).

B. Pharmacology

Valaciclovir provides a substantial increase in the plasma concentration of acyclovir and may prove to be highly efficacious in varied clinical situations.

Herpes simplex virus is very sensitive to acyclovir, but in the treatment of HSV infections, frequent oral dosing of acyclovir is mandated. With enhanced bioavaibility of valaciclovir, equal or greater clinical efficacy might be realized with a less frequent dosing schedule. Occasionally, HSV demonstrates resistance to acyclovir that can be overcome by high plasma concentration of acyclovir delivered by the intravenous route. Valaciclovir may be effective in this setting.

Varicella zoster virus is less sensitive to acyclovir, necessitating a frequent dosing schedule, a dramatic increase in the dose of acyclovir, and often the institution of intravenous treatment. Valaciclovir at 1000 mg TID, as compared with acyclovir, 800 mg five times a day, in the treatment of acute herpes zoster has been shown in a large multinational double-blind study to significantly reduce duration of pain (91).

Acyclovir has shown efficacy in the suppression of cytomegalovirus (CMV) infections in bone marrow recipients (92). The relative resistance that CMV displays for acyclovir requires very high and frequent dosing schedules that might be obviated by valaciclovir.

C. Adverse Effects

Valaciclovir has been shown to have the same side effects profile as acyclovir (93).

III. EPSTEIN-BARR VIRUS

Epstein-Barr virus (EBV) also belongs to the herpesvirus family of DNA viruses (94). EBV is associated with a number of human illnesses, including infectious mononucleosis (IM), African Burkitt's lymphoma, nasopharyngeal carcinoma, lymphomas and lymphoproliferative diseases in immunocompromised patients, and chronic fatigue syndrome (95). Rashes occur in 3–16% of patients with IM; this number increases dramatically in patients treated with certain penicillin derivatives such as ampicillin. Heterophile antibodies are present in 90% of IM patients, and the remaining 10% can be diagnosed with EBV-specific antibodies. By cytology of peripheral blood, there is evidence of lymphocytosis and atypical lymphocytes. In HIV-infected patients, EBV is associated with oral hairy leukoplakia, which serves as a diagnostic marker for AIDS (96). Although acyclovir does manage to decrease EBV replication in cases of oropharyngeal EBV infections, acyclovir is generally ineffective in the treatment of EBV-induced lesions (97). Furthermore, a vaccine using a recombinant gp350 envelope glycoprotein of EBV has shown preliminary in vivo success in animals (98).

IV. CYTOMEGALOVIRUS

Cytomegalovirus (CMV) is also a DNA virus belonging to the herpesvirus family. CMV is ubiquitous in the human population. CMV rarely causes disease in immunocompetent individuals, while immunocompromised individuals commonly have CMV-associated diseases. The most common mode of CMV transmission in adults is sexual intercourse. Among AIDS patients, almost 90% have CMV at the time of death. Although CMV has few cutaneous manifestations, the most common is perianal ulcerations (99). Histologically a basophilic intranuclear inclusion (i.e., owl's eye) nonspecifically indicates a CMV infection. The FDA has approved ganciclovir and foscarnet in the treatment of CMV retinitis. In transplant patients, IFN-α or CMV hyperimmune globulin have shown partial protection (100). Currently, there are ongoing clinical trials using a live attenuated CMV vaccine; however, the results have been mixed (101).

V. HUMAN HERPESVIRUS TYPE 6

Human herpesvirus type 6 (HHV-6) is yet another member of the herpesvirus family. HHV-6 has been recognized as the causative agent in exanthem subitum (roseola infantum), otherwise known as sixth disease (102). Exanthem subitum is highly contagious, and presents with 3–5 d of fever, followed by 1–2 d of a maculopapular rash, commonly on the neck and trunk. The preferred treatment is symptomatic relief. However, preliminary data show that ganciclovir and foscarnet have significant in vitro efficacy (103).

VI. B VIRUS

B virus herpesvirus simiae is also a member of the herpesvirus family of DNA viruses, however, it normally resides in primates and more commonly infects individuals handling macaque monkeys. This zoonosis initially induces erythema and vesicular lesions (104). However, the symptoms soon become generalized, affecting the nervous system, at times developing into a fatal case of encephalitis. The treatment of choice is intravenous acyclovir (105).

VII. HUMAN HERPESVIRUS 8

Kaposi's sarcoma (KS) lesions have been found to contain a new virus with homology with the herpesviridae (106). The DNA sequence identified represents roughly 2% of the whole virus. The DNA sequence has been identified in HIV-related KS, Mediterranean KS, iatrogenic KS, and African KS (107). This virus has also been identified in body cavity-based lymphomas of HIV-positive patients. Furthermore, HHV-8 DNA sequences have been detected in squamous cell carcinomas, basal cell carcinomas, and other lesions from HIV-negative transplant patients (108). The exact role of HHV-8 in causing disease or malignancy is not known. Although HHV-8 is present in KS lesions, more studies are needed in order to substantiate an etiological role (109).

VIII. HUMAN PAPILLOMAVIRUS

The human papillomaviruses (HPV) are DNA viruses belonging to the papovaviruses. There are over 70 different HPV genotypes, and they induce warts on different sites of the body. Certain HPV are trophic for nongenital regions (110) (e.g., HPV-1,-2,-3,-4,-10,-28,-29, and -57), while others are trophic for genital-mucosal regions (111) (e.g., HPV-6,-11,-16,-18,-31,-33, and -35); the third category includes HPV-5 and-8, which induce epidermodysplasia verruciformis (112). The first category of HPV trophic for nongenital regions includes common warts (verruca vulgaris), which present on hands and pressure surfaces, plantar warts, and flat warts. The preferred treatment for common warts is cytodestructive, using agents such as liquid nitrogen, cantharidin, salicylic acid, and lactic acid in flexible colloidin. The treatment for plantar warts includes liquid nitrogen, salicylic acid, or lactic acid in flexible colloidin. The treatment for flat warts includes topical retinoids, liquid nitrogen, salicylic acid in propylene glycol, and tissue cautery (113). Immunomodulators promise an expanded treatment armament against warts in the future (114). Although interferon is FDA approved for use only for genital warts, some investigators report successful treatment of nongenital warts using interferon. Furthermore, cimetidine, which also has immunomodulatory activities, has shown marginal success in the treatment of such warts (113).

The second category of HPV trophic for genital regions is comprised of HPV that can have differential malignant potential. HPV-6 and-11, which cause condylomata acuminata, have a very low malignant potential. HPV-31,-33, and -35 are examples of genotypes with intermediate malignant potential. However, HPV-16 and-18, which occur in genital tract dysplasia and carcinoma, cervical carcinoma, vulvar carcinoma, and bowenoid papulosis, have a very high malignant potential. There are three major modalities of treatment for genital warts. Cytodestructive measures use lasers, cryotherapy, or surgery (115). Chemodestructive measures use 5-fluorouracil cream, podofilox, bichloracetic acid, or trichloroacetic acid. Finally, intralesional injection of IFN-α has been shown to be efficacious in treating condylomata acuminata that are resistant to other forms of therapy (114). Interferon use is potentially most efficacious in combination with a cytodestructive or chemodestructive form of therapy. The specific choice of therapy is contingent on the location, number, size, and exact type of warts.

IX. MEASLES

Measles (rubeola) is caused by a virus belonging to the paramyxovirus family of RNA viruses (116). The typical symptoms include fever, cough, coryza, conjunctivitis, Koplik's spots, and as the disease progresses, a generalized macular and papular rash. Measles occurs in early childhood in more urban settings and is commonly seen in children 5–10 y old in rural areas. The FDA licensed the use of a live attenuated measles virus in 1963. However, treatment of measles is solely supportive, and not curative (117).

X. RUBELLA

Rubella (German measles) is also caused by a RNA virus and can infect both children and adults. Rubella presents with lymphadenopathy and rash, which lasts approximately 2–3 d. While the disease is self-limited, in utero, it can cause severe birth defects. The vaccine for rubella is administered in conjunction with the mumps and measles vaccine (118).

XI. PARVOVIRUS B19

Erythema infectiosum is caused by parvovirus B19. Erythema infectiosum presents with a low-grade fever, which is followed by a rash on the face, commonly refered to as "slapped cheek." In conjunction, there is a general erythematous rash on the trunk, neck, and extensor surfaces of the extremities (119). In adults, the most common sequela is acute arthropathy. However, aplastic crisis, chronic anemia, and fetal hydrops have been associated with parvovirus B19 infections. The treatment is nonspecific and supportive (120).

XII. POXVIRUSES

The most common pox virus infection of humans is molluscum contagiosum (MC), caused by the MC virus (MCV). Although two different isolates of MCV are recognized, their clinical presentations are identical (121). The mode of spread of MCV is person to person. In children MC is caused by fomite spread of MCV, while in adults it is commonly sexually transmitted (122). Therefore, MC seen on the genital region of children should raise the suspicion of sexual abuse. The lesion of MC is a dome-shaped papule with a central umbilication that appears on mucocutaneous regions. The course of MC is much more severe in immunocompromised patients. The treatment of MC lesions includes the use of liquid nitrogen, curetting, or both. Recently the intralesional injection of IFN-α has shown efficacy in immunocompetent patients, but the results are less impressive in immunocompromised AIDS patients.

Orf (contagious ecthyma or contagious pustular dermatitis) is a virally induced zoonosis. The clinical presentation on humans begins with cutaneous nodules that heal within 35 d. Therefore, there is no specific treatment for orf (123).

Milker's nodules (MN) is similarly a zoonosis seen in individuals that handle cattle (124). However, person-to-person spread has not been documented. MN lesions commonly occur on hands and forearms and are one to four in number. MN is similarly self-limited and does not require any specific treatment (125).

XIII. ENTEROVIRUSES

Different enteroviruses are known to cause hand-foot-and-mouth disease (HFMD). Coxsackie virus A16 and enterovirus 71 are associated with epidemic cases of HFMD, while sporadic cases have other Coxsackie viruses as etiological agents. HFMD primarily affects individuals prior to age 15, presenting with vesicular lesions on the extremities and mouth. HFMD is self-limited and has no specific treatment (126).

Coxsackie viruses A2, A4, A5, A6, A8, and A10 are believed to cause herpangina. Herpangina presents with gray-white papulovesicular lesions on the mucous membranes, especially around the soft palate, tonsillar pillars, and fauces, that eventually ulcerate (127). Herpangina is self-limited and does not have a specific treatment (128).

XIV. HUMAN RETROVIRUSES

Retroviruses are a family of viruses with an RNA genome that is reverse-transcribed to DNA upon infection. The important disease-causing human retroviruses are the human T-cell leukemia virus (HTLV) types I and II and human immunodeficiency virus (HIV) types 1 and 2. HTLV-I is highly correlated with the presentation of adult T-cell leukemia (ATL) and less associated with the presentation of cutaneous T-cell lymphoma (CTCL) (129). HTLV-II is not correlated with a particular disease, but the virus has been isolated from cells obtained from a patient with hairy cell leukemia. ATL presents with multiple cutaneous manifestations, most notably erythematous patches, papular and nodular tumors, or erythroderma (130).

XV. HUMAN IMMUNODEFICIENCY VIRUS

The human immunodeficiency virus (HIV) is known to infect human $CD4^+$ cells and monocytes/macrophages. HIV is believed to be the causative agent in acquired immunodeficiency syndrome (AIDS). HIV infection leads to a systematic disarmament of the immune system, leading to multiple presentations. Over 90% of HIV-positive patients have cutaneous lesions as a secondary manifestation of HIV infection. The cutaneous lesions can be grouped as having either a neoplastic, infectious, or noninfectious, nonneoplastic etiology (131).

The most common neoplastic lesion in HIV-positive patients is Kaposi's sarcoma (KS). KS is seen predominantly in homosexual and bisexual HIV-positive patients. This, and the fact that KS is more common in female sex partners of bisexual men, has indicated a possible infectious origin to KS. KS appears as erythematous macules or papules that develop into violaceous nodules or plaques. This presentation can coexist with edema in the lower extremities (132). Preferred treatment for KS is usually local radiotherapy, cytodestructive measures, or intralesional injections of bleomycin, vincristine sulfate, or IFN-α. Other neoplastic lesions in HIV-positive patients are more rare; B-cell and T-cell lymphomas appear in AIDS patients, with B-cell lymphomas being relatively more common. Still other cutaneous cancers that afflict AIDS patients include squamous cell carcinoma, basal cell carcinoma, and melanoma (133).

Infectious manifestations account for the majority of skin lesions in AIDS patients. Herpesviruses, HPV, and molluscum contagiosum are the most common opportunistic viral pathogens (134). *Staphylococcus aureus* is the most common bacterial pathogen. However, the most common mucocutaneous infection afflicting AIDS patients is candidiasis (135).

Noninfectious manifestations include autoimmune and idiopathic conditions. Seborrheic dermatitis is seen in 5–12% of the general population, while it is present in 20–80% of HIV-positive patients. Similarly, Reiter's syndrome and psoriasis are much more common in the HIV-positive population (136).

Zidovudine (AZT) is the first line of treatment for HIV infection. AZT works by acting as a thymidine analog, inhibiting reverse transcriptase. However, in AZT nonresponders, didanosine (ddI), which acts similarly to AZT but not identical, is sometimes efficacious. In those patients who have very low $CD4^+$ counts and have multiple HIV-related illnesses, zalcitabine (ddC) in combination with AZT is indicated. Stavudine and lamivudine, the fourth and fifth approved nucleoside analog inhibitors of reverse transcriptase, are indicated for patients who are intolerant to or have failed therapy with AZT. Most recently, the first protease inhibitor, saquinavir, was approved for treatment of HIV infection.

XVI. CONCLUSION

There are many viruses that cause cutaneous lesions. The appearance, distribution, length of presentation, route of reaching the skin, mechanism of causing skin lesions, and the viral etiological agent responsible differ widely between these cutaneous lesions. The art of medicine has given us appreciation for the patterns and appearances of such lesions and illnesses. However, it is the science of medicine, with the ever-expanding armaments of probing, detecting, and identifying that will uncover yet unknown organisms in lesions otherwise known as idiopathic. Recently, studies of Kaposi's sarcoma identified HHV-8 as the eighth human herpesvirus. Such improvements in technology similarly promise better therapeutics for previously untreatable viral infections. Partial fulfillment of this promise has been seen for many of the herpesviruses, with acyclovir being the prototype of specific and safe drugs. By dissecting and learning the basic life cycle of the virus and interaction of the virus with the host immune system, research promises a future of effective treatments for viral infections.

REFERENCES

1. Bryson YJ, Dillon M, Lovett M, Acuna G, Taylor S, Cherry JD, Johnson BL, Weismeier E, Growdon W, Creagh-Kirk T, Keeney R. Treatment of first episodes of genital herpes simplex virus infection with oral acyclovir: a randomized double-blind controlled trial in normal subjects. N Engl J Med 1983; 308:916–921.
2. Mertz GJ, Critchlow CW, Benedetti J, Reichman RC, Dolin R, Connor J, Redfield DC, Savoia MC, Richman DD, Tyrrell DL, Miedzinski L, Portnoy J, Keeney RE, Corey L. Double-blind placebo-controlled trial of oral acyclovir in first-episode genital herpes simplex virus infection. JAMA 1984; 252:1147–1151.
3. Nilsen AE, Aasen T, Halsos AM, Kinge BR, Tjotta EA, Wikstrom K, Fiddian AP. Efficacy of oral acyclovir in the treatment of initial and recurrent genital herpes. Lancet 1982; 2:571–573.
4. Corey L, Fife KH, Benedetti JK, Winter CA, Fahnlander A, Connor JD, Hintz MA, Holmes KK. Intravenous acyclovir for the treatment of primary genital herpes. Ann Intern Med 1983; 98:914–921.
5. Peacock JE Jr, Kaplowitz LG, Sparling PF, Durak DT, Gnann JW, Whitley RJ, Lovett M, Bryson YJ, Klein RJ, Friedman-Kien AE, Knowlton GM, Davis LG. Intravenous acyclovir therapy of first episodes of genital herpes: a multicenter double-blind, placebo-controlled trial. Am J Med 1988; 85:301–306.
6. Mindel AM, Adler W, Sutherland S, Fiddian AP. Intravenous acyclovir treatment for primary genital herpes. Lancet 1982; 1(8274):697–700.
7. Corey L, Nahmias AJ, Guinan ME, Benedetti JK, Critchlow CW, Holmes KK. A trial of topical acyclovir in genital herpes simplex virus infections. N Engl J Med 1982; 306:1313–1319.
8. Corey L, Beneditti J, Critchlow C, Mertz G, Douglas J, Fife K, Fahnlander A, Remington ML, Winter C, Dragavon J. Treatment of primary first-episode genital herpes simplex virus infections with acyclovir: results of topical, intravenous and oral therapy. J Antimicrob Chemother 1983; 12(suppl B):79–88.
9. Corey L, Mindel A, Fife KH, Sutherland S, Benedetti J, Adler MW. Risk of recurrence after treatment of first episode genital herpes with intravenous acyclovir. Sex Transm Dis 1985; 12:215–218.

10. Mindel A, Weller IV, Faherty A, Sutherland S, Fiddian AP, Adler MW. Acyclovir in first attacks of genital herpes and prevention of recurrences. Genitourin Med 1986; 62:28–32.
11. Reichman RC, Badger GJ, Guinan ME, Nahmias AG, Keeney RE, Davis LG, Ashikaga T, Dolin R. Topically administered acyclovir in the treatment of recurrent herpes simplex genitalis: a controlled trial. J Infect Dis 1983; 147:336–340.
12. Luby JP, Gnann JW Jr, Alexander WJ, Hatcher VA, Friedman-Kien AE, Klein RJ, Keyserling H, Nahmias A, Mills J, Schachter J, Douglas JM, Corey L. Sacks SL. A collaborative study of patient-initiated treatment of recurrent genital herpes with topical acyclovir or placebo. J Infect Dis 1984; 150:1–6.
13. Reichman RC, Badger GJ, Mertz GJ, Corey L, Richman DD, Connor JD, Redfield D, Savoia MC, Oxman MN, Bryson Y, Tyrrell DL, Portnoy J, Creigh-Kirk T, Keeney RE, Ashikaga T, Dolin R. Treatment of recurrent genital herpes simplex infections with oral acyclovir: a controlled trial. JAMA 1984; 251:2103–2107.
14. Sibrack CD, Gutman LT, Wilfert CM, McLaren C, St. Clair MH, Keller PM, Barry DW. Pathogenicity of acyclovir-resisitant herpes simplex virus type 1 from an immunodeficient child. J Infect Dis 1982; 146:673–682.
15. Straus SE, Seidlin M, Takiff HE, Rooney JF, Felser JM, Smith HA, Roane P, Johnson F, Hallahan C, Ostrove JM, Nusinoff-Lehrman S. Effect of oral acyclovir treatment of symptomatic and asymptomatic virus shedding in recurrent gential herpes. Sex Transm Dis 1989; 16:107–113.
16. Rooney JF, Felser JM, Ostrove JM, Straus SE. Acquisition of genital herpes from an asymptomatic sexual partner. N Engl J Med 1986; 314:1561–1564.
17. Straus SE, Croen KD, Sawyer MH, Freidfeld AG, Felser JM, Dale JK, Smith HA, Hallahan C, Lehrman SN. Acyclovir suppression of frequently recurring gential herpes: efficacy and diminishing need during successive years of treatment. JAMA 1988; 260:2227–2230.
18. McLaren C, Ellis MN, Hunter GA. A colorimetric assay for the measurement of the sensitivity of herpes simplex viruses to antiviral agents. Antiviral Res 1983; 3:223–234.
19. Clive D, Turner NT, Hozier J, Batson AG, Tucker WE Jr. Preclinical toxicology studies with acyclovir: genetic toxicity tests. Fund App Toxicol 1983; 3:587–602.
20. Clive D, Corey L, Reichman RC, Davis LG, Hoszier JC. A double-blind, placebo-controlled cytogenetic study of oral acyclovir in patients with recurrent gential herpes. J Infect Dis 1991; 164:753–757.
21. Douglas JM, Critchlow C, Benedetti J, Mertz GJ, Connor JD, Hintz MA, Fahnlander A, Remington M, Winter C, Corey L. A double-blind study of oral acyclovir for suppression of recurrences of genital herpes simplex virus infection. N Engl J Med 1984; 310:1551–1556.
22. Sacks SL, Fox R, Levendusky P, Stiver HG, Roland S, Nusinoff-Lehrman S, Keeney R. Chronic suppression for six months compared with intermittent lesional therapy of recurrent genital herpes using oral acylclovir: effects on lesions and nonlesional prodromes. Sex Transm Dis 1988; 15: 58–62.
23. Mattison HR, Reichman RC, Benedetti J, Bolgiano D, Davis LG, Bailey-Farchione A, Remington M, Winter C, Corey L. Double-blind, placebo-controlled trial compar-

ing long-term suppressive with short-term oral acyclovir therapy for management of recurrent genital herpes. Am J Med 1988; 85(2A):20–25.

24. Gold D, Ashley R, Solberg G, Abbo H, Corey L. Chronic-dose acyclovir to suppress frequently recurring genital herpes simplex virus infection: effect on antibody response to herpes simplex virus type II proteins. J Infect Dis 1988; 158:1227–1234.
25. Douglas JM Jr, Davis LG, Reminton ML, Paulsen CA, Perrin EB, Boodman P, Conner JD, King D, Corey L. A double-blind placebo-controlled trial of the effect of chronically administered oral acyclovir on sperm production in men with frequently recurrent genital herpes. J Infect Dis 1988; 157;588–593.
26. Straus SE, Takiff HE, Seidlin M, Bachrach S, Lininger L, Digiovanna JJ, Western KA, Smith HA, Lehrman SN, Creagh-Kirk T, Alling DW. Suppression of frequently recurring genital herpes. A placebo-controlled double-blind trial of oral acyclovir. N Engl J Med 1984; 310:1545–1550.
27. Molin L, Ruhnek-Forsbeck M, Svennerholm B. One year acyclovir suppression of frequently recurring genital herpes: a study of efficacy, safety, virus sensitivity and antibody response. Scan J Infect Dis 1991; 80(Suppl):33–39.
28. Mertz GJ, Jones CC, Mills J, Fife KH, Lemon SM, Stapleton JT, Hill EL, Davis LG. Long term acyclovir suppresson of frequently recurring genital herpes simplex virus infection. A multicenter double-blind trial. JAMA 1988; 260:201–206.
29. Nusinoff Lehrman S, Douglas JM, Corey L, Barry DW. Recurrent genital herpes and suppressive oral acyclovir therapy: relation between clinical outcome and in-vitro drug sensitivity. Ann Intern Med 1986; 104:786–790.
30. Collins P. Viral sensitivity following the introduction of acyclovir. Am J Med 1988; 85(2A):129–134.
31. Mindel A. Prophylaxis for genital herpes. Should it be used routinely? Drugs 1991; 41:319–325.
32. Price RW, Khan A. Resistance of peripheral autonomic neurons to in-vivo productive infection by herpes simplex virus mutants deficient in thymidine kinase. Infect Immunol 1981; 34:571–580.
33. Darby G, Field HJ, Salisbury SA. Altered substrate specificity of herpes simplex virus thymidine kinase confers acyclovir-resistance. Nature (Lond) 1981; 289:81–83.
34. Spruance SL, Stewart JC, Rowe NH, McKeough MB, Wenerstrom G, Freeman DJ. Treatment of recurrent herpes simplex labialis with oral acyclovir. J Infect Dis 1990; 161:185–190.
35. Rooney JF, Straus SE, Mannix ML, Wohlenberg CR, Banks S, Jagannath S, Braver JE, Notkins AL. UV light-induced reactivation of herpes simplex virus type 2 and prevention by acyclovir. J Infect Dis 1992; 166:500–506.
36. Spruance SL, Hamill ML, Hoge WS, Davis LG, Mills J. Acyclovir prevents reactivation of herpes simplex labialis in skiers. JAMA 1988; 260:1597–1599.
37. Schadelin J, Schilt HU, Rohner M. Preventative therapy of herpes labialis associated with trigeminal surgery. Am J Med 1988; 85(2A):46–48.
38. Green JA, Spruance LS, Wenerstrom G, Piepkorn MW. Post-herpetic erythema multiforme prevented with prophylactic oral acyclovir. Ann Intern Med 1985; 102:632.

39. Lemak MA, Duvic M, Bean SF. Oral acyclovir for the prevention of herpes-associated erythema multiforme. J Am Acad Dermat 1986; 15:50–54.
40. Molin L. Oral acyclovir prevents herpes simplex virus-associated erythema multiforme. Br J Dermat 1987; 116:109–111.
41. Leigh IM, Macey M, Newland A. Treatment of recurrent erythema multiforme. Br J Dermat 1988; 119 (suppl 33):20.
42. Legge RH, Thompson AB, Linder J, Woods GL, Robbins RA, Moulton AL, Rennard SI. Acyclovir-responsive herpetic tracheobronchitis. Am J Med 1988; 85:561–563.
43. Shepp D, Newton B, Dandiliker P, Flournoy N, Meyets J. Oral acyclovir therapy of mucocutaneous herpes simplex virus infections in immunocompromised marrow transplant recipients. Ann Intern Med 1985; 102:783–785.
44. Niimura M, Nishikawa T. Treatment of eczema herpeticum with oral acyclovir. Am J Med 1988; 85(2A):49–52.
45. Robinson GE, Underhill GS, Forster GE, Kennedy C, McLean K. Treatment with acyclovir of genital herpes simplex virus infection complicated by eczema herpeticum. Br J Vener Dis 1984; 60:241–242.
46. Swart RNJ, Vermeer BJ, van der Meer JWM, Enshchede FAJ, Versteeg J. Treatment of eczema herpeticum with acyclovir. Arch Dermat 1983; 119:13–16.
47. Field LM. Avoiding dermabrasion-induced herpes activation. JAAD 1986; 14:144.
48. Balfour HH Jr, Bean B, Laskin OL, Ambinder RF, Meyers JD, Wade JC, Zaia JA, Aeppli D, Kirk LE, Segreti AC, Keeney RE. Acyclovir halts progression of herpes zoster in immunocompromised patients. N Engl J Med 1983; 308:1448–1453.
49. Shepp DH, Dandliker PS, Meyers JD. Treatment of varicella-zoster virus infection in severely immunocompromised patients: a randomized comparison of acyclovir and vidarabine. N Engl J Med 1986; 314:208–212.
50. Wood MJ, Ogan PH, McKendrick MW, Care CD, McGill JI, Webb EM. Efficacy of oral acyclovir treatment of acute herpes zoster. Am J Med 1988; 85(2A):79–83.
51. Huff JC, Bean B, Balfour HH Jr, Laskin OL, Connor JD, Corey L, Bryson YJ, McGuirt P. Therapy of herpes zoster with oral acyclovir. Am J Med 1988; 85(2A):84–89.
52. Pedersen A. Varicella zoster virus and recurrent aphtous ulceration. Lancet 1989; 1:1203.
53. Wormser GP, Mack L, Lenox T, Hewlett D, Goldfarb J, Yarrish RL, Reitano M. Lack of effect of oral acyclovir on prevention of aphtous stomatitis. Otolaryngol Head Neck Surg 1988; 98:14–17.
54. Pedersen A. Acyclovir in the prevention of severe aphtous ulcers. Arch Dermat 1992; 128:119.
55. Preblud SR. Varicella: complications and costs. Pediatrics 1986; 78(suppl):728–735.
56. Felser JM, Freifeld A. The epidemiology, natural history, and complications of varicella. In: Straus SE, mod. Varicella-zoster virus infections: biology, history, treatment and prevention. Ann Intern Med 1988;108:223–229.
57. Preblud SR. Age-specific risks of varicella complications. Pediatrics 1981; 68:14–17.
58. Straus SE, Ostrove JM, Inchauspe G. Varicella-zoster virus infections. Biology, natural history, treatment and prevention. Ann Int Med 1988; 108:221–237.

59. Shulman ST. Acyclovir treatment of disseminated varicella in childhood malignant neoplasms. Am J Dis Child 1985; 139:137–140.
60. Nyerges G, Meszner Z, Gyarmati E, Kerpel-Fronius S. Acyclovir prevents dissemination of varicella in immunocompromised children. J Infect Dis 1988; 157:309–313.
61. Nyerges G, Meszner Z. Treatment of chickenpox in immuncocompromised children. Am J Med 1988; 85(2A):94–95.
62. Balfour HH Jr. Varicella zoster virus infections in immunocompromised host. A review of natural history and management. Am J Med 1988; 85(2A):68–73.
63. Morales JM. Successful acyclovir therapy of severe varicella hepatitis in an adult renal transplant recipient. Am J Med 1991; 90:401.
64. Balfour HH Jr, Kelly JM, Suarez CS, et al. Acyclovir treatment of varicella in otherwise healthy children. J Pediatr 1990; 116:633–639.
65. Dunkle LM, Arvin AM, Whitley RJ, et al. A controlled trial of acyclovir for chickenpox in normal children. N Engl J Med 1991; 325:1539–1544.
66. Balfour HH Jr, Rotbart HA, Feldman S, Dunkle LM, Feder HM, Prober CG, Hayden GF, Steinberg S, Whitley RJ, Goldberg L, McGuirt PV, and the collaborative Acyclovir Varicella Study Group. Acyclovir treatment of varicella in otherwise healthy adolescents. J Pediatr 1992; 120:627–633.
67. American Academy of Pedicatrics Committee on Infectious Diseases. The use of oral acyclovir in otherwise healthy children with varicella. Pediatrics 1993; 91:674–676.
68. Andersson J, Britton S, Ernberg I, Andersson U, Henle W, Skoldenberg B, Tisella A. Effect of acyclovir on infectious mononucleosis: a double-blind, placebo-controlled study. J Infect Dis 1986; 153:283–290.
69. Resnick L, Herbst JS, Ablashi DV, Atherton S, Frank B, Rosen L, Horwitz SN. Regression of oral hairy leukoplakia after orally administered acyclovir therapy. JAMA 1988; 259:384–388.
70. Saliba F, Eyraud D, Samuel D, David MF, Arulnaden JL, Dussaix E, Mathieu, D, Bismuth H. Randomized controlled trial of acyclovir for the prevention of cytomegalovirus infection and disease in liver transplant recipients. Transplant Proc 1993; 25:1444–1445.
71. Nakazato PZ, Burns W, Moore P, Garcia-Kennedy R, Cox K, Esquivel C. Viral prophylaxis in hepatic transplantation: preliminary report of a randomized trial of acyclovir and gancyclovir. Transplant Proc 1993; 25:1935–1937.
72. Kizilisik TA, Preiksaitis JK, Kneteman NM. Cytomegalovirus disease in liver transplant recipients: impact of acyclovir prophylaxis. Transplant Proc 1993; 25:2282–2283.
73. Perren TJ, Powles RL, Easton D, Stolle K, Selby PJ. Prevention of herpes zoster in patients by long-term oral acyclovir after allogeneic bone marrow transplantation. Am J Med 1988; 85(2A):99–101.
74. Wade JC, Newton B, Flournoy N, Meyers JD. Oral acyclovir for prevention of herpes simplex virus reactivation after marrow transplantaion. Ann Intern Med 1984; 100:823–828.

75. Saral R, Burns WH, Laskin OL, Santos GW, Lietman PS. Acyclovir prophylaxis of herpes-simplex-virus infections. A randomized, double-blind, controlled trial in bone-marrow-transplant recipients. N Engl J Med 1981; 305:63–67.
76. Andrews EB, Yankaskas BC, Cordero JF, Schoeffler K, Hampp S. Acyclovir in pregnancy registry: six years' experience. The Acyclovir in Pregnancy Registry Advisory Committee. Obstet Gynecol 1992; 79:7–13.
77. Centers for Disease Control. Sexually transmitted diseases; treatment guidelines. Atlanta: Centers for Disease Control, 1989; 15–16.
78. Burroughs Wellcome Co. Zovirax (acyclovir) ointment 5%. Package insert. April 1991.
79. Valsecci R, Imberti G, Cainelli T. Contact allergy to acyclovir. Contact Dermatitis 1990; 23:372–373.
80. Goday J, Aguirre A, Ibarra NG, Eizaguirre X. Allergic contact dermatiitis from acyclovir. Contact Dermatitis 1991; 24:380–381.
81. Burroughs Wellcome Co. Zovirax (acyclovir) capsules, tablets, suspension. Package insert. February 1992.
82. Hisler BM, Daneshvar SA, Aronson PJ, Hashimoto K. Peripheral edema and oral acyclovir. J Am Acad Dermat 1988; 18:1142–1143.
83. Eck P, Silver SM, Clark EC. Acute renal failure and coma after a high dose of oral acyclovir. N Engl J Med 1991; 325:1178–1179.
84. Hernandez E, Prega M, Moreno F, Montoyo C. Acute renal failure induced by oral acyclovir. Clin Nephrol 1991; 36:155–156.
85. Burroughs Wellcome Co. Zovirax sterile powder (acyclovir sodium). Package insert. September 1991.
86. Sylvester RK, Ogden WB, Draxler CA, Lewis FB. Vesicular eruption. A local complication of concentrated acyclovir infusions. JAMA 1986; 255:385–386.
87. Sawyer MH, Webb DE, Balow HE, Straus SE. Acyclovir-induced renal failure. Clinical course and histology. Am J Med 1988; 84:1067–1071.
88. Peterslund NA, Larsen ML, Mygind H. Acyclovir crystalluria. Scand J Infect Dis 1988; 20:225–228.
89. Krigel RL. Reversible neurotoxicity due to oral acyclovir in a patient with chronic lmphocytic leukemia. J Infect Dis 1986; 154:189.
90. MacDiarmaid-Gordon AR, O'Connor M, Beaman M, Ackrill P. Neurotoxicity associated with oral acyclovir in patients undergoing dialysis. Nephron 1992; 62:280–283.
91. Friedman D, Weller S, Dix L. Acyclovir plasma concentrations and duration of herpes zoster pain: higher levels associated with the greater efficacy achieved with valtrex (valacyclovir HCI). 34th Interscience Conference on Antimicrobial Agents and Chemotherapy, Orlando, Fla. Abstract no. A72 (1994).
92. Meyers JD, Reed EC, Shepp DH, Thornquist M, Dandliker PS, Vicary CA, Flournoy N, Kirk LE, Kersey JH, Thomas ED, Balfour HH Jr. Acyclovir for the prevention of cytomegalovirus infecton and disease after allegenic marrow transplantation. N Engl J Med 1988; 318:70–75.
93. Weller S., Blum MR, Doucette M, Burnette T, Cederberg DM, de Miranda P, Smiley ML. Pharmacokinetics of the acyclovir pro-drug valaciclovir after escalating single-

and multiple-dose administration to normal volunteers. Clin Pharm Ther, 1993; 54:595–605.

94. Niederman JC. Epstein-Barr virus infections. In: Fitzpatrick TB, Eisen AZ, Wolff K, et al., eds. Dermatology in general medicine, 4th ed. New York: McGraw-Hill, 1993; 2581–2586.
95. Straus SE, Cohen JI, Tosato G, Meier J. NIH conference. Epstein-Barr virus infections: biology, pathogenesis, and management. Ann Intern Med 1993; 118:45–58.
96. Liebowitz D, Kieff E. Epstein-Barr virus. In: Roizman B, Whitley RJ, Lopez C, eds. The human herpesviruses. New York: Raven Press, 1993; 107–172.
97. Ernberg I, Andersson J. Acyclovir efficiently inhibits oropharyngeal secretion of Epstein-Barr virus in patients with acute infectious mononucleosis. J Gen Virol 1986; 67:2267–2272.
98. Pearson GR, Levine PH. Epstein-Barr virus vaccine: the time to proceed is now. In: Roizman B, Whitley RJ, Lopez C, eds. The human herpesviruses. New York: Raven Press, 1993; 349–356.
99. Lesher JL Jr. Cytomegalovirus infections and the skin. J Am Acad Dermat 1988; 18:1333–1338.
100. Griffiths PD. Current management of cytomegalovirus disease. J Med Virol 1993; (suppl 1):106–111.
101. Alford CA, Britt WJ. Cytomegalovirus. In: Roizman B, Whitley RJ, Lopez C, eds. The human herpesviruses. New York: Raven Press, 1993; 227–255.
102. Caserta MT, Hall CB. Human herpesvirus-6. Annu Rev Med 1993; 44:377–383.
103. Asano Y, Yoshikawa T, Suga S, Kobayashi I, Nakashima T, Yazaki T, Kajita Y, Ozaki T. Clinical features of infants with primary human herpesvirus 6 infection (exanthem subitum, roseola infantum). Pediatrics 1994; 93:104–108.
104. Benson PM, Malane SL, Banks R, Hicks CB, Hilliard J. B virus (*Herpesvirus simiae*) and human infection. Arch Dermat 1989; 125:1247–1248.
105. Whitley RJ. The biology of B virus (cercopithecine virus 1). In: Roizman B, Whitley RJ, Lopez C, eds. The human herpesviruses. New York: Raven Press, 1993; 317–328.
106. Chang Y, Cesarman F, Pessin MS, Lee F, Culpepper J, Knowles DM, Moore PS. Identification of herpesvirus-like DNA sequences in AIDS-associated Kaposi's sarcoma. Science 1994; 266:1865–1869.
107. Huang YQ, Li JJ, Kaplan MH, Poiesz B, Katabira E, Zhang WC, Feiner D, Friedman-Kien AE. Human herpesvirus-like nucleic acid in various forms of Kaposi's sarcoma. Lancet 1995; 345:759–761.
108. Rady PL, Yen A, Rollefson JL, Orengo I, Bruce S, Hughes TK, Tyring SK. Kaposi's sarcoma associated herpesvirus-like DNA sequences in various forms of skin lesions from organ transplant patients. Lancet 1995; 345:1339–1340.
109. Memar OM, Rady PL, Tyring SK. Human herpesvirus-8: detection of novel herpesvirus-like DNA sequences in Kaposi's sarcoma and other lesions. J Mol Med 1995; 73:603–609.
110. Bolton RA. Nongenital warts: classification and treatment options. Am Fam Physician 1991; 43:2049–2056.

111. Brown DR, Fife KH. Human papillomavirus infections of the genital tract. Med Clin N Am 1990; 74:1455–85.
112. Memar OM, Arany I, Tyring SK. Skin-associated lymphoid tissue in human immunodeficiency virus-1, human papillomavirus, and herpes simplex virus infections. J Invest Dermat 1995; 105:99s–104s.
113. Lowy DR, Androphy EJ. Warts. In: Fitzpatrick TB, Eisen AZ, Wolff K, et al., eds. Dermatology in general medicine, 4th ed. New York: McGraw-Hill, 1993; 2611–2621.
114. Browder JF, Araujo OE, Myer NA, Flowers FP. The interferons and their use in condyloma acuminata. Ann Pharmacother 1992; 26:42–45.
115. Wright TC, Richart RM, Ferenczy A. Electrosurgery for HPV-related diseases of the lower genital tract: a practical handbook for diagnosis and treatment by loop electrosurgical excision and fulguration procedures. Anjou, Quebec: Bio Vision Inc. and Arthur Vision, Inc., 1992.
116. Robbins FC. Measles: clinical features, pathogenesis, pathology and complications. Am J Dis Child 1962; 103:266–273.
117. Cooper LZ. Measles. In: Fitzpatrick TB, Eisen AZ, Wolff K, Freedberg IM, Austen KF, eds. Dermatology in general medicine, 4th ed. New York: McGraw-Hill, 1993; 2516–2520.
118. Bialecki C, Feder HM Jr, Grant-Kels JM. The six classic childhood exanthems: a review and update. J Am Acad Dermat 1989; 21:891–903.
119. Chorba T, Anderson LJ. Erythema infectiosum (fifth disease). Clin Dermat 1989; 7:65–74.
120. Thurn J. Human parvovirus B19: historical and clinical review. Rev Infect Dis 1988; 10:1005–1011.
121. Epstein WL. Molluscum contagiosum. Semin Dermat 1992; 11:184–189.
122. Janniger CK, Schwartz RA. Molluscum contagiosum in children. Cutis 1993; 52:194–196.
123. Huerter CJ, Alvarez L, Stinson R. Orf: case report and literature review. Cleve Clin J Med 1991; 58:531–534.
124. Moscovici C, Cohen EP, Sanders J, et al. Isolation of a viral agent from pseudocowpox disease. Science 1963; 141:915–916.
125. Lowy DR. Milker's nodules and molluscum contagiosum. In: Fitzpatrick TB, Eisen AZ, Wolff K, Freedberg IM, Austen KF., eds. Dermatology in general medicine, 4th ed. New York: McGraw-Hill, 1993; 2606–2610.
126. Thomas I, Janniger CK. Hand, foot, and mouth disease. Cutis 1993; 52:265–266.
127. Haring JI. Case #12. Herpangina. RDH 1991; 11:10.
128. Cherry JD. Herpangina. In: Feigin RD, Cherry JD, eds. Textbook of pediatric infectious diseases, 3rd ed. Philadelphia: W.B. Saunders, 1992; 230–232.
129. Chan HL, Su IJ, Kuo TT, Kuan YZ, Chen MJ, Shih LY, Eimoto T, Maeda Y, Kikuchi M, Takeshita M. Cutaneous manifestations of adult T cell leukemia/lymphoma. J Am Acad Dermat 1985; 13:213–219.
130. Lisby G, Lisby S, Wantzin GL. Retroviruses in dermatology. Int J Dermat 1988; 27:463–467.

131. Memar O, Cerelli R, Lee P, Tyring SK. Cutaneous manifestations of HIV-1 infection. J Am Pediat Med Assoc 1995; 85:362–374.
132. Strickler MC, Friedman-Kien AE. Kaposi's sarcoma. Clin Dermat 1991; 9:39–47.
133. Kaplan MH, Sadick N, McNutt NS, et al. Dermatologic findings and manifestations of acquired immunodeficiency syndrome (AIDS). J Am Acad Dermat 1987; 16:485–506.
134. Fletcher CV. Treatment of herpesvirus infections in HIV-infected individuals. Ann Pharmacother 1992; 26:955–962.
135. Berger TG. Treatment of bacterial, fungal, and parasitic infections in the HIV-infected host. Semin Dermat 1993; 12:296–300.
136. Zall MJ, Su WP, Fransway AF. Dermatologic manifestations of human immunodeficiency virus infection. Mayo Clinic Proc 1992; 67:1089–1108.

as examples of such serious conditions. The majority of conditions requiring systemic drugs with an element of risk justify this risk through the inherent propensity for significant irreversible morbidity or based on a marked effect of the disease on the patient's lifestyle. The psychosocial impact of severe psoriasis or acne vulgaris can be profound. Likewise, the impact on day-to-day functioning that the ulcerations of pyoderma gangrenosum present easily justifies therapy with drugs such as cyclosporine in selected cases. The bottom line is that the clinician must carefully balance the disease and drug risks to ensure that the patient is far more likely to benefit from the proposed drug therapy than to suffer significant adverse effects from this therapy.

The priority sequence of systemic drug choice should be individualized for each specific patient. Using psoriasis as an example, factors such as drug cost, patient time schedule, distance to travel for medical care, gender and childbearing potential, and preexisting risk factors have a tremendous impact on systemic drug choice for patients with extensive skin involvement. The above issues and many others will influence the choice between options such as PUVA, etretinate, methotrexate, and cyclosporine in these severe psoriasis cases. The net result is that for all dermatoses, safety can be optimized with careful attention to the individual features of each patient.

Be cognizant of important drug-drug interactions when prescribing systemic drugs for various skin diseases. Methotrexate and cyclosporine are two examples of systemic drugs with numerous potential interactions with other medications. A significant number of adverse effects from these drugs result from inadequate attention to these potential interactions. The clinician should systematically record and review all medications the patient takes to minimize these prescribing errors.

When possible one should minimize the risk of systemic drug therapy through adjunctive therapy with other systemic drugs, with topical or local therapy, or by reducing/eliminating disease precipitators. The need for "steroid-sparing" measures for patients receiving chronic oral corticosteroid therapy is routinely addressed utilizing drugs such as azathioprine and cyclosporine. This mind-set should be expanded to any dermatosis requiring systemic drug therapy in order to lessen the dose and/or duration of therapy required.

III. GENERAL PRINCIPLES FOR MONITORING SYSTEMIC THERAPY

Informed consent is a communication process, not just a signature on a piece of paper. Furthermore, the informed consent communication is the cornerstone for active patient involvement in the monitoring process, particularly when the information is reinforced with a thorough, well-written patient education handout. (The handout should not be relied upon as a substitute for direct oral communication between the patient and physician.) The result of these steps, when done properly, is a patient who is well informed about what symptoms to report to the physician, what preventative measures to take to minimize the risk of specific adverse effects, and what monitoring steps are required. Because this information is generally difficult to retain, the patient education handout is useful on an ongoing basis to reinforce key elements of this process. The overall benefits are improved delivery of medical care and improved medicolegal risk management.

Virtually all tests and examinations to be used in the monitoring process should have a baseline determination. In many situations a preexisting abnormality in a given organ will preclude use of the intended systemic drug. An example would be significantly abnormal renal function in a patient to be treated with cyclosporine. In other clinical situations an abnormal baseline test result will necessitate more careful monitoring. Mildly abnormal baseline liver function tests often allow methotrexate therapy to proceed; however, frequent testing in the early weeks of therapy will be required. Finally, the clinician may avoid blame for a preexisting condition (e.g., leukopenia) that was subclinical, although the implications after therapy has started may be significant, particularly when prescribing cytotoxic drugs.

"Critical toxicities" are defined as any drug-induced adverse effect that can result in loss of life or in potentially irreversible, significant morbidity. These potentially serious adverse effects are the primary focus of the monitoring process. Examples of "critical toxicities" are hepatotoxicity, agranulocytosis/aplastic anemia, malignancy induction, teratogenicity, and renal toxicity. These adverse effects are be the primary examples discussed in this chapter. No doubt other adverse effects such as opportunistic infections, hyperlipidemia, and pneumonitis meet the above definition, but the major principles can be thoroughly illustrated with the first five major side effects listed above. Of particular importance are the critical toxicities, which are idiopathic and have the potential for rapid, dramatic changes in the test values. Agranulocytosis and hepatocellular toxicity leading to toxic hepatitis are important examples that will be discussed in detail later.

The primary goal of monitoring is risk reduction through detection of drug-induced abnormalities at an early, reversible stage. Frequently this early, reversible stage will have no clinical findings detectable by the patient or physician. Moderate leukopenia (3500–4000 WBC/mm^3) and mild transaminase elevations (abnormal, but less than two times the upper normal value) mandate careful attention, although the great majority of cases do not progress to agranulocytosis or toxic hepatitis, respectively (2). It is the absence of such appropriate careful follow-up that has led to some of the serious outcomes in the literature (3–6). Abnormal renal function tests in patients receiving cyclosporine serve as another example of a potentially serious, yet completely reversible, adverse effect when recognized in an early, subclinical stage (7).

Risk reduction can be optimized through use of well-defined monitoring guidelines available in the literature. More frequent surveillance is required for high-risk patients and/or abnormal test results. Monitoring guidelines for methotrexate, cyclosporine, azathioprine, cyclophosphamide, and the retinoids can be found in several key resources (5,8–11). When initially gaining experience in prescribing these drugs, one should adhere relatively closely to the published guidelines. As greater clinical experience is attained, the clinician may get a feel regarding scenarios that allow greater flexibility. Importantly, one should note that overall monitoring guidelines are designed for relatively low-risk patients with normal test results. More careful follow-up testing is justifiable for higher-risk patients due to preexisting conditions or abnormal baseline or subsequent test results.

Share the responsibility of monitoring for systemic drug adverse effects with other appropriate specialists. Many referrals for tests or examinations performed by consultants are built into the published monitoring guidelines. Examples are the ophthalmological consultation required for patients receiving antimalarial agents (12,13) and PUVA therapy (14) and the referrals for liver biopsy in psoriatic patients receiving methotrexate (5). I would propose regular involvement of the patient's primary physician for ongoing surveillance in patients receiving cytotoxic drugs with even a theoretical potential for malignancy induction. In addition, the current climate of medical practice warrants liberal involvement of nondermatological consultants when abnormal laboratory test results are beyond the expertise of the dermatologist, even if only phone consultation is required to settle the issue.

IV. SPECIFIC ADVERSE EFFECTS

A. Hepatotoxicity

The major categories of drug-induced hepatotoxicity are hepatocellular, obstructive, and steatosis (fatty liver) (2,15). Steatosis may progress to fibrosis and subsequent cirrhosis. Of the above categories, hepatocellular toxicity and steatosis are most relevant to dermatology.

Severe hepatocellular toxicity may occasionally be due to methotrexate and azathioprine (5,16,17). Cyclosporine and etretinate may rarely cause significant hepatocellular toxicity (18–20). This category of liver toxicity is initially characterized by elevated transaminase values (SGOT and SGPT), although later in the disease progression alkaline phosphatase and eventually bilirubin elevations typically occur. Transaminase elevations up to two times the upper normal laboratory value mandate careful follow-up. If this elevation occurs rapidly, temporary cessation of drug therapy, with subsequent dose reduction after the laboratory values normalize, is recommended. Indefinite cessation of drug therapy is prudent when transaminase values exceed three times the upper normal value (2). Toxic hepatitis is generally accompanied by abdominal pain, nausea, anorexia, and fatigue, with clinical findings of jaundice when significant bilirubin elevations are present.

More commonly dermatologists are faced with the potential for indolent liver toxicity from methotrexate in the form of steatosis in the absence of significant transaminase elevations. The potential for this subclinical progression to fibrosis and cirrhosis is the basis of current recommendations for periodic liver biopsies, even with normal liver function tests (5,21). Roenigk grade IIIa (mild fibrosis) liver biopsy changes necessitate careful follow-up, with a repeat liver biopsy in about 6 mo (5). Grade IIIb changes (moderate-severe fibrosis) or grade IV changes (cirrhosis) require cessation of methotrexate therapy.

Several additional points are worth highlighting. In many cases of mild transaminase elevation, the abnormality will correct itself without stopping the drug therapy. The trend of the laboratory values is the key to the decision making. Stable or improving transaminase values, along with normal alkaline phosphatase and bilirubin values, and the absence of symptoms of toxic hepatitis allow continuation of drug therapy with close surveillance until the test results normalize. Compared with leukopenia leading to agranulocytosis, there is a much greater "warning period" prior to progression to toxic hepatitis with mild-moderate transaminase elevations.

B. Agranulocytosis and Aplastic Anemia

Agranulocytosis and aplastic anemia are part of a continuum of severe abnormalities in circulating levels of leukocytes (agranulocytosis) possibly accompanied by thrombocytopenia and severe anemia (aplastic anemia). Agranulocytosis is defined by a white blood cell count of less than $1500/mm^3$ and/or neutrophils/granulocytes less than $500/mm^3$. Typically a reduction to these troublesome levels is preceded by less severe leukopenia and/or neutropenia. As discussed above, this warning period of less severe reduction in white blood cell (WBC) counts may be relatively brief.

Dapsone is the systemic dermatological agent most commonly responsible for agranulocytosis (22,23). Of the drugs covered in this book azathioprine, methotrexate, and cyclophosphamide have the greatest potential for agranulocytosis (2,10,19,24–26). One advantage of cyclosporine therapy for immunosuppression is the virtual absence of hematological toxicity (18,19). Azathioprine generally produces a gradual dose-dependent WBC count reduction to a range of $3500–4500/mm^3$ (2,9,24). Methotrexate has a less predictable effect on WBC counts (25,26).

My general recommendation is to temporarily discontinue the drug therapy when the WBC count is less than $3500–4000/mm^3$, particularly if there is a rapid decrease from the previous test result. Levels significantly below this range necessitate indefinite drug discontinuation. When there is agranulocytosis by the above definition, subsequent rechallenge with the responsible drug when the WBC count normalizes is contraindicated.

With the majority of drugs with the potential for causing agranulocytosis or aplastic anemia, the risk is greatest in the initial months of therapy or with significant dose escalations. Likewise, the monitoring should be most frequent during these circumstances. Finally, patients should be advised to report any signs or symptoms of infection during therapy with drugs having the potential to induce agranulocytosis. Fortunately, with the current technology leading to the availability of ultrasterile hospital rooms and, if necessary, bone marrow transplantation, early recognition of these serious hematological toxicities can generally lead to eventual normalization of these rare complications of systemic drug therapy.

C. Renal Toxicity

Renal toxicity from the systemic drugs discussed in this book is primarily an issue with cyclosporine therapy. Even with "low-dose" cyclosporine therapy (up to 5 mg/kg/d), significant, yet reversible, alteration in renal function is relatively common (7,8). The mechanism can be due to either prerenal azotemia (vasoconstriction of afferent renal arterioles) or acute tubular necrosis. In either case, early detection of laboratory features of a decreased glomerular filtration rate and appropriate cyclosporine dose reduction will virtually always allow complete resolution of test abnormalities.

Methotrexate presents a different clinical scenario. The drug is not inherently toxic to the kidney; however, even a relatively small decrease in glomerular filtration will impair methotrexate excretion by the kidney. This reduction allows persistent therapeutic drug levels, markedly increasing other important adverse effects such as hepatotoxicity and hematological toxicity.

Creatinine values will fairly reliably estimate the glomerular filtration rate in younger patients. A 24 h urine collection for creatinine clearance is generally considered to be more reliable in patients over 50 y old, especially for thin individuals (5,8,27). There are no symptoms reliably present with early renal function impairment, making regular renal function testing imperative in patients receiving cyclosporine or methotrexate.

D. Malignancy Induction

There are two widely divergent viewpoints on the risk of malignancy induction from systemic dermatological agents. There is no doubt that prolonged, high-dose, combination immunosuppressive therapy in the transplantation setting significantly increases the risk of selected malignancies (28,29). Statistically significant increases in lymphomas, Kaposi's sarcoma, and squamous cell carcinomas of the skin and female cervix have been regularly documented in this population. It is of interest that the most common malignancies in the general population are not increased by immunosuppressive therapy (28,29). This includes breast, lung, colorectal, and prostate carcinomas. Fortunately there is no increase in melanomas in this population (28,29). Although there are conflicting results, there appears to be a small increase in lymphoma incidence in rheumatoid arthritis patients (30–32).

In contrast, the largest dermatological population receiving immunosuppresive therapy is psoriasis patients on low-dose cyclosporine in investigative protocols. There have been only two patients developing non-Hodgkin's B-cell lymphomas in about 1000 psoriasis patients who have been treated with cyclosporine to date (19,33). Furthermore, these lymphomas have been reversible upon cessation of cyclosporine therapy. There is no increase in Kaposi's sarcoma or squamous cell carcinoma in this psoriasis population either.

There have been multiple theories to explain the discrepancy in the incidence of immunosuppressive therapy malignancy induction in the various populations described above. It is generally believed that the depth of immunosuppression correlates with the malignancy risk (34–36). Transplantation of solid organs or bone marrow requires sustained relatively high-dose, combination drug therapy for a successful outcome. Psoriasis patients typically receive cyclosporine for a relatively brief duration (ideally 3–4 mo) and at much lower doses (5 mg/kg/d or less) than transplantation patients. Additional issues such as presence of a persistent foreign antigen source (organ transplantation) and immune dysregulation in autoimmune disorders (rheumatoid arthritis) may also explain in part the differences in malignancy incidence when comparing transplantation cases, rheumatoid arthritis patients, and the psoriasis population. There is insufficient data on autoimmune bullous dermatoses such as pemphigus vulgaris and bullous pemphigoid, which may require relatively aggressive combination immunosuppressive therapy, to draw any clear conclusions on malignancy risk in these patients.

The above discussion is necessary to intelligently address the necessity of surveillance for selected malignancies in dermatological patients. Until the final answer is in for the malignancy risk in dermatological patients receiving immunosuppressive therapy, the prudent approach is to be aware of selected malignancies that are increased in some settings of therapeutic immunosuppression. Surveillance directed at detection of lymphomas (primarily non-Hodgkin's B-cell type), Kaposi's sarcoma (cutaneous and oral), and squamous cell carcinomas of the skin and female genital tract is logical. It is appropriate to involve the patient's primary physician in surveillance for systemic lymphomas and Pap smears for cervical carcinomas. For now, it appears that most of these malignancies are reversible upon cessation of therapy, given reasonably early detection.

As a final issue, it appears that conventional immunosuppression with azathioprine, compared with full-dose cyclosporine, produces the same risk of malignancy and the same spectrum of malignancies described above. Alkylating agents such as cyclophosphamide and chlorambucil present the additional increased risk of leukemias, particularly acute nonlymphocytic leukemias (37–39). Furthermore, cyclophosphamide therapy markedly increases the risk of bladder carcinoma (40). These points should be considered when selecting immunosuppressive drugs for dermatological conditions.

E. Teratogenicity

The approach to this category of adverse effects differs in that absolute and complete prevention is essential. There are no cytotoxic or immunomodulatory drugs that have an official FDA approval for use in pregnancy. These drugs should be used in pregnancy only with serious conditions in which the mother's life is in jeopardy.

The well-defined retinoid embryopathy syndrome needs only brief mention (41,42). Serious fetal malformations and fetal loss make stringent contraception guidelines when using isotretinoin in women of childbearing potential the standard of care. Etretinate should be avoided altogether in women of childbearing potential due its long-term persistence in circulation.

Reviews on methotrexate suggest a significant risk of teratogenesis, although documented teratogenicity in humans is uncommon (5,43). Cyclosporine has potential for fetal malformations, although evidence of human teratogenesis is lacking (18). Regardless, both drugs should be used for dermatological conditions during pregnancy in only the rarest of circumstances. Extreme caution should be exercised with azathioprine and cyclophosphamide as well.

F. Other Critical Toxicities

Only three other adverse effects meeting the definition of "critical toxicities" will be briefly discussed as they pertain to cytotoxic and immunomodulatory drugs. Overall the risk of these adverse effects is much less than the five categories previously discussed.

Opportunistic infections are surprisingly infrequent in the immunosuppressive treatment of dermatological conditions. Perhaps the relative paucity of these serious infections is due to the less aggressive immunosuppression in dermatology than that utilized in the transplantation setting. One would expect a very high risk of opportunistic infections when treating extensive bullous conditions such as toxic epidermal necrolysis (TEN) and pemphigus vulgaris. Indeed the risk of sepsis from corticosteroid therapy of extensive TEN has led to burn unit management without immunosuppressive therapy as the current standard of care (44).

Combination immunosuppressive therapy is still commonly required in advanced cases of pemphigus vulgaris, with surprisingly little risk of serious infections. The clinician should instruct the patient to quickly report any significant fever or other symptoms or signs of infection to allow early, aggressive treatment of infectious complications.

Pneumonitis is an infrequent complication of methotrexate, azathioprine, and cyclophosphamide therapy (45,46). The risk of pneumonitis from methotrexate is much greater in rheumatoid arthritis patients than for psoriasis patients. This discrepancy is probably due to the inherent tendency of rheumatoid arthritis patients to develop a restrictive pulmonary disorder ("rheumatoid lung") in the absence of immunosuppressive therapy (2,47). With the above three drugs it is important to have the patient report any pulmonary symptomatology such as dyspnea, cough, or pleuritic chest pain. Routine chest radiographs are currently not the standard of care in following these patients (5).

Hypertension is primarily a risk of cyclosporine therapy (19,48). As with cyclosporine-induced renal toxicity, early detection and dosage adjustments leaves hypertension as a reversible, relatively mild complication of cyclosporine therapy. At times the hypertension may be persistent. In these cases calcium channel blockers are the drugs of choice for blood pressure control (49). Regular blood pressure checks are a central part of cyclosporine monitoring guidelines.

V. SPECIFIC DRUG MONITORING GUIDELINES

A. Methotrexate

There are multiple sources of protocols for monitoring methotrexate therapy for psoriasis and other cutaneous conditions, with the most recent Roenigk guidelines being the "gold standard" (5). The focus of these guidelines is early detection of hepatocellular toxicity, steatosis leading to fibrosis and cirrhosis, leukopenia possibly leading to agranulocytosis, and monitoring of renal function. There is a well-written, understandable patient education handout available through the National Psoriasis Foundation, that can serve to reinforce the patient's role in the monitoring process.

Although the above references are thorough sources on methotrexate monitoring guidelines and general principles, several issues are worth highlighting:

Despite trends in other fields, the liver biopsy is still the standard of care for following dermatological patients on methotrexate therapy (5). The well-documented potential for significant hepatic fibrosis and cirrhosis in the absence of liver function test changes is the basis for the liver biopsy role. Deaths from cirrhosis (5,6,50) and several cases requiring liver transplantation in patients who were not followed with liver biopsies (51) underscores the role of this procedure. Currently noninvasive imaging techniques do not adequately discriminate fat from fibrosis (2,52).

A creatinine clearance is an appropriate baseline test in patients over 50 y old, especially with relatively thin patients (5,8,27).

Baseline liver biopsies are necessary for all patients at high risk for prior liver disease. A delayed "baseline" liver biopsy can be done 3–4 mo into therapy on patients with normal liver function tests and no risk factors for liver diseases (2,27). This delay allows time to determine if the patient responds to and tolerates methotrexate. A word of caution: A substantial number of patients with psoriasis and no risk factors will show abnormal liver architecture on biopsy. Some will even show class III liver disease with no previous exposure to methotrexate.

Laboratory testing is optimally performed 5–6 d after a previous methotrexate dose to allow normalization of the expected transient, mild methotrexate effects on hematological and liver function test parameters.

In contrast to the most recent guidelines by Roenigk and colleagues (2), I tend to follow the CBCs less frequently than the recommended long-term monthly determinations in patients on long-term therapy receiving a stable weekly dose (generally every 2–3 mo after dose stabilization). On the other hand, liver function testing should be done more frequently than the recommended interval of every 3–4 mo, especially early in therapy and with dose escalations.

Routine chest radiographs are not indicated in the absence of pulmonary symptoms. Prior guidelines recommended yearly chest radiographs (53).

B. Cyclosporine Guidelines

There are multiple sources of guidelines for monitoring cyclosporine therapy. The most helpful single source is a British Journal of Dermatology monograph on all aspects of cyclosporine therapy for psoriasis (8), with a more recent brief update (33). The major focus of monitoring is on surveillance for renal toxicity and hypertension. As previously discussed, there may be a small increase in malignancy risk for dermatological patients receiving cyclosporine. I am not aware of a published patient education handout for this drug.

Issues of cyclosporine monitoring to highlight include the following:

Older patients should have at least one baseline creatinine clearance determination, along with periodic assessment of creatinine clearance if long-term therapy is needed (8). The reality is that with the emphasis on short-term cyclosporine "crisis" therapy for 3–4 mo in psoriasis patients, the baseline creatinine clearance testing will likely be all that is necessary.

A serum creatinine increase of 30% over the baseline value requires a dosage reduction of at least 1 mg/kg/d (8). Should subsequent creatinine values not improve substantially on repeat testing another similar dosage reduction is in order, or one should consider withholding cyclosporine. Many dermatologists will involve an internist or nephrologist in this renal monitoring.

Whole blood trough cyclosporine levels do not reliably predict efficacy or toxicity (2,18). It is reasonable to check the cyclosporine level once or twice early in therapy and with possible drug interactions that may effect the circulating drug levels.

Dermatologists should periodically perform a total skin and oral examination on patients receiving long-term (more than 3–4 mo) cyclosporine (2). Likewise, regular examination of major lymph node groups, examination of the liver and spleen, and periodic chest radiographs (every 6–12 mo) will screen for immunosuppression-induced lymphomas. Pap smears and pelvic examinations will assist in early detection of premalignant cervical changes. A team approach with the patient's primary physician is in order here.

Fortunately there is minimal if any hematological toxicity or hepatotoxicity from this drug (18,19). Still occasional testing of these parameters is required.

Recent studies demonstrated the need for a greater concern regarding hyperlipidemia from low-dose cyclosporine than originally appreciated (54). I would suggest checking both triglyceride and cholesterol values at the same time as testing other chemistries such as potassium, magnesium, and uric acid.

C. Azathioprine Guidelines

The last drug covered in significant detail is azathioprine. Published sources of monitoring guidelines are relatively few in number (9,10). The most troublesome adverse effects are agranulocytosis and aplastic anemia, with a lesser concern for hepatocellular toxicity. The issue of azathioprine-induced lymphomas and other malignancies is not settled yet. In my experience opportunistic infections are quite infrequent at doses up to 2 mg/kg/d in dermatological patients.

The most noteworthy development in azathioprine monitoring is thiopurine methyltransferase testing to determine who is at greatest risk for severe hematological complications (55,56). Patients who are homozygous recessive for this enzyme's activity (0.3% of the population) are at increased risk for serious complications due to delayed metabolism of the parent compound. In addition, testing for thiopurine methyltransferase activity can help predict which patients will metabolize the parent drug quickly (90% of the population) and thus can easily tolerate full doses of azathioprine. Until testing for the activity of this enzyme is the widespread clinical practice, careful surveillance of hematological parameters, as desribed in the above references, is the standard of care.

The same principles for addressing the malignancy induction controversy as discussed with cyclosporine are pertinent with azathioprine therapy.

Patient education regarding important signs of possible opportunistic infections is important in patients receiving azathioprine therapy, even though the actual risk of these infections is quite low.

D. Other Drugs and Sources for Monitoring Guidelines

A few other drugs deserve brief mention here. Cyclophosphamide is prescribed by a relatively small number of mostly academic dermatologists. Published guidelines primarily focus on the acute hematological toxicities and screening for bladder carcinoma. I would advise careful attention to the malignancy induction issue, including the unique risk of leukemia and bladder carcinoma in patients receiving cyclophosphamide (37–40).

Chlorambucil has recently been described as effective for selected cases of pyoderma gangrenosum and dermatomyositis (57,58). An approach to monitoring this drug can be found in the references above in addition to other sources. Given that chlorambucil is an alkylating agent as well, the clinician should exercise similar caution in surveillance for additional toxicities (especially leukemia) as is done with cyclophosphamide therapy.

Retinoids such as isotretinoin and etretinate are discussed elsewhere in this book. Monitoring guideline sources are numerous, providing adequate background information to help ensure safe use of these drugs (2,11,59).

Many other cytotoxic and immunomodulatory agents are discussed in this book. The reader is advised to consult the individual chapters for approaches to monitoring for adverse effects from these drugs.

REFERENCES

1. Wolverton SE. Systemic drug therapy for psoriasis: the most critical issues. Arch Dermat 1991; 127:565.
2. Wolverton SE. Monitoring for adverse effects from systemic drugs used in dermatology. J Am Acad Dermat 1992; 26:661.
3. Lewis JH, Zimmerman HJ, Benson GD, et al. Hepatic injury associated with ketoconazole therapy: analysis of 33 cases. Gastroenterology 1984; 86:503.
4. Janssen PAJ and Symoens JE. Hepatic reactions during ketoconazole treatment. Am J Med 1983; 74(1B):80.
5. Roenigk HH Jr, Auerbach R, Maibach HI, et al. Methotrexate in psoriasis: revised guidelines. J Am Acad Dermat 1988; 19:145.
6. Pai SH, Wertheimer S, and Zak FG. Severe liver damage caused by treatment of psoriasis with methotrexate. NY J Med 1973; 73:2585.

7. Mason J. Renal side-effects of cyclosporin A. Br J Dermat 1990; 122(suppl 36):71.
8. A consensus report: cyclosporin A therapy for psoriasis. Br J Dermat 1990; 122(suppl 36):1.
9. Rapini RP, Jordon RE, Wolverton SE. Cytotoxic agents. In: Wolverton SE, Wilkin JK, eds. Systemic drugs for skin diseases. Philadelphia: W.B. Saunders, 1991:125.
10. McDonald CJ. Use of cytotoxic drugs in dermatologic diseases. II. J Am Acad Dermat 1985; 12:965.
11. Ellis CN, Voorhees JJ. Etretinate therapy. J Am Acad Dermat 1987; 16:267.
12. Easterbrook M. Ocular effects and safety of antimalarial agents. Am J Med 1988; 85(4A):23.
13. Rynes RI, Bernstein HN. Ophthalmologic safety profile of antimalarial drugs. Lupus 1993; 2(suppl 1):517.
14. Bickers DR. Position paper—PUVA therapy. J Am Acad Dermat 1983; 8:265.
15. Pessayre D, Larrey D. Acute and chronic drug-induced hepatitis. Baillières Clin Gastroenterol 1988; 2:385.
16. Sterneck M, Wiesner R, Ascher N, et al. Azathioprine hepatotoxicity after liver transplantation. Hepatology 1991; 14:806.
17. Tolman KG. Hepatotoxicity of antirheumatic drugs. J Rheumatol 1990; 22(suppl):6.
18. Gupta AK, Brown MD, Ellis CN et al. Cyclosporine in dermatology. J Am Acad Dermat 1989; 21:1245.
19. Krupp P, Monka C. Side-effect profile of cyclosporin A in patients treated for psoriasis. Br J Dermat 1990; 122(suppl 36):47.
20. Roenigk HH Jr. Liver toxicity of retinoid therapy. J Am Acad Dermat 1988; 19:199.
21. Newman M, Auerbach R, Feiner H, et al. The role of liver biopsies in psoriatic patients receiving long-term methotrexate treatment. Arch Dermat 1989; 125:1218.
22. Ognibene AJ. Agranulocytosis due to dapsone. Ann Intern Med 1970; 72:521.
23. Hörnsten P, Keisu M, Wiholm B-E. The incidence of agranulocytosis during treatment of dermatitis herpetiformis with dapsone as reported in Sweden, 1972 through 1988. Arch Dermat 1990; 126:919.
24. Min DI, Monaco AP. Complications associated with immunosuppressive therapy and their management. Pharmacother 1991; 11:1195.
25. Shupack JL, Webster GF. Pancytopenia following low-dose oral methotrexate therapy for psoriasis, JAMA 1988; 259:3594.
26. Kevat SG, McCarthy PJ, Hill WR, et al. Pancytopenia induced by low-dose methotrexate for rheumatoid arthritis. Aust NZ J Med 1988 18:697.
27. Callen JP, Kulp-Shorten CL. Methotrexate. Wolverton SE, Wilkin JK, eds. In: Systemic drugs for skin diseases. Philadelphia: W.B. Saunders, 1991:152.
28. Cockburn IT, Krupp P. The risk of neoplasms in patients treated with cyclosporine A. J Autoimmun 1989; 2:723.
29. Penn I, Brunson ME. Cancers after cyclosporine therapy. Transplant Proc 1988; 20(suppl 3):885.
30. Silman AJ, Petrie J, Hazleman B, et al. Lymphoproliferative cancer and other malignancies in patients with rheumatoid arthritis treated with azathioprine: a 20-year follow-up study. Ann Rheum Disc 1988; 47:988.

31. van Wanghe P, Dequeker J. Compliance and long-term effect of azathioprine in 65 rheumatiod arthritis cases. Ann Rheum Dis. 1982; 41(suppl 1):40.
32. Whisnant JK, Pelkey J. Rheumatiod arthritis: treatment with azathioprine (IMURAN®): clinical side-effects and laboratory abnormalities. Ann Rheum Dis 1982; 41(suppl 1):44.
33. Mihatsch MJ, Wolff K. Consensus conference on cyclosporin A for psoriasis February 1992. Br J Dermat 1992; 126:621.
34. Wilkinson AH, Smith JL, Hunsicker LG, et al. Increased frequency of posttransplant lymphomas in patients treated with cyclosporine, azathioprine, and prednisone. Transplantation 1989; 47:293.
35. Shah B, First MR, Munda R, et al. Current experience with renal transplantation in older patients. Am J Kidney Dis 1988; 12:516.
36. Ryffel B. The carcinogenicity of cyclosporin. Toxicology 1992; 73:1.
37. Haas JF, Kittelmann B, Mehnert WH, et al. Risk of leukemia in ovarian tumor and breast cancer patients following treatment by cyclophosphamide. Br J Cancer 1987; 55:213.
38. Ellis M, Lishner M. Second malignancies following treatment in non-Hodgkins lymphoma. Leuk Lymph 1993; 9:337.
39. Palmer RG, Denman AM. Malignancies induced by chlorambucil. Cancer Treat Rev 1989; 11:121.
40. Pedersen-Bjergaard J, Ersboll J, Hansen VL, et al. Carcinoma of the urinary bladder after treatment with cyclophosphamide for non-Hodgkin's lymphoma. N Engl J Med 1988; 318:1028.
41. Stern RS. When a uniquely effective drug is teratogenic: the case of isotretinoin. N Engl J Med 1989; 320:1007.
42. Lammer EJ, Chen CT, Hoar RM, et al. Retinoic acid embryopathy. N Engl J Med 1985; 313:837.
43. Kozlowski RD, Steinbrunner JV, MacKenzie AH, et al. Outcome of first-trimester exposure to low-dose methotrexate in eight patients with rheumatic disease. Am J Med 1990; 88:589.
44. Halebian PH, Madden MR, Findlestein JL, et al. Improved burn center survival of patients with toxic epidermal necrolysis managed without corticosteroids. Ann Surg 1986; 204:504.
45. Phillips TJ, Jones DH, Baker H. Pulmonary complications following methotrexate therapy. J Am Acad Dermat 1987; 16:373.
46. Drugs that cause pulmonary toxicity. Med Lett Drugs Ther 1990; 32:88.
47. Sostman HD, Matthay RA, Putman CE, et al. Methotrexate-induced pneumonitis. Medicine 1976; 55:371.
48. Porter GA, Bennett WM, Sheps SG. Cyclosporine-associated hypertension. Arch Intern Med 1990; 150:280.
49. Weir MR. Therapeutic benefits of calcium channel blockers in cyclosporine-treated organ transplant recipients: blood pressure control and immunosuppression. Am J Med 1991; 90(5A):325.
50. Coe RO, Bull FE. Cirrhosis associated with methotrexate treatment of psoriasis. JAMA 1968; 206:1515.

51. Gilbert SC, Klintmalm G, Menter A, et al. Methotrexate-induced cirrhosis requiring liver transplantation in three patients with psoriasis. Arch Intern Med 1990; 150:889.
52. Mitchell D, Johnson RD, Testa HJ, et al. Ultrasound and radionuclide scans—poor indicatiors of liver damage in patients treated with methotrexate. Clin Exp Dermat 1987; 12:243.
53. Roenigk HH, Auerbach R, Maibach HI, et al. Methotrexate guidelines—revised. J Am Acad Dermat 1982; 6:145.
54. Stiller MJ, Pak GH, Kenny C, et al. Elevation of fasting serum lipids in patients treated with low-dose cyclosporine for severe plaque-type psoriasis. J Am Acad Dermat 1992; 27:434.
55. Lennard L, van Loon JA, Weinshilboum RM. Pharmacogenetics of acute azathioprine toxicity: relationship to thiopurine methyltransferase genetic polymorphism. Clin Pharmacol Ther 1989; 46:149.
56. Snow JL, Gibson LE. The role of genetic variation in thiopurine methyltransferase activity and the efficacy and/or side effects of azathioprine therapy in dermatologic patients. Arch Dermat 1994; .
57. Sinway PA, Callen JP. Chlorambucil. An effective corticosteroid-sparing agent for patients with recalcitrant dermatomyositis. Arthr Rheum 1993; 36:319.
58. Caller JP, Case JD, Sager D. Chlorambucil—an effective corticosteroid-sparing agent for pyoderma gangrenosum. J Am Acad Dermat 1989; 21:515.
59. Dicken CH. Retinoids: a review. J Am Acad Dermat 1984; 11:541.

Index

About the Editor

CHARLES J. McDONALD is Professor and Chairman of the Department of Dermatology, Brown University, Providence, Rhode Island, as well as a Director-at-large and National Officer of the American Cancer Society. A pioneer in the use of immunomodulatory and cytotoxic agents in dermatological disease, he is a member of the American Academy of Dermatology, the American Medical Association, the American Society for Clinical Oncology, the American Association for the Advancement of Science, and the American Venereal Disease Association, among other organizations. Dr. McDonald received the B.S. degree (1951) in chemistry from North Carolina Agricultural and Technical University, Greensboro, North Carolina, the M.S. degree (1952) in biology from the University of Michigan, Ann Arbor, and the M.D. degree (1960) from the Howard University School of Medicine, Washington, D.C. He later received postgraduate training in dermatology and clinical pharmacology (oncology) at the Yale University School of Medicine, New Haven, Connecticut.